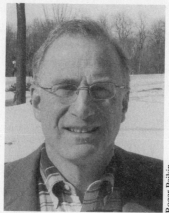

Roger Peikin

About the Author

STEVEN R. PEIKIN, M.D., is professor of medicine and head of
gastroenterology at the University of Medicine and Dentistry
of New Jersey Robert Wood-Johnson Medical School at Camden, Cooper Hospital/University Medical Center. He has been
a fellow at Massachusetts General Hospital and Harvard Medical School, and a clinical associate at the National Institutes of
Health. Dr. Peikin is the author of *The Complete Book of Diet
Drugs*. He lives in Chestnut Hill, New Jersey, with his wife and
children.

D0354058

Gastrointestinal Health

THIRD EDITION

The Proven Nutritional Program to Prevent, Cure, or Alleviate Irritable Bowel Syndrome (IBS), Ulcers, Gas, Constipation, Heartburn, and Many Other Digestive Disorders

STEVEN R. PEIKIN, M.D.

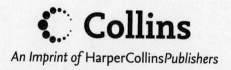
Collins

An Imprint of HarperCollinsPublishers

This book is intended to help people better understand gastrointestinal symptoms and disorders. It should not be used as a means of self-diagnosis, since symptoms of relatively innocuous disorders are often confused with those of more serious diseases. A definitive diagnosis should always be made by a qualified physician.

As with all dietary regimens, the Self-Help Nutritional Program should be used in the context of a broader course of treatment as determined by a physician. The reader is advised that this dietary approach may not be appropriate in treating certain symptoms and disorders. In particular, the meal plans in the nutritional program are not recommended for people with acute pancreatitis, acute cholecystitis, intestinal obstruction, diverticulitis, or moderately or very active stages of Crohn's disease and ulcerative colitis.

The over-the-counter and prescription drugs mentioned throughout the book should be used only when approved by your personal physician. Any drug may cause side effects, which at times can be severe.

The first edition of this book was published in hardcover in 1991 by HarperCollins Publishers.

Revised Perennial edition published 1999.
First Perennial Currents edition published 2004.

Library of Congress Cataloging-in-Publication Data

Peikin, Steven R.
    Gastrointestinal health : the proven nutritional program to prevent, cure, or alleviate irritable bowel syndrome (IBS), ulcers, heartburn, and many other digestive disorders / Steven Peikin.—Rev. ed.
        p. cm.
    Previously published: New York : HarperPerennial, 1999.
    Rev. ed. of 1999 publication.
    Includes index.
    ISBN 0-06-058532-3
        1. Gastrointestinal system—Diseases—Popular works. I. Title.

RC806.P456 2004
616.3'30654—dc22   2004050756

        07 08 09 RRD 10 9 8 7 6 5

To Lori with love

Contents

PART SEVEN
Weight Considerations

PART EIGHT
Your Gastrointestinal Maintenance Plan

PART NINE
Gastrointestinal-Healthy Recipes

Acknowledgments

I would like to thank my colleagues at Jefferson Medical College of Thomas Jefferson University for their help in preparing the first edition; and for the second and third editions, my colleagues at Cooper Hospital/University Medical Center and Robert Wood Johnson Medical School in Camden, New Jersey. Special thanks to Adam B. Elfant, M.D., Cynthia Greich-McCleery, M.D., Christopher Deitch, M.D., Thomas Judge, M.D., Generosa Grana, M.D., Omar Perez-Jimenez, M.D., Scott Cohen, D.O., and Shahbaz Qureshi, M.D., for their thoughtful comments and review of the manuscript; special thanks to Laura Hill, R.D., Barbara Whedon, R.D., and Nancy Baggett, noted recipe writer and author of several cookbooks, for their help in recipe development; special thanks to Liz Emery, M.S., R.D., for assistance in preparation of the manuscript and to N. Joyce Scott, Marjorie Varneke, Mychelle Brown, and Kathleen Little for technical assistance in the preparation of the manuscript.

For their help in developing specific chapters of *Gastrointestinal Health*, my special thanks to former fellow in gastroenterology David Stampfl, M.D.; Vicki Schwartz, M.S., R.D.; Brenda Byrne, M.D., for her signification contribution and authorship of chapter 18; and the late Patricia Vogel, B.A., for her contribution to chapter 34. It was a pleasure working with Louis Chaptini, M.D., who coauthored chapters 11, 12, 13, and 15 in the third edition; Brian Berberian, M.D. who coauthored chapters 6 and 9 in the third edition; Gregory Lessor, M.D., who coauthored chapter 16 in the third edition; and Liz Emery, M.S., R.D., who authored Part Four in the third edition.

A note of thanks to my agent Barbara Lowenstein and also Bridget Sweeney, Gail Winston, and Lia Pelosi at HarperCollins, who helped with the second and third editions of *Gastrointestinal Health*.

A note of appreciation to Tom Culp, Chip Butler, Herb Rappaport, Bill Miller, and George Connelly for keeping me focused on the important things in life.

I wish to express a debt of gratitude to Josleen Wilson, author of *Woman: Your Body, Your Health* and many other health books, for her valuable help in the preparation of the first edition of *Gastrointestinal Health* and to Lori Snodgrass, for assistance in the preparation of the second edition. Finally, special thanks to Cheryl Clifford Marco, R.D., Manager of Outpatient Nutrition, Thomas Jefferson University Hospital, and author of the recipe section of *Gastrointestinal Health*.

Preface

Since the release of *Gastrointestinal Health* in 1991, there have been many new and exciting developments in the field of gastroenterology. Most notable is confirmation of the discovery that many diseases of the upper gastrointestinal tract (ulcers, gastritis, stomach cancer) are caused by a bacterial infection. It may surprise some people that almost a third of American adults are currently infected with the bacteria *Helicobacter pylori* and this may, in part, explain why so many people suffer from upper gastrointestinal diseases. The reader will learn of new ways to diagnose (one which can give you an answer in four minutes using just a drop of blood) and new ways to treat *Helicobacter pylori* infection.

In the second edition I added a chapter on colon cancer and in the third edition this has been expanded to include many ways to avoid developing colon cancer, the second most-common cause of death in the United States, and how to diagnose it early while it is still curable. I discuss a new blood test that can tell certain individuals who have a family history of colon cancer whether they are likely to develop the disease. A new stool test can predict who has polyps and cancer.

Important information recently has been published about irritable bowel syndrome, the most common gastrointestinal disease affecting young women. New theories on what causes irritable bowel syndrome and the latest ways to improve symptoms of diarrhea, constipation, and abdominal pain are discussed.

Millions of Americans suffer from ulcerative colitis and Crohn's disease, and the new edition of *Gastrointestinal Health* contains an expanded chapter on inflammatory bowel disease. The latest information on combination drug regimens to treat inflammatory bowel disease and dietary recommendations for each stage of ulcerative colitis and Crohn's disease have been added.

Many new over-the-counter and prescription drugs have reached the market since 1991. Four new over-the-counter and one new prescription drug have been approved by the Federal Drug Administration (FDA) for the management of gastroesophageal reflux. All but a few people can now be rid of their heartburn by taking medications and following the nutritional advice outlined in this book. Eight drug regimens designed to eradicate *Helicobacter pylori* have been approved by the FDA since 1991 and are outlined in the chapter on peptic ulcer disease.

Several new endoscopic procedures are included in the third edition. Many are used to treat acid reflux and one (videocapsule endoscopy) involves the swallowing of a pill containing a camera to investigate disorders of the small intestine.

Since 1991, several old drugs have been shown to be useful in treating new diseases. The use of tricyclic antidepressant medication in the treatment of noncardiac chest pain, non-ulcer dyspepsia, and irritable bowel syndrome; high doses of pancreatic enzymes to treat the pain of chronic pancreatitis; better antibiotic regimens to treat patients with Crohn's disease and ulcerative colitis, are just a few examples of the great strides that have been made recently in the pharmacologic management of gastrointestinal symptoms.

The third edition of *Gastrointestinal Health* contains new information on dietary supplements and herbal treatments for those individuals with gastrointestinal problems since many more Americans are treating their symptoms with alternative medicine remedies. In this section Liz Emery, M.S., R.D., has outlined those tinctures, supplements, and probiotics beneficial in treating gastrointestinal disorders. The third edition continues to express the importance of nutritional management for most gastrointestinal problems. The reader is offered the latest up-to-date nutritional recommendations. Meal plans and recipes are included for your convenience.

It was my intention in writing *Gastrointestinal Health* that the book be practical, useful, and easy to refer to when you or a family member develops heartburn, abdominal pain, diarrhea, constipation, hemorrhoids, or any of the other myriad yet common problems that affect almost all of us from time to time.

Introduction

*Y*ou have a problem that's driving you crazy. Stomach pain, cramps or spasms, queasiness, frequent constipation or intermittent diarrhea, heartburn—all are signs that something is out of whack with your digestive system. Maybe you've been told you have irritable bowel syndrome (IBS) or "colitis," a catch-all term used to describe bouts of severe spasm followed by diarrhea or constipation or both. Perhaps when you're under stress you suddenly double over with stomach cramps and have to race to the bathroom. You might wake up in the mornings with what a patient of mine calls a "grungy" stomach. Or maybe in the middle of the night you feel acid rise in your throat, waking you out of a sound sleep. Or maybe, like many people who come to me at Cooper Hospital/University Medical Center in Camden and Voorhees, New Jersey, you have been diagnosed with more than one gastrointestinal (GI) problem—perhaps diverticulitis and constipation. Your doctor has told you to adhere to a low fiber diet for your diverticulitis but the low fiber content of that diet has aggravated your constipation. GI disturbances often trigger each other, and perhaps the most frustrating part of solving these problems is that what's soothing for one set of symptoms seems to aggravate another.

Virtually everyone, even people with cast-iron stomachs, suffers a bout of gastrointestinal distress from time to time as a reaction to stressful living, erratic diet, or temporary illness. Generally, as the event that triggered the symptom passes, so does the symptom. For many people, however, digestive problems are long-standing, provoked by almost anything, and often unrelieved, or only partly relieved by medication.

More than 80 million Americans live with and suffer from chronic digestive problems. These sufferers may be of any age and background, for GI problems cross all barriers of age and economics, but a surprising number of sufferers are between twenty-five and forty-five years of age. More than 60 percent are women. Next to the common cold, *digestive ailments*

1

account for more absences from work and more visits to the doctor than any other condition. Symptoms may be continuous, with daily pain or discomfort, or they may subside for days or weeks at a time, only to come back again, without seeming provocation. Symptoms may be always mild or always severe, or they may swing from bad to worse.

GI symptoms are impossible to ignore, often revolving around meals, business lunches, and social occasions. The pleasure/pain syndrome becomes integrated into daily life: you enjoy eating something, then suffer the consequences. Chronic GI symptoms don't just go away. In fact, many tend to worsen with age: the longer you have them, the more aggravating they become.

Most treatments for GI problems involve medication. Year after year, GI drugs top the pharmaceutical bestseller lists. The cost of ulcer disease in America is more than $10 billion annually. Omeprazole (Prilosec), a drug used to treat heartburn and ulcers, sold worldwide well in excess of $6 billion last year. Americans spend almost half a billion dollars a year on laxatives.

For many people gastrointestinal medications are miracle cures: Protonix and Nexium to treat heartburn; Asacol, Pentasa, Prednisone, Imuran, and Remicade to treat inflammatory bowel disease; Metaclopramide to treat heartburn, regurgitation, nausea, and vomiting related to a sluggish stomach; Imodium A-D, Kaopectate, and Sandostatin to treat difficult diarrhea; Metamucil, Zelnorm, or Konsyl to treat constipation. Yet, overall, drug therapy for many GI problems has been notoriously unreliable. The most common and troublesome conditions, such as IBS, respond poorly to drugs of any kind. Although some GI drugs seem to correct problems virtually overnight, many are only partly effective and laden with potentially serious side effects. And often, the relief offered by drugs is only temporary, so taking the medication becomes a steady routine.

The Link Between Nutrition and Disease

It has taken science a long time to make the connection between diet and disease. Only in recent years has the medical field made a strong case for dietary treatment of some of our most severe medical problems, including heart disease.

The current interest in nutrition as treatment began with a scientific study initiated nearly forty years ago in Framingham, Massachusetts. The National Heart Institute selected a community of 28,000 people for a study that has since provided the most important, well-documented evidence of the role diet and exercise play in heart disease.

The results of the first batch of statistics, which were collected and analyzed over a period of fourteen years, documented for the first time the major risk factors for heart disease besides age and heredity: obesity, smoking, lack of physical exercise, and *high levels of cholesterol and other fats in the blood*.

The Framingham study continues today, and many more studies have sprung from this early work, linking nutrition to many of our more common ailments. It is now generally accepted that diet can play an important role in countering high blood pressure, heart disease, and some cancers.

Ironically, little work has been done on the effect of diet on GI diseases. Diet—the first thing people think about when they suffer digestive symptoms—is also the last thing most people, including some physicians, know anything about. We are so confused about the effect of diet on the GI tract, that until very recently, doctors believed that people suffering from peptic ulcer disease should consume milk and cream—the exact opposite of what we now know to be true (the calcium in milk stimulates acid secretion, worsening the condition). Even gastroenterologists, who specialize in digestive disease, are often poorly trained in diet and nutrition. Physicians treat GI symptoms, if they treat them with diet at all, with general "tips": "Eat more fiber" or "Stay away from fatty foods." It is up to the patient to figure out how to apply this advice. This means that most fail to take advantage of new advances in diet therapy that could greatly improve symptoms.

Some of us follow spartan diets in an attempt to reduce symptoms. Others eat foods that actually make the condition worse, or resign themselves to suffering in silence. Many people with chronic heartburn, for example, never know which foods cause the stomach to produce more acid or allow the acid to back up into the esophagus. Many people suffer from bloating, belching, or flatulence without knowing exactly which foods produce excessive gas. Others suffer unnecessarily from diarrhea, constipation, or ulcer attacks. Hundreds of thousands of people walk around with packets of antacid in their pockets at all times.

Yet, a logical way to treat GI disorders is by diet. GI problems are aggravated by what we eat because food comes into direct contact with the GI tract. If the wrong food causes the problem, the right foods may solve the problem, or at least help.

The main reason doctors have been slow to recommend diet therapy is that it's complicated and hard for both physician and patient. Each patient with a GI disorder has a slightly different problem. There are many different kinds of disorders, and each has its own set of food responses. Different parts of the GI system react to different foods, and some foods affect the digestive tract in more than one site. As a result, it is common for people to have multiple GI problems. For example, a person with IBS, which affects the lower GI tract, may also suffer from upper GI symptoms, including gas pains, nausea, and heartburn. Even those of us experienced in nutritional therapy may have trouble designing a menu plan that offers good nutrition and at the same time detours around troublesome foods for every patient.

For these reasons, a comprehensive nutritional program to relieve many common GI problems is a difficult undertaking. There are hundreds of weight loss books and dozens of heart disease diets—but no single GI program.

The Self-Help Nutritional Program

In my GI practice at Cooper Hospital/University Medical Center in Camden and Voorhees, New Jersey, I used to design (with the help of dietitians) an individual nutritional program for each patient—a time-consuming process. I realized that we could help many more people if we could come up with one program that almost everyone could follow.

We began by listing all the common gastrointestinal disorders and their primary symptoms. We then identified the foods and eating habits associated with each symptom. We soon saw that many of the same factors were involved with most troublesome symptoms. We reviewed the list and finally isolated the six most notable culprits, the factors responsible for a long list of symptoms.

Applying the latest nutritional research to these six diverse factors, we turned them into nutritional principles. These principles, in turn, became the foundation of a nutritional program that almost all of our GI patients could use to help themselves. It is a program designed to treat the full spectrum of common digestive disorders, from heartburn to constipation to gas to irritable bowel syndrome. It can also help prevent diverticulitis, appendicitis, hemorrhoids, and gallstones; help heal ulcers and prevent ulcer recurrence; help conquer obesity; and may lessen the likelihood of developing bowel cancer.

The six principles of the program are:

High fiber

Low fat

Low lactose

Low spice

Low gas-forming legumes

Low calories

The six principles have been incorporated into a Two-Week Master Program. Each recipe in the Master Program incorporates all six principles, and is precisely calculated to fit the nutritional specifications of the Program. Each has been analyzed for macronutrient content, fiber, and calories.

The initial Two-Week Master Program is for everyone. After that, you can continue to repeat the Master Program, interchanging the recipes with any that appear in Part Nine of this book, and you can adapt your own recipes, using the six concepts of the program described in Part Six.

All of the recipes in *Gastrointestinal Health* were developed and tested by Cheryl Clifford Marco, R.D., manager of Thomas Jefferson University Hospital's outpatient nutritional counseling service, and a superb recipe writer. Each menu is designed to be easy on your digestive tract while offering flavor and variety.

This Self-Help Nutritional Program represents a breakthrough in the treatment of digestive problems, because it is not a one-note theory. It doesn't depend on drugs or on severe restriction of many foods. It is a high-fiber, low-fat, totally balanced diet that works in harmony with your digestive tract. It takes into account your appetite and your cravings for "comfort" foods. It also regulates the delicate biochemical balance between the brain and the digestive system so that you feel satisfied and gratified. It recognizes that foods are chemicals and that certain ratios must be maintained to soothe the digestive system, satisfy hunger, and meet nutritional needs.

The Self-Help Nutritional Program cannot always be individualized. For instance, some people with irritable bowel syndrome actually do better with a low-residue diet than a high-fiber diet. Most diseases of the small intestine, such as adhesions that cause kinks in the intestine, are not helped by using a high-fiber diet. Nutritional advice for patients with inflammatory bowel disease depends on the severity of their colitis and ileitis. For instance, when the disease is mild, a high-fiber diet seems to help, whereas, when the disease is severe, a low-residue diet is preferable. These conditions require medical treatment and special dietary planning. Where possible I have customized the Self-Help Nutritional Program to help those individuals with more complex problems, but there is always the chance that the dietary recommendations outlined in the Self-Help Nutritional

Program could worsen your symptoms rather than improve them. If you feel this is happening, you should stop the program and consult your physician.

Immediate Help

Learning how to treat your GI problem properly with diet does not mean blindly following a nutritional regimen for years in the hope that it is helping you. Rather, it means that your symptoms are almost immediately relieved. This quick response is rarely seen with other chronic ailments that have a dietary component. For instance, diet has no direct effect on the symptoms of coronary artery disease. Eating fatty foods does not cause chest pain, nor will avoiding fatty foods alleviate chest pain. In the long run (twenty to thirty years), if you eat a heart-healthy diet you may avoid clogged arteries and you may live longer, but at the time you're eating it you can't tell that it's helping you.

In addition to quick relief of GI symptoms, the long-term benefits of changing your diet can also be impressive: fewer incapacitating attacks; help in controlling serious diseases such as diverticulitis; and, over years, help in the prevention of colon cancer. Such a preventive approach now could spare much grief in the future.

The Self-Help Nutritional Program makes it easy for you to change your eating habits. The initial Two-Week Master Program will prove to you just how beneficial a change in diet can be for your symptoms. After that, it is up to you to make the program work by incorporating each of the six principles into your daily meals. Relief of symptoms will be your greatest motivator: if you go back to your old habits, the symptoms will often quickly return.

Because you will continue to feel well, you may soon forget what it was like to wake up every day with nausea, or to strain every time you went to the bathroom, or to have burning pain in your chest at night when you were trying to sleep. If you start slipping on the diet and begin to eat indiscriminately again, your symptoms could recur in a hurry. The GI complaints we're talking about are "diet responsive," which means that they are not usually permanently cured. So your symptoms will be your own built-in motivators.

The goal of this book is to help you minimize your dependence on drugs and maximize your control over your own health. Just as new information about the effect of nutrition on disease has steered potential heart-disease patients away from coronary bypass operations, the goal of the program is to reduce your GI symptoms without drugs whenever possible.

This is a new way of thinking about treating GI problems. And not only is it good for your GI symptoms, it's good for your heart, good for your blood pressure, good for your blood sugar, and good for your cholesterol count. By all modern nutritional standards, it would be difficult to devise a healthier diet regimen.

Finally, you have the upper hand over your digestive problems. This is a program to live with; the only lifetime diet you should need. Rigid self-discipline is not central to the program. When we speak of a high-fiber, low-fat diet, we're not talking about eating bagfuls of crude bran. We are speaking of shifting the ratio of fat to fiber and fat to carbohydrates, lowering the one, while raising the other.

Dietary therapy for gastrointestinal disorders has been dramatically effective for scores of patients, some of whom have suffered for years from GI complaints that responded to no other therapy. For many people, following the principles of the program is enough to relieve all digestive symptoms; flare-ups occur rarely if at all. For those with serious underlying disease, the Self-Help Nutritional Program can be used as an adjunct to a drug therapy program prescribed by your physician (information about most over-the-counter and prescription GI drugs is included throughout Part Two). In these instances, following the program's principles may allow you to reduce the amount of medication you take and gain a greater measure of control over your problem.

Whether you've been plagued by GI symptoms for years and nothing has ever helped, or whether your ailment is so minor that you think you can live with it, you should try a dietary approach. Dietary management of GI problems really works for real people. If you suffer from any common digestive problem, this may be the program you've been waiting for.

PART ONE

Gastrointestinal Health

1

The Self-Help Nutritional Program: A Healing Diet

*T*he science of nutrition is a changing field, and different concepts become fashionable almost weekly. New reports seem to contradict what has gone before and, invariably, new fads based on incomplete data emerge.

Amid the confusion, American eating habits have undergone profound changes. Today, one-third of our meals are consumed outside the home; when we do eat at home, we often resort to prepared convenience foods. All of us have to struggle harder to maintain nutritional balance, and the struggle is more difficult for people with GI disorders who are subject to severe and debilitating symptoms.

Many become fixated on their next meal, worrying in advance about their reactions. They know instinctively that some foods make their problems worse, but don't know how to establish a nutritional routine they can depend on. In frustration, some people end up eating almost nothing. Existing on too little food, smoking too much for oral gratification, which makes the GI disorder worse, they are often irritable and frustrated.

Double Trouble

One patient of ours was a twenty-eight-year-old ballet dancer who constantly yo-yoed on and off weight-loss diets to maintain a perfectly slim body. At the same time, she was under high performance stress. While still in her teens Margo began to have severe and sudden stomach cramps, followed by diarrhea; she had her first ulcer attack on her twenty-first birthday. She had suffered on and off from both problems ever since. Although Margo had taken many different drugs in an effort to control the various symptoms, she was still vulnerable to sudden, painful attacks that

Some Myths and Facts

Here are a few more of our common misconceptions about diet and GI disorders.

Myth: A bland diet relieves ulcer symptoms. The traditional ulcer diet includes milk, cream, rice, fish, and other bland food. It was believed that eating small, tasteless meals would help ulcers heal by reducing acid secretion and setting up a buffer against stomach acid.

Fact: A diet high in milk products can actually be harmful to ulcers because milk and cream *increase* acid production in the stomach, which can delay ulcer healing. A bland diet is often a low-fiber diet. Fiber is now thought to aid ulcer healing. Fiber may also help prevent relapse of duodenal ulcers by slowing the rate at which the stomach empties. The only foods to be avoided by someone with ulcer pain are specific "Flag Foods" (see chapter 26).

Myth: Constipation is a normal part of life, especially as you grow older, and is best treated by laxatives as needed.

Fact: Many people have become dependent on laxatives or enemas, claiming that this is the only way they can move their bowels. After long-term laxative abuse, many people develop "lazy bowel," and the bowel ceases to function normally. Stimulant laxatives also cause colicky pain by strengthening bowel contractions against dry, hard stool. For the great majority of people, the best way to treat and prevent constipation is by a high-fiber diet.

Myth: Heartburn is caused by eating spicy foods.

Fact: Many foods that are not spicy can promote heartburn, including chocolate, tea, coffee, and fatty foods. Spicy foods by themselves will not cause inflammation of the esophagus or the stomach, but can make symptoms worse if the lining is already inflamed.

sometimes lasted weeks at a time. And as so commonly happens with GI patients, the foods recommended for one condition were problems for the other.

Margo came to us after a long bout of cramps and diarrhea that had left her frustrated and weak. We diagnosed her symptoms as irritable bowel syndrome, and recommended that she follow the Two-Week Master Program. We also suggested that she join a stop-smoking group because we felt certain that cigarettes were aggravating her symptoms.

Even though Margo had voluntarily sought our help, she seemed ambivalent about taking our advice. I wondered if there was something about her illness that she was keeping from me. After talking with her about her profession it became obvious that Margo liked one of the side effects of her GI disorder—it helped keep her weight down. Margo's symptoms were often so severe that she couldn't eat anything at all. She would go to parties and dinners and smoke cigarettes—but never touch a morsel of food. The cigarettes, which raised her already high rate of metabolism even further, supplied the oral gratification she missed from food.

There was another element working against any program to treat her disorder—she had a high tolerance for pain. Her profession sometimes required that she endure extreme muscle pain, and dance through periods of exhaustion. Physical suffering seemed fairly normal to her.

The magic words that finally convinced Margo to get serious about the Self-Help Nutritional Program were "You can eat three meals a day on the Two-Week Program and you will not gain weight."

Margo was a hard case. Interestingly enough, however, once she "got" it—once she accepted the fact that she could eat real food and be free from pain without gaining weight—it was a snap for her to start the program and stick to it. She was so naturally disciplined that she thought nothing of following the regimen.

One element of the program especially appealed to her. Even though the Two-Week Master Program is recommended for most common digestive disorders, each problem has its own set of "triggers"—foods or other factors that make the disorder flare—because specific foods irritate specific parts of the GI system. We call these triggers *Flag Foods*. When we developed the Self-Help Nutritional Program we identified Flag Foods for each GI disorder. (Lists of Flag Foods for each disorder are given in chapter 26.)

Knowing which Flag Foods affect your particular problem(s) lets you fine-tune the Self-Help Nutritional Program to your individual needs. Some people have to be wary of only one or two Flag Foods, while others have to avoid a whole list of Flag Foods to keep their symptoms under control. Flag Foods give you an easy way to loosen or tighten the reins on the Self-Help Nutritional Program.

Margo quickly learned all of her Flag Foods. When faced with a rushed lunch hour or late-night snack after the theater she could pick out her Flag Foods and avoid them. She selected the lowest-calorie recipes from recipes low in calories to begin with, and she ate them regularly.

Margo's abdominal cramps subsided almost immediately, and she had no counterresponse from the ulcers. No one was more surprised than we were when she came in for a routine follow-up visit and told us she had stopped smoking—cold turkey. That was Margo's nature. Once she made up her mind, it was done. Ultimately, Margo became one of our greatest success stories. To date, she has gone a full year without an attack from either of her GI disorders.

*F*or some people who lead hectic lives, switching to new eating habits can seem impossible. Not everyone is as self-disciplined as Margo.

I remember George, a young trial attorney who popped antacid tablets throughout the day to try to cope with overwhelming heartburn. If he had an attack while in court he would suffer through it without the antacid because he didn't want the opposing lawyer or the jury to know he had a problem. Often his attacks occurred at night when he went to bed, especially after grabbing a late-night snack on his way home from the office.

Finally, his symptoms were nonstop, and he came for treatment. He wanted me to give him a bigger and better antacid tablet. George didn't have a clue about why he had heartburn. "I think it's because I'm a few pounds overweight," he told me. He was partly right, but there were other reasons as well.

George's life was complicated. He lived alone. He often worked around the clock, consuming chocolate shakes, hamburgers, and French fries at his desk in the middle of the night. If he had time off he went out partying with his friends. If George knew where his kitchen was he gave no sign of it.

I explained the mechanisms that caused his heartburn and told him there was no way to control his attacks in the courtroom or in the middle of the night—short of chronic heavy doses of drugs—unless he changed his destructive eating habits. I explained the principles of the Self-Help Nutritional Program, and also gave him a list of the Flag Foods known to aggravate heartburn.

George seemed overwhelmed by the prospect of these changes, but I insisted he give the program a try. George's mother helped him get started by going grocery shopping for him and stocking his kitchen pantry with enough high-fiber, low-fat foods to last a month. She prepared some of the entrees recommended in the Two-Week Master Program and put them in his freezer. Then she taped his list of Flag Foods to the door of his refrigerator. Under this she added a hand-lettered poster citing one of George's worst heartburn-provoking habits. It said, DO NOT EAT BEFORE GOING TO BED. She then browbeat her son into trying the first week of the Two-Week Master Program.

Within forty-eight hours George felt 100 percent better. Without ever resorting to drug therapy and taking only occasional antacids, George felt immediate relief of his symptoms. By the end of the week his roll of Tums was gathering dust on top of his dresser. His excellent response was typical of the remarkable improvement that can be achieved with proper dietary treatment of heartburn.

George's mother wasn't in the mood to baby him forever, however. After the first week, George had to manage the nutritional program on his own. Fortunately, the guidelines and recipes for the program are so simple that even George was able to incorporate them into his hectic life. One year later, he is still following the program. He slips from time to time, but renewal of the old heartburn symptoms quickly puts him back on track. Overall, George says the program isn't nearly as difficult as he expected. For him, the rewards far outweigh the effort needed to change his eating habits.

Even if you think "culinary" is a foreign word, you can manage the Self-Help Nutritional Program. Even if you're like George, who would

GI Problems the Self-Help Nutritional Program Can Help

Condition	Helps Prevent	Heals	Helps Control or Reduce
Appendicitis	X		
Colon cancer	X		
Constipation	X	X	X
Crohn's disease			X
Diverticulitis	X		
Diverticulosis	X		X
Esophagitis	X	X	X
Gallstones	X		X
Gastroparesis			X
Heartburn	X	X	X
Hemorrhoids	X	X	X
IBS (irritable bowel syndrome)			X
Intestinal gas	X	X	X
Pancreatitis			X
Ulcerative colitis			X
Ulcers	X		X

rather have a magic pill to make it all go away, you can get with the program and personally take control of your health.

The Self-Help Nutritional Program lends itself particularly to the treatment of the most common GI problems—heartburn, peptic ulcers, chronic pancreatitis, gallbladder disease, gas, constipation, mild diarrhea, hemorrhoids, IBS, and diverticulosis.*

The program is designed for people who already have significant digestive symptoms, which means that it is much more than a healthy diet. It is a *healing* diet. It is naturally low in calories. It avoids excessive caffeine and keeps alcohol to a minimum. It tells you to stop smoking because smoking makes most GI disorders worse. Most importantly, the Self-Help Nutritional Program shows you how to identify the Flag Foods that trigger GI problems in *you*.

---

*The diet is not recommended for people with acute diverticulitis and moderate to severe inflammatory bowel disease (Crohn's disease; ulcerative colitis) unless directed by a physician.

2 *How the GI Tract Works*

*T*he digestive tract is a long, intricate system that comprises many separate organs, each performing different functions. To successfully treat a GI problem with diet means understanding the complex workings of the gastrointestinal system, and how the food you eat affects it.

The body runs itself by absorbing nutrients processed by the digestive system. At the center of the digestive system is the alimentary canal, or gastrointestinal tract, which travels from mouth to anus in 30 feet of tightly packed coils. From beginning to end, food is ingested and processed, nutrients are absorbed, and residue is propelled to the end of the tract and finally eliminated.

Your GI tract will digest about 23,000 pounds of solid food in your lifetime, which makes it a very efficient, hard-working system. It takes between twelve and fifteen hours for a single morsel of food to be fully processed, although it can take much longer, depending on the kind of morsel it is. Meat goes slower, grain goes faster.

From top to bottom, the GI tract is made up of the mouth, pharynx, esophagus, stomach, small intestine, and large intestine.

Mouth, Pharynx, and Esophagus

Digestion begins in the mouth. When you chew, salivary glands in the cheek and glands at the back of the tongue produce enzymes that break the food into fragments. Specific enzymes break down carbohydrates and fats respectively.

When you swallow, complex controlling mechanisms within the pharynx, the common passageway for food and air, ensure that food goes into the esophagus, instead of into the windpipe (trachea).

The esophagus is the passageway between the mouth and the stomach. The delicate lining of the esophagus is the site of heartburn, the most common GI complaint. Swallowed food quickly passes through the esophagus into the stomach, where it is temporarily stored.

Stomach

The stomach is a large, tough organ with three layers of muscle, running up and down, across, and crosswise. As these muscles contract, the food mixture is churned up. The stomach adds quantities of the digestive enzyme pepsin and strong hydrochloric acid to the churning mixture, which help to break down dietary protein. The stomach lining normally withstands the noxious acid by forming a mucus barrier against it. If acid production is excessive, however, or if the barrier is weak, the stomach lining may be eroded. The result is an ulcer.

Although a few substances, such as aspirin, may enter the bloodstream directly through the stomach walls, most food is stored here until contractions of the smooth muscle wall pump it into the small intestine. It may take between two and four hours or longer for an average-sized meal to be pumped into the small intestine. Even when the stomach is empty, the muscles continue their steady pumping action. The wavelike contractions, called peristalsis, create the familiar pangs that signal "hunger" to the brain. The growling sound made by the continuous contractions tends to be louder when the stomach is empty. Anxiety causes an even louder noise because the smooth muscle is responsive to stress.

Small Intestine

Most of the serious business of digestion and absorption occurs in the long, narrow, small intestine. The food mixture first enters the duodenum, another likely place for ulcers to develop because the mixture is still acidic. The major work of digestion begins here with action from certain hormones. One hormone, called cholecystokinin, or CCK, draws in bile from the gallbladder to make fat more digestible. This same hormone also draws juices from the pancreas to calm the acidity left in the food mixture and to aid digestion of fat, protein, and carbohydrates.

The food mixture travels along the small intestine allowing time for refined processing and absorption. Proteins are split by various enzymes into individual amino acids; carbohydrate becomes simple sugar; and fat becomes glycerol and fatty acid. In this form, food can be absorbed by the body. Millions of tiny fingerlike projections called villi line the interior of the small intestine, increasing its surface area. As the nutrients pass by, the villi pick them out and transport them into the bloodstream.

The digestive system now begins to interact with another body system, the circulatory system. Nutrients travel through the bloodstream to the liver, a giant chemical factory that is the key organ of human metabolism.

The liver works around the clock to secrete bile, make various proteins, and remove toxic substances from ingested food. Blood that has circulated through the liver is ready to be used as fuel by body cells. If the liver fails, the body dies.

Large Intestine

After all possible nutrients have been absorbed through the walls of the small intestine, a watery mix of undigested material is left. This residue of fecal matter is propelled toward the large intestine, or colon. The large intestine, which is shorter (only 3 feet, compared to the 20-foot length of the small intestine) and fatter than the small intestine, absorbs excess water from the fiber residue and stores the feces. Eventually the feces are evacuated by the last portion of the colon, the rectum, and discharged through a muscular canal called the anus.

Beside fiber, feces also contain large quantities of living and dead bacteria, along with debris shed by the lining of the intestines. People who consume highly refined, low-fiber foods may have little actual fiber residue in the feces. Those who eat substantial quantities of vegetables and grains will have much more residue.

Many digestive problems arise here in the lower GI tract. Diverticulosis, a condition in which little ballooned sacs of intestinal membrane have been forced outward by high pressure, is one of the most common lower GI tract disorders. Appendicitis, although not a digestive disorder per se, is another problem that arises here. The appendix is a fingerlike projection hanging from the large intestine that helps certain animals digest plant matter. In humans, the appendix is probably useless. However, when it collects bacteria and undigested food, it can swell and may even burst, which is a life-threatening situation. People who consume a high-fiber diet are much less likely to develop appendicitis. The reason is that fiber keeps the food moving through the intestines, and this regular, fairly rapid transit prevents the accumulation of trapped food residue.

GASTROINTESTINAL TRACT
by Stuart Eisenberg, M.D.

1. Hypopharynx (throat)
2. Upper esophageal sphincter
3. Esophagus
4. Lower esophageal sphincter
5. Stomach
6. Pylorus (pyloric valve or channel)
7. Duodenum
8. Pancreas
9. Liver
10. Gallbladder
11. Common bile duct
12. Spleen
13. Small intestine (jejunum)
14. Small intestine (ileum)
15. Terminal ileum
16. Cecum
17. Appendix
18. Ascending (right) colon
19. Transverse colon
20. Descending (left) colon
21. Sigmoid colon
22. Diverticuli
23. Rectum
24. Anus

Colon cancer, second in prevalence only to lung cancer when statistics for men and women are combined, is another potentially dangerous condition that arises in the lower GI tract.

Despite its complexity, the digestive system works in a remarkably smooth fashion for most people most of the time. When all is well with the GI tract, the only thing you have to think about is eating when you are hungry and moving your bowels when pressure builds up in the rectum. You may hear your stomach growl when you are hungry or hear gurgling as peristaltic contractions propel food along the GI tract, but you should not actually feel these actions. Digesting and absorbing food should be as effortless and comfortable as breathing. At least that's what nature intended.

How Civilization Has Altered Digestion

In our evolutionary past it's unlikely that our ancestors ever had many of the types of digestive problems we frequently experience today. Cave dwellers and some of their descendants had cast-iron stomachs, which processed anything put into them. Our earliest ancestors ate nuts, seeds, roots, and wild plants. They brought every animal that ever moved to the dinner table—game and birds, as well as ants and bees, grubs and worms, snakes and mice. As they became agriculturists and began to grow their own plants and raise domestic livestock, some built villages along the coastlines and rivers and added quantities of fish and shellfish to their diets. Our prehistoric food pattern may not have been ideal in every respect, but it served the human body reasonably well because it contained extensive nutrients and minimal pollutants.

In different cultures, in different parts of the world, at different times in history, humans have eaten a startlingly wide array of materials. Joseph Addison, who lived in England in the sixteenth century, observed, "Every animal, but man, keeps to one dish. Man falls upon everything that comes in his way; not the smallest fruit or excrescence of the earth, scarce a berry or a mushroom can escape him."

One thing this wide variety of foods had in common was that it came in its natural state: stems and roots, husks and skins, seeds and pits. Once inside the GI tract it required quite a bit of processing to digest. Over several million years the human body developed a highly efficient processing plant that could squeeze every possible nutrient from the items we ate. Anything left over after the processing plant did its job was efficiently eliminated through the colon.

Then a sudden drastic change occurred in our diet, with no time allowed for evolutionary adjustment. A real machine took over the processing job. With the development of the rolling mill in the nineteenth century, the bran and germ of cereal grains was removed in the processing of flour. Sugar was processed from cane; oil was processed from seeds. Bread consumption fell by two-thirds.

Losing Nutrition

Food went through a sudden evolution of its own, and began to arrive on store shelves in small boxes instead of bushel baskets. Soon processed foods turned into Twinkies and Oreos, and "junk foods" proliferated in both supermarkets and restaurants. The small amount of fiber remaining in foods was lost.

Of all the many weird and spectacular creatures and plants that humans had consumed, none ever came close to resembling a chocolate shake or a hamburger bun topped with a fatty beef patty, processed cheese, mayonnaise, pickles, and catsup. None ever looked like soda pop or a sugar-coated doughnut with custard or jelly filling. Even our remarkable adaptability could not deal with the steady stream of refined sugar, bleached white flour, hydrogenated fat, and salt that poured into the typical American diet. Even rats could not survive on white bread, which was (and is) the most commonly eaten food in America.

The change in our eating habits was akin to suddenly starting to pour paste through a highly complex engine. Our GI engine became clogged and sluggish. Functioning was impaired. Constipation became common and caused much unnecessary discomfort, along with the pain associated with hemorrhoids, diverticulosis, and varicose veins.

The incidence of appendicitis doubled. The appendix tends to collect debris when there is not enough bulk to keep residue moving rapidly through the colon. This leads to clogging and infection. One study that analyzed the diets of 135 children with appendicitis and 212 children without it showed that children who consumed low-fiber diets were twice as likely to develop appendicitis.

At the same time, our consumption of alcohol, tobacco, and caffeine has also increased. In an era when the body needed more nutrients to fight environmental toxins, stress, drugs, alcohol, and tobacco, we were getting even less.

The radical shift in diet and environment over the past hundred years is directly related to the GI ailments that we face today. Everyone of us has a GI upset sometimes, and many Americans—in fact, 80 million—have chronic symptoms.

3 *What Your Symptoms Mean*

*P*ressure, burning pain, and spasm are the primary symptoms of digestive disorders that you may *feel*. Other symptoms that you may experience, but don't necessarily feel, are constipation, diarrhea, bleeding, belching, flatulence, and weight loss.

Although the range of symptoms appears limited, the number of possible disorders is long. It's not always easy to identify a GI disorder by the symptom it produces. Nor is the degree of pain always an indication of the severity of the disorder. Some serious disorders produce relatively little pain, while minor problems can create pain out of proportion to their importance.

You may mistakenly believe you have one kind of GI problem, and really have another. Or more than one. Spasms, for example, can occur anywhere along the digestive tract. When spasm occurs in the esophagus it is often indistinguishable from a heart attack. Spasm of the esophagus may also cause difficulty in swallowing. It can occur suddenly without cause, or in response to cold or hot liquids, acid reflux, or stress.

A spasm farther down the GI tract may produce a sharp pain in the abdomen that makes you double over. Spasm here may be associated with diarrhea, blockage of the bowel, gallstones, or irritable bowel syndrome (IBS).

So, location of the symptom can sometimes help determine the cause. Burning pains usually involve the upper GI tract. Burning may be felt in the middle of the chest just beneath the breastbone (heartburn) or in the upper abdomen (ulcers or pancreatitis).

Feelings of abdominal distension and cramping are symptoms often involving the middle and lower GI tract (small and large intestines). Irritable bowel syndrome, diverticulitis, and excessive intestinal gas are typical problems that arise in this region.

What Your Symptoms Mean

Symptom	Location	Possible Cause	Helped by the Self-Help Nutritional Program? Yes	No
Burning pain	Below breastbone	Heartburn	X	
	Pit of stomach	Peptic ulcers	X	
		Pancreatitis	X	
	Anus	Hemorrhoids	X	
Spasm or cramping	Below breastbone	Esophageal spasm	X*	
		Heart attack		X
	Right upper abdomen	Gallstones	X	
	Pit of stomach	Stress	X	
		Gas	X	
	Around umbilicus	Gas	X	
		Constriction of blood vessel		X
		Bowel obstruction		X
		Early appendicitis		X
	Lower abdomen	IBS	X	
		Constipation	X	
		Diarrhea	X	
	Right lower abdomen	Ileitis (Crohn's disease)	X†	
		Appendicitis		X
	Left lower abdomen	Diverticulosis	X	
		Diverticulitis		X

*Often helpful in preventing triggers of spasm (acid reflux, spicy foods).

†Often helpful in mild cases; can be contraindicated in severe Crohn's disease. Always consult your doctor before starting the Self-Help Nutritional Program if you have Crohn's disease.

Note: Unexplained weight loss, difficulty swallowing, rectal bleeding, frequent urge to move your bowels, and recent onset of constipation are symptoms that should receive prompt attention and diagnosis from your physician as they may be signs of serious disease.

Find Your Gut Reaction Quotient

If you suffer from GI distress but have never had your symptoms properly diagnosed by a physician it is important to do so before embarking on the Self-Help Nutritional Program. The program is a healthy diet for almost everyone, but digestive symptoms can sometimes signal serious disease that requires medical therapy. Relying solely on self-diagnosis is risky because symptoms of a mild disorder such as irritable bowel syndrome may be identical to symptoms of a life-threatening disease such as bowel cancer. Only your physician can make a specific diagnosis of your GI problem. Often diagnosis can be made during a regular office visit, but sometimes further tests are required.

The following quiz can help you inventory your GI complaints. Many GI sufferers ultimately come to accept as normal levels of distress that healthier individuals would find unacceptable. The quiz will let you gain a sense of control over what may seem to be an escalating range of symptoms. Answering yes to any of the questions listed below means that you should see your physician for specific diagnosis. If the diagnosis falls within the range of the common digestive disorders discussed in this book, you are a good candidate for the Self-Help Nutritional Program.

1 Do you frequently have a sour taste in your mouth when you lie down or bend over? (This means acid has refluxed from the stomach up the esophagus to your mouth.)

2 Do you occasionally regurgitate undigested food? (You may have a defective sphincter [valve] at the end of your esophagus, which allows gastric contents to reflux back up into the esophagus.)

3 Do you frequently wake up in the middle of the night coughing? (This could be caused by acid reflux being aspirated into the lungs when you lie down. If you have this particular symptom your physician will first rule out a heart or lung problem.)

4 Do certain foods such as citrus juice burn on the way down to your stomach? (Burning indicates that the esophagus is inflamed, usually caused by acid reflux. If you are immune compromised in any way—if you take drugs that suppress the immune system or if you have advanced cancer or AIDS—your physician will first rule out infection of the esophagus caused by yeast or herpes simplex.)

5   Do you experience heartburn, that burning feeling underneath the breastbone, more than twice a month?

6   Do you frequently belch? (If the belching occurs because you are swallowing air, therapy such as counseling or relaxation techniques can help treat the underlying cause of anxiety. If the belching is caused by reflux problems, the Self-Help Nutritional Program is for you.)

7   Do you have trouble swallowing solids or liquids? (Your esophagus may be obstructed or it may not be contracting properly. See your physician before embarking on any dietary changes.)

8   Do you get a burning or gnawing pain in the upper abdomen between the breastbone and the navel? (This could be a symptom of gastric ulcers, gastritis [inflammation of the stomach lining], duodenal ulcers, duodenitis [inflammation of the duodenum], or pancreatitis. Much less commonly this symptom is associated with cancer of the stomach.)

9   Do you ever get black, tarry bowel movements? (You may have a bleeding ulcer. See your doctor immediately.)

10   Do you feel full right after you start eating? (This so-called "early satiety" may indicate significant stomach problems, especially if it is recent in onset. Slow stomach emptying, called gastroparesis, or even a stomach tumor can cause early satiety. See your doctor as soon as possible.)

11   Have you recently had an episode of waxing and waning sharp or dull pain just below your rib cage on the right side? (This symptom suggests gallstones. After correct diagnosis, the Self-Help Nutritional Program can help relieve symptoms.)

12   Do you have a yellowish tinge to your skin or the whites of your eyes (best seen in natural sunlight)? This may be associated with itching, dark amber urine, and light clay-colored stools. (These symptoms may mean you have liver disease or your bile duct system is blocked. See your doctor right away.)

13 Do you have frequent episodes of pain in both sides of the lower abdomen? (If your doctor says you have irritable bowel syndrome, start the Self-Help Nutritional Program.)

14 Do you have frequent episodes of pain in the left lower abdomen? (If your doctor says you have IBS or diverticulosis, start the Self-Help Nutritional Program. If the diagnosis is *diverticulitis,* meaning that the little pouches, or diverticula, are inflamed, postpone the program until you have received appropriate medical treatment for the acute inflammation.)

15 Do you have frequent episodes of pain in your right lower abdomen? (See your doctor. You may have appendicitis, ovarian cysts, or ileitis [Crohn's disease]. If your physician rules out these conditions and makes a diagnosis of IBS, you can start the Self-Help Nutritional Program.)

16 Do you have a history of chronic diarrhea and rectal bleeding? (You could have inflammatory bowel disease [ulcerative colitis or Crohn's disease], colon polyps, hemorrhoids, or dysentery [bacterial infection of the bowel]. See your doctor.)

17 Do you have a long history of loose stools, constipation, or constipation alternating with diarrhea? (This is a likely case of IBS, which responds well to the Self-Help Nutritional Program. If this is a new symptom, however, it's important to see your doctor for diagnosis.)

18 Have you recently become constipated? (This could signal a tumor blocking the colon, especially if you are more than forty years old. Other possible causes of constipation are recent travel, irritable bowel syndrome, and side effects of drugs such as Procardia and Carafate. See your doctor as soon as possible.)

19 Are your stools pencil-thin in shape? (Again, this could reflect a blockage of the colon by a tumor. See your doctor.)

20 Do you constantly feel the need to move your bowels, even if you can't, or even if you've just had a bowel movement? (This symptom, called tenesmus, is sometimes caused by partial blockages of the colon. See your doctor right away.)

21 Do you experience frequent episodes of flatulence that bother you? (Some flatulence is normal, but some people have excessive flatulence. The Self-Help Nutritional Program can help. See chapters 10 and 26.)

22   Are you losing weight without trying? (Unexplained weight loss is associated with several potentially serious diseases. See your doctor as soon as possible.)

23   Do you suffer from hemorrhoids or anal fissures? (The Self-Help Nutritional Program can definitely help you, but your doctor will first want to make certain that you do not have an associated colon problem.)

24   Do you notice blood on the surface of the stool? (This usually means you have hemorrhoids or a fissure. Occasionally, inflammatory bowel disease confined to the rectum known as proctitis can cause this symptom. See your doctor.)

25   Do you notice blood mixed in the stool? (This usually means that the blood has entered the stool higher up in the colon. You could have a polyp, tumor, bleeding diverticulum, or inflammatory bowel disease. See your doctor.)

26   Do you have itching around the anus? (You could have hemorrhoids, but pinworms is another possibility, especially if you have small children. See your doctor.)

In most cases, having GI symptoms does not necessarily mean that you have a serious disease. Nevertheless, I recommend that you see your doctor so your problem can be diagnosed properly.

How a Doctor Diagnoses Your Problem

On the initial visit the physician usually makes a working diagnosis based on the most likely cause of your symptoms. Often there is also a "differential diagnosis," a list of various possibilities that could also account for your symptoms. For example, if you are a young woman with long-standing constipation occasionally alternating with diarrhea and cramps in the lower abdomen, but no sign of fever, weight loss, or blood in the stool, then the most likely diagnosis is irritable bowel syndrome. But other possibilities would include inflammatory bowel disease (ulcerative colitis or Crohn's disease), bowel cancer, endometriosis, and several other less likely possibilities.

Your physician may recommend treatment based on the symptoms alone. Or, if there is a possibility of serious underlying disease, he or she is likely to carry out one or more GI tests to clearly pinpoint the diagnosis and rule out other diseases.

Here are some of the common tests used to evaluate the GI tract.

Upper GI Series (Barium Swallow).   You swallow barium, a radiopaque liquid (a substance is radiopaque when it cannot be penetrated by X-rays and will therefore show up as a white area on an X-ray film), and a radiologist uses a fluoroscope connected to a TV monitor to observe the progress of barium through your digestive tract. The radiologist takes individual X-rays to review. The upper GI series examines the esophagus, stomach, and the first part of the small intestine (duodenum). The test may also include a small bowel follow-through, performed immediately afterward, to examine the entire length of the small intestine. Sometimes the procedure is carried out using "double contrast" media, meaning that you also swallow tablets to release gas in your stomach. The gas helps show the stomach lining in greater detail.

The upper GI series is performed if you have one or more of the following symptoms: difficulty swallowing, ulcer symptoms, heartburn, gastrointestinal bleeding. It can help diagnose narrowing of the esophagus, inflammation or strictures of the esophagus, hiatal hernia, or spasms. It can identify gastric and duodenal ulcers or tumors. The small bowel follow-through may reveal ileitis (Crohn's disease).

Sometimes additional studies are needed to directly visualize the upper GI tract (see below).

Endoscopy.*   Endoscopy allows direct visualization of the upper GI tract. The endoscope is a long thin tube containing a powerful light source that works on the principle of fiber optics, or as a video camera. The endoscope is inserted through your mouth (after appropriate sedation) and then gently advanced down into the esophagus, stomach, and duodenum.

This allows the physician to look directly into the upper GI tract for ulcers, inflammation, tumors, or bleeding. Tissue samples can be collected by biopsy through the endoscope. Polyps can be removed, and bleeding can often be stopped by applying an electrical current to the site (electrocautery).

Endoscopic Retrograde Cholangiography and Pancreatography (ERCP).*   A special side-viewing endoscope is passed through the mouth

*Sedative required.

and the tip is placed in the duodenum (first portion of the small intestine) where the common bile duct and pancreatic duct empty through a valve called the sphincter of Oddi. A catheter connected to a syringe containing radiopaque dye is inserted through the endoscope. The physician then tries to thread the tip of the catheter through the sphincter of Oddi into the common bile duct and/or pancreatic duct. Dye is injected and X-rays obtained that outline the duct(s). ERCP is useful in detecting common bile duct stones, chronic pancreatitis, and cancers of the bile duct and pancreas. ERCP can be used to treat problems as well as diagnose them. Stones can be extracted from ducts (see chapter 7) and blocked ducts can be opened by placing a special tube known as a stent through the obstructed area.

Bernstein Test.   Sometimes this test is used to distinguish heart pain from heartburn. A small tube is inserted through the nose into the esophagus so that one end rests near the end of the esophagus. First saltwater is infused through the tube into the esophagus, and then a weak solution of hydrochloric acid follows. If you feel the typical burning sensation of heartburn or chest pain only with the acid solution, but feel nothing unusual with the saline solution, the test is considered positive for reflux esophagitis.

pH Probe.   A thin tube that can measure pH (acid content) is inserted through the nose into the esophagus and left in place for twelve to twenty-four hours. The pH study is performed on a day while you are working, eating, and sleeping, to determine how many episodes of acid reflux you have and how long each lasts. When a symptom such as chest pain correlates on a temporal basis with a drop in the pH of the esophagus, then the pain is caused by acid reflux.

Esophageal Motility Study.   A small tube that can measure pressure is passed through the mouth and into the esophagus. The patient is asked to swallow sips of water and the pressure caused by the contracting esophagus is recorded. Esophageal motility abnormalities like nutcracker esophagus, diffuse esophageal spasm, achalasia, scleroderma esophagus, and nonspecific motor disorder of the esophagus that cause trouble swallowing and/or chest pain can be diagnosed.

Electrocardiogram.   Sometimes an electrocardiogram (EKG) is done to rule out heart problems and distinguish heartburn from angina.

Lower GI Series.   After an overnight fast and a bowel-cleansing regimen that includes laxatives and enemas, barium is placed by enema into the colon and X-rays are taken. This test is used to detect polyps, inflammation of the colon, and colon cancer. The test may be single (barium only) or double contrast (barium and air).

Flexible Sigmoidoscopy.   The flexible sigmoidoscope is a 2-foot-long tube similar in principle to the endoscope (see above). The instrument allows a physician to directly examine the lining of the rectum and a portion of the lower colon. The procedure is used to investigate unexplained rectal bleeding, change in bowel habits, or rectal pain. Sigmoidoscopy is also used to evaluate abnormalities found on barium X-rays, and to monitor progress of inflammatory bowel disease. The physician can also remove small polyps and tissue samples through the sigmoidoscope.

Colonoscopy.*   This procedure is similar to sigmoidoscopy, but the entire length of the colon is investigated. It is most often used to evaluate unexplained blood in the stool, abdominal pain, persistent diarrhea, or polyps found on barium X-rays or at the time of sigmoidoscopy. Sometimes colonoscopy is used to determine the type and extent of inflammatory bowel disease (ulcerative colitis and Crohn's disease) and to screen patients who are known to be at high risk for colon cancer, such as patients with a long history of ulcerative colitis or a family history of colon cancer. Colonoscopy is recommended to screen for colon cancer if you are over 50 years old.

Gallbladder Studies.   Imaging of the gallbladder may be carried out by using radiopaque tablets and X ray (oral cholecystography), ultrasound, or nuclear medicine (HIDA) scan.

Oral Cholecystography. After a high-fat dinner, special radiopaque tablets are swallowed. The tablets get absorbed, taken up by the liver, secreted into bile, and stored in the gallbladder. The patient eats no food after dinner and the next morning gets a series of X-rays of the abdomen (right upper quadrant) that will demonstrate the gallbladder. Stones appear as lucencies (dark circles) within the whitened gallbladder. If the gallbladder is severely inflamed and not functioning well, or if a stone is blocking the duct to the gallbladder (cystic duct), the gallbladder will not show up on the X-ray.

Ultrasound. Disease of the gallbladder, liver, and sometimes the pancreas can be found by imaging these organs by ultrasound. An ultrasound probe that looks like a microphone or a wand is pressed over the

*Sedative required.

abdomen. Gallstones, liver cysts and tumors, blockage of the bile duct, and pancreatic tumors and cysts can be seen. The test is best at diagnosing gallstones and liver cysts and poor in evaluating pancreatic disease.

HIDA. After an overnight fast a slightly radioactive substance (tracer) is injected intravenously, taken up by the liver, secreted into the bile and stored in the gallbladder. A machine then scans the abdomen for radioactivity. If a stone is blocking the cystic duct, no tracer will be found in the gallbladder. If a stone is blocking the common bile duct, no tracer will be found in the small intestine. After the gallbladder is imaged, the person may be given the hormone cholecystokinin (CCK) to contract the gallbladder. The amount of radioactivity (counts) before and after gallbladder contraction is determined and the gallbladder ejection fraction calculated. A low ejection fraction means the gallbladder is contracting poorly due to chronic inflammation (chronic cholecystitis).

Computerized Tomography (CT scan).   CT scan is an excellent way to image the liver and pancreas. After administration of a radiopaque substance by mouth and intravenously, the patient is placed in a large tubelike structure and multiple X-rays are taken and computer synthesized to form a clear image of the internal organs.

Magnetic Resonance Imaging (MRI).   The body is placed in a tubelike structure containing a strong magnetic field. Radiowaves transmitted by the machine "excite" hydrogen nuclei in the body, which in turn give off their own radiowaves. The body's radiowaves are detected by a special antenna called a coil and the signal processed by a high-speed computer to generate a clear image of the internal organs. No radiation is involved. Patients with certain implanted metal devices (for example, pacemaker) cannot have an MRI. The MRI constructs incredibly clear images of the liver and pancreas.

Endoscopic Ultrasound (Echoendoscopy).   The echoendoscope contains an ultrasound probe built into the tip of an endoscope. Depending on the area of interest the tube is either inserted through your mouth or through the anus. The ultrasound probe can be placed next to a rectal, esophageal, stomach, or pancreatic tumor and the size and depth of the tumor can be determined (tumor staging). Abnormal appearing lymph nodes and tumors lying beneath the lining of the esophagus, stomach, and intestine can be biopsied (fine needle aspiration or FNA) through some echoendoscopes. The echoendoscope is also very good at finding small stones in the gallbladder and common bile duct that cannot be detected by conventional (transabdominal) ultrasound.

Video Capsule Endoscopy.   Video capsule endoscopy is intended to diagnose disorders of the small intestines. Upper endoscopy can reach only the duodenum; enteroscopy can usually reach the mid-jejunum; colonoscopy can reach only the most distal portion of the ileum. There is a large area in between the mid-jejunum and distal ileum that cannot be seen endoscopically.

Upper GI and small bowel follow-through (see above) looks at this area but is not as sensitive as endoscopy and could miss small lesions such as arteriovenous malformations (AVM). Patients undergoing video capsule endoscopy swallow a large pill that contains a TV camera, which sends images by telemetry every three seconds to sensors placed on the surface of the abdomen. The sensors are connected to a recording device, which the patient wears around his or her waist. The patient performs activities of daily life for the next eight hours until the procedure is stopped by taking off the sensors. The capsule eventually passes through the digestive system and is excreted during a bowel movement and not recovered. Images received are downloaded onto a computer and read by a gastroenterologist. These images can detect extremely small lesions that can be missed by radiographic procedures and are out of the reach of more standard endoscopic procedures.

A proper diagnosis will allow you to receive treatment targeted specifically to your condition. Read on to find out what it means when all of the diagnostic tests turn out to be normal.

4

Is Your GI Disorder Psychosomatic?
The Brain-Gut Connection

*M*any people get the idea that their GI complaints aren't "real" because their doctor can't find any reason for their trouble.

Digestive disorders are classified as either *functional* or *organic*. Disorders like gastroesophageal reflux (esophagitis), inflammatory bowel disease (Crohn's disease; ulcerative colitis), and colon cancer are defined as organic. "Organic" means that the problem arises from a disease state, such as an inflamed colon or large intestine, which causes structural damage that can be detected with various tests.

For instance, when I insert a colonscope into the colon of a patient with active ulcerative colitis, I can readily see the damage. Instead of the usual normal pinkish color, the lining of the colon is bright red, there is a sore or break in its surface, and it bleeds easily.

"Functional" means that something isn't working properly, but there is no recognizable organic or structural damage. In the case of functional GI disorders, something is amiss with the fine-tuning of the system, even though the individual parts appear normal. Subtle biochemical defects may be causing the problem. Or perhaps the parts are poorly coordinated, so that the system doesn't function optimally.

Functional and organic problems may produce similar symptoms, but may not respond to the same kind of treatment. Organic disorders, for example, often require drug therapy, along with dietary changes. Functional disorders, which are usually less dangerous, often do not respond well to drug therapy, but they may respond remarkably well to dietary change.

Many of my patients seem to be disappointed when no organic cause is found on the diagnostic tests and relieved when something is found, even when the problem is potentially serious. This seems unreasonable—I would much rather learn that my lower abdominal cramps are caused by irritable bowel syndrome than by ulcerative colitis or bowel cancer. The functional disorder is relatively harmless; the others are more serious. But many people are afraid they might be labeled as nuts, crocks, or hypochondriacs if they have a functional disorder. In truth, the functional label does not mean that your GI problem is all in your head or that you brought the symptoms upon yourself.

When a patient's symptoms are evaluated and all the tests ordered come back normal, some doctors might say the symptoms are *psychosomatic.* "Psychosomatic," as the word implies, means that in some way the mind or brain is causing dysfunction of the body. This may imply to the patient that the doctor feels the problem is not "real." That's why doctors don't use the term very much anymore. Although there is little evidence that the mind can actually cause disease, it can certainly make preexisting GI conditions worse. The so-called brain-gut connection is very real.

There are nerves that travel from the brain to the esophagus, stomach, gallbladder, pancreas, small intestine, and colon. That is why just looking at or smelling food can stimulate stomach and intestinal contractions, as well as stomach acid and pancreatic enzyme secretion.

It's no wonder that in periods of stress, when nervous discharge is on overload, excessive gastrointestinal motility can cause cramps, excessive acid secretion, and burning abdominal pain in certain predisposed individuals. Many people can handle stress without experiencing gut-wrenching problems, but if you have irritable bowel syndrome, your pain threshold may be lower.

In fact, it appears that the brain has an important effect not only on functional bowel problems but on organic problems as well. Stress can make symptoms worse in organic disorders such as inflammatory bowel disease, peptic ulcer disease, and gastroesophageal reflux disease. Studies have even shown that stress and mental attitude can have a negative effect on survival from cancer.

So don't be too upset if your doctor can't find an organic cause for your symptoms, and don't worry if your symptoms act up under periods of stress. Having a functional problem or having a psychosomatic component to your disorder should not carry a stigma.

One of our patients, a thirty-two-year-old woman named Sara, suffered from severe cramps in the lower abdomen. She had pain at various times during the month, which did not appear to be associated with her menstrual periods. Sara did notice a correlation between her symptoms and episodes of stress in her job selling computer software. The gut-twisting cramps were often followed by severe bouts of diarrhea; then she might have several days of constipation. The constipation made her feel bloated and she said her waistline seemed to increase by two or three inches. Her symptoms became so severe at times that they interfered with her job and her social life.

Sara had been to several doctors who performed many tests, including a barium enema, upper GI series, sigmoidoscopy, and pelvic exam with ultrasound. All test results were normal. According to the tests there was nothing organically wrong with Sara. One doctor told her that her symptoms were psychosomatic. Another finally told her that she had a condition called irritable bowel syndrome (IBS), or spastic colon, for which there is no identifiable cause. IBS affects almost three out of every ten young women. It isn't a life-threatening problem, but unfortunately drugs rarely work to control symptoms.

Since IBS appears to be stress related, Sara's doctor had suggested she relax more. Good advice, but not always easy to follow. Sara didn't know how to relax. And she resented the doctor's implication that she was causing her own problem. But she tried. She went on a European vacation and experienced IBS symptoms almost every day she was away. Catching trains and planes, moving from one hotel to another, along with an erratic diet, was producing enough stress to keep her GI symptoms in full force.

When Sara came to us, she said she knew she should probably change her diet, but she didn't know what to change. It seemed that no matter what she ate, she got sick. We started Sara on the Two-Week Master Program. Even though the program is naturally high in fiber, which has been shown to be effective against IBS, we added some supplemental Metamucil, which is a natural fiber. After years of suffering, Sara saw a marked improvement in her symptoms in one week. Her swings from diarrhea to constipation straightened out, and the episodes of cramps became fewer and milder.

It's unlikely that we will understand the true cause of IBS any time soon. We know that some people seek medical help for IBS while others live with their symptoms. Researchers have tried to make something of this, distinguishing between psychological patterns of patients and nonpatients and attributing the disease to those patterns. But this has led us no closer to the answer. Why mostly young women? If stress is experienced at work, what kind of stress? If muscles contract irregularly in the bowel, is it caused by a genetic factor? If a biochemical factor is involved, what kind is it?

For the time being, we can at least relieve the symptoms. The Self-Help Nutritional Program is designed to help people suffering from both functional and organic digestive disorders. In many cases, particularly for a functional problem like IBS, the nutritional program alone is enough to completely eliminate symptoms. When serious underlying disease is present, the nutritional program can be a useful adjunct to drug therapy, often permitting lower drug doses and helping to speed recovery and prevent recurrence. For the most part, all of the disorders that follow can be improved by following the Self-Help Nutritional Program.

PART TWO

Gastrointestinal Problems— and How to Alleviate Them

5 GERD: Heartburn and Other Symptoms of Gastroesophageal Reflux Disease

*H*eartburn, a burning sensation or pressure in the middle of the chest, usually occurs within an hour after eating, and is often brought on by certain types of food. According to a Gallop poll about 36 percent of all Americans suffer heartburn at least once a month, and about 7 percent experience it daily. For some people heartburn is so severe that it becomes incapacitating. Most heartburn sufferers feel it right behind the breastbone, but occasionally a "referred" burning is felt in the back between the shoulder blades or in the jaw and teeth.

Why are some people bothered by heartburn while others are not? Heartburn is a symptom of a disorder called GERD (gastroesophageal reflux disease). The cause of the disorder is a small one-way valve, called the lower esophageal sphincter (LES), located between the esophagus and the stomach. When functioning properly, the LES allows food and water to pass into the stomach, but prevents backward flow. If the LES is loose or weak, ferocious stomach acids can back up into the esophagus, causing a powerful burning sensation as the acid comes in contact with the sensitive lining of the esophagus. Over time the esophagus may become inflamed, a condition called reflux esophagitis.

Sometimes heartburn is caused, in part, by a hiatal hernia, an oversized opening in the diaphragm that allows the stomach to protrude into the chest cavity, making reflux of acid easier. Although there is a connection between hiatal hernia and acid reflux, many people with a hiatal hernia have no symptoms at all and many people with heartburn do not have a hiatal hernia.

Not everyone with heartburn has a persistently weak LES. Normally the LES relaxes completely after a swallow in order to let food or saliva pass into the stomach. In some people the LES relaxes for no reason at all. These so-called transient lower esophageal sphincter relaxations (TLESRs) are now thought to be an important cause of acid reflux.

Certain foods are known to weaken or "relax" the valve, making reflux more likely. For instance, greasy or fatty foods cause release of the hormone cholecystokinin (CCK), which causes the LES to relax. Caffeinated beverages not only relax the LES but also stimulate acid secretion. Chocolate contains both fat and caffeine (a double whammy!). Peppermint oil, which contains menthol, is a calcium channel blocker similar to verapamil and diltiazem used to treat high blood pressure. Since gut muscle needs calcium to contract, calcium blockers can relax the LES.

Excessive pressure on the abdomen can also make it easier for stomach acid to flow back into the esophagus. As a rule, anything that increases the pressure on the abdomen—obesity, straining, or tight-fitting garments—can promote backflow of stomach contents to the esophagus. For this reason, heartburn is especially common during pregnancy. And some people experience heartburn only when weight passes a particular limit. Certain drugs may also contribute to heartburn by relaxing the LES or stimulating acid secretion by the stomach (see box).

For some sufferers of heartburn the burning sensation is the only problem. Although heartburn is the most common symptom of GERD, regurgitation is also frequently present. Regurgitation is caused by stomach contents flowing backward up the esophagus all the way to the mouth. Sour-tasting material in the back of your throat usually brought on by bending over (which increases abdominal pressure) is what we call regurgitation.

Less frequent but by no means rare GERD symptoms include chest pain indistinguishable from heart pain known as angina (see noncardiac chest pain at the end of this chapter) and so-called extraesophageal (outside the esophagus) symptoms including hoarseness, throat clearing, the feeling that

Drugs That Can Cause Heartburn

Drug	Brand Name	Disease Treated	Relaxes LES	Stimulated Acid
dicyclomine	(Bentyl)	spastic colon	X	
aminophylline	(Theodur)	asthma	X	X
propranolol	(Inderal)	hypertension: angina	X	
diltiazem	(Cardizem)	hypertension	X	
verapamil	(Calan)	hypertension	X	
isosorbide	(Isordil)	angina	X	

something is sticking in your throat (also known as globus), cough (especially at night), and asthma. Regurgitation of acid to the throat can inflame the sensitive laryngeal and pharyngeal (throat) tissues leading to hoarseness, vocal cord polyps, and, rarely, laryngeal cancer. Frequent throat clearing and a feeling that something is present in the throat is also caused by inflamed throat tissue. Patients who have these symptoms often see otolaryngologists (ENT doctors) who can diagnose GERD by looking directly at the larynx and throat with a thin flexible instrument called a nasopharyngoscope.

People who have a chronic cough or asthma are often seen by lung specialists (pulmonologists). Pulmonologists recognize that acid reflux to the throat and larynx is a common cause of cough. Pulmonologists also recognize that GERD treatment (see below) may benefit some asthma patients, especially those who develop asthma in adulthood and have more wheezing at nighttime and after eating.

The Significance of Nighttime Heartburn

Two large published surveys have shown that about 75 percent of heartburn sufferers experience nighttime heartburn. Most episodes of acid reflux occur during the daytime because that is when we usually eat. Refluxed acid is usually cleared rapidly back into the stomach by several of our body's defense mechanisms.

First of all, during the daytime we are erect and gravity helps to empty the esophagus of acid. Second, while we are awake we swallow approximately two times per minute and this allows swallowed saliva, which is rich in bicarbonate to neutralize any acid present in the esophagus. Third, the mechanical contractions of the esophagus associated with swallowing (see peristalsis below) push the contents in the esophagus back into the stomach. At nighttime these defense mechanisms barely work at all.

During sleep we make very little saliva or else we would be choking all the time. The frequency of swallowing goes way down and gravity is now working against us because we are supine. The result is that nighttime acid reflux lingers in the esophagus causing more injury to the cells lining the esophagus. People with nighttime heartburn are more likely to have esophageal ulcerations and other complications of GERD.

Complications of GERD

Although the majority of GERD sufferers do not go on to develop any serious problems, in some people acid reflux can lead to serious complications.

• Reflux Esophagitis

Repeated exposure to acid can inflame the lining of the esophagus, making it so sensitive that sometimes swallowing is painful. The irritated lining may start to bleed, or an ulcer may develop in the esophagus. Bleeding may cause the person to vomit fresh, bright red blood or old "coffee ground" blood. Sometimes the bleeding goes unnoticed until the individual passes black, tarry bowel movements, indicating the presence of blood. Or blood may show up when the stool is tested by a physician.

Continuous inflammation over a long period of time may cause scar tissue to build up in the esophagus, narrowing the opening. Such a stricture makes it difficult to swallow solid food, and the esophagus will have to be dilated by a special nonsurgical procedure. Strictures are sometimes malignant (cancerous). Fortunately, reflux esophagitis is only rarely associated with cancer of the esophagus (see Barrett's esophagus, below). Cancer of the esophagus can also be caused by smoking and alcohol. So, even if you think you can live with the discomfort of daily heartburn, it's important for your future health to try to bring symptoms under control.

• Barrett's Esophagus

When heartburn goes on unabated and untreated over a long period of time, acid reflux from the stomach can cause the lining of the esophagus to look like the lining of the small intestine. This so-called Barrett's esophagus—initiated by acid reflux—can at times (less than 10 percent of the time) turn to cancer. Adenocarcinoma of the esophagus arising from Barrett's esophagus is the most common form of esophageal cancer in Caucasian men.

Since the risk of cancer is increased in people with Barrett's esophagus, they require regular checkups. Checkups include endoscopy (see chapter 3) at which time biopsies of the esophagus affected by Barrett's are obtained. If the biopsies show no evidence of dysplasia (not quite cancer but getting there), then endoscopy is usually repeated at three-year intervals. Endoscopy is repeated at more frequent intervals in those patients whose biopsies show mild to moderate dysplasia.

If endoscopic biopsy demonstrates severe dysplasia (cancerous changes in the lining of the esophagus but not yet invading deeper into the wall), then surgical removal of the Barrett's esophagus may be recommended. *It is always a good idea to get a second opinion from another pathologist and gastroenterologist before having surgery for Barrett's esophagus.*

A procedure using a laser called photodynamic therapy may someday replace surgery. It currently is used in people who are poor candidates for surgery (for example, those with a bad heart). Research studies are now under way to see if it can be effectively used for any person with severe dysplasia or even in patients with Barrett's without dysplasia.

Treating Barrett's esophagus with medical or even surgical intervention (fundoplication—see below) will not usually reverse the changes in the lining. Nevertheless, many gastroenterologists recommend using a strong prescription anti-acid medication such as Protonix or Nexium (proton pump inhibitors—see below) indefinitely for people with Barrett's esophagus in an attempt to prevent further damage and even the development of cancer.

Diagnosis

There is no relationship between reflux esophagitis and heart disease, although sometimes the symptoms seem similar. Because part of the esophagus is located just behind the heart, heartburn can be confused with angina, chest pain caused by inadequate blood flow to the heart. There are certain distinct differences in symptoms, however.

Heartburn is usually made worse by lying down and by eating fatty foods and chocolate; on the other hand, it is made better by antacids. None of these things is true for angina. Angina is usually brought on by exercise and is not helped by antacids. Even so, it is not always easy to distinguish between the two problems, and anyone experiencing chest pain should see a physician for correct diagnosis (see noncardiac chest pain below for other causes of chest discomfort).

Symptoms alone are usually enough to diagnose heartburn. However, many doctors will want the suspected diagnosis confirmed by an upper GI series (barium swallow) or endoscopy. A hiatal hernia can also be seen with these procedures. A barium swallow or endoscopy is always ordered when an individual has difficulty or pain in swallowing.

Many gastroenterologists advise a "once in a lifetime endoscopy" to diagnose Barrett's esophagus especially in people over the age of 50 who have had long-standing GERD symptoms.

To distinguish heartburn from angina, a Bernstein test may be ordered. A 24-hour pH probe and EKG may also be recommended (see chapter 3).

• Treatment

Heartburn often responds extremely well to the dietary guidelines established by the Self-Help Nutritional Program. Nutrition along with some valuable changes in lifestyle, is excellent treatment for heartburn. The dietary program is naturally low in fat, a major culprit behind heartburn. High-fat foods are retained in the stomach longer and also tend to relax the LES valve between the esophagus and the stomach, which makes it easier for acid to back up. (For more tips on preventing heartburn, see chapter 26.)

If you have a sudden attack of heartburn, sit up or stand up. Loosen restrictive clothing such as a belt or waistband. Take a dose of a liquid antacid such as Mylanta, Maalox, or Riopan. You can start with two tablespoons and go up to six tablespoons, if needed. Antacids work almost immediately to neutralize acid and are therefore preferable to Tagamet HB, Zantac 75, Pepcid AC, Axid AR, and their prescription-dose equivalents in treating an acute attack of heartburn. The exception is Pepcid Complete, which contains an antacid for quick relief, and Pepcid to maintain heartburn relief. Don't smoke or drink alcohol or coffee.

People who suffer from frequent heartburn can make the following lifestyle changes to ease the discomfort. They may also need to take medication to either treat or avert attacks of heartburn.

Meals.   Avoid lying down for at least three hours after meals.

Sleeping Habits.   Many people who suffer from heartburn sleep with a pile of pillows under their head to keep stomach acid from backing up. Sleeping on pillows is not always effective because only your head and neck are elevated while your chest and torso remain flat. Sleeping on extra pillows can also cause your body to jackknife, actually increasing pressure on the abdomen and making reflux worse.

Heartburn can be vastly relieved if you permanently elevate the head of your bed on 6-inch blocks. Elevating the head of the bed means that your body is in a comfortable position while your whole torso is raised; to back up into the esophagus, stomach acid would have to flow uphill.

Clothing.   Avoid wearing tight clothing

Weight.   If you are overweight, especially if the excess weight is around your waist, lose some weight. The Self-Help Nutritional Program will naturally keep your weight under control, but you may first need to cut calories and increase exercise to establish your ideal weight (see Part Seven).

Flag Foods.   Pay special attention to Flag Foods for heartburn (see chapter 26). The idea is to avoid the foods that relax the LES valve and increase stomach acid. The big culprits are fat, chocolate, peppermints, nuts, and caffeine-containing beverages.

Medication.   A lot of heart medication such as calcium channel blockers, nitrates, and beta-blockers decrease LES pressure and aggravate heartburn. If you take OTC or prescription medications for any medical problems, check with your physician to make sure they are not making your heartburn worse by inadvertently causing the LES valve to relax.

Antacids.   You can further neutralize the acid in your stomach by taking antacids. Antacids are usually taken on an "as needed" basis whenever you experience heartburn. The bad news about antacids is that they are only modestly effective and the effect is often short-lived.

Over-the-Counter H_2 Blockers.   The chemical histamine is a potent stimulus for stomach acid secretion. Several drugs currently available in both over-the-counter (OTC) and prescription strengths can prevent or treat heartburn by preventing histamine from attaching to the stomach cells that make acid. These so-called H_2 blockers can be added when diet and antacids alone are not sufficient to control symptoms.

Some people prefer to take pills rather than stick to a diet. People with daily predictable heartburn often find it useful to take one of the OTC H_2 blockers before bedtime or before a meal that is expected to contain all the no-no foods that cause heartburn. When taken before bedtime or a meal, Pepcid AC, Tagamet HB, Zantac 75, or Axid AR may prevent the development of heartburn.

Pepcid Complete is a unique product because it is a combination of an antacid and an H_2 blocker. The antacid portion offers quick relief by immediately neutralizing any acid in the esophagus or stomach and the H_2 blocker portion (Pepcid) inhibits further secretion of acid from the stomach, giving a longer relief of heartburn than would be seen with an antacid acting alone. Because it acts immediately to relieve heartburn, Pepcid Complete can be taken like antacids on an "as needed" basis to treat heartburn episodes. A monograph on GERD published by the American Gastroenterological Association in 2002 listed combination antacid/H_2 blockers as the most effective OTC medication for the treatment of heartburn.

Most OTC H_2 blockers are one-half the dose of their prescription equivalents. The exception is Extra Strength Pepcid AC, which is the same dose as prescription-strength Pepcid (20 mg). Extra Strength Pepcid AC is recommended when the other H_2 blockers do not control all GERD symptoms. You can also try the 20 mg dose right off the bat if you want.

Over-the-Counter Proton Pump Inhibitors.   Proton pump inhibitors block the enzyme that pumps protons or hydrogen ions (H+) from special cells in the stomach. Hydrogen ions combine with chloride to form hydrochloric acid. By blocking the so-called proton pump these drugs can effectively shut down acid production in the stomach.

Prilosec OTC is the first OTC proton pump inhibitor. This class of drug inhibits acid secretion more effectively than H_2 blockers and this usually translates into more effective heartburn relief. However, Prilosec's onset of action is quite slow: hours or days as opposed to 30 minutes to one hour for H_2 blockers and literally a minute or less for antacids and Pepcid Complete. Prilosec OTC can be given once a day for a 14-day course, which can be repeated a second time in individuals who have frequent episodes of heartburn. Prilosec OTC is not intended to be used to prevent a heartburn episode after a greasy meal (use OTC H_2 blockers instead) or to treat an episode of heartburn (use antacids or Pepcid Complete). If you experience an episode of heartburn while taking Prilosec OTC you can take an antacid. You should not take an H_2 blocker for several hours before taking Prilosec OTC because H_2 blockers can decrease the effectiveness of proton pump inhibitors. Prilosec OTC works best when taken 30 minutes to one hour before the first meal of the day. Prilosec OTC is the same strength as prescription omeprazole (generic Prilosec). Some people who have prescription plans with a low co-pay may find prescription omeprazole cheaper than Prilosec OTC.

• Advanced Measures

The measures mentioned above are all things you can do yourself to relieve the daily discomfort of heartburn. If you still experience heartburn after following the Self-Help Nutritional Program for four weeks and incorporating these recommendations, see your physician. When the OTC H_2 blockers fall short, your doctor can give you a prescription for Tagamet, Zantac, Pepcid, or Axid (usually twice the strength of the OTC drugs, except for Extra Strength Pepcid AC, which contains the same dose of Pepcid as the 20 mg prescription strength). Many doctors use H_2 blockers as a first-line treatment for heartburn because of their overall safety and effectiveness. Frequently the recommended dosage of these drugs—for example, 150 mg twice a day for Zantac—has to be doubled (300 mg twice a day or 150 mg four times a day) in order to relieve symptoms. Rather than double the dose of the H_2 blocker, which also doubles the expense, I personally feel it is cheaper and more effective to switch from an H_2 blocker to a so-called proton pump inhibitor (Prilosec, Prevacid, Aciphex, Protonix, or Nexium, see below).

Although blocking acid secretion is a useful strategy to treat heartburn and esophagitis, another strategy is to fix the actual problem by strengthening the LES valve. Promotility drugs (Reglan and Propulsid) work by increasing the tone of the LES. They also improve esophageal contractions so that any refluxed acid gets cleared quickly back to the stomach. Finally, they hasten emptying of stomach contents into the small intestine so there is less acid to reflux into the esophagus when you lie down. These drugs work about as well as the H_2 blockers but not as well as the proton pump inhibitors and can be used as a first-line treatment of GERD. These drugs can also be used in combination with a proton pump inhibitor for those individuals who do not respond to Prilosec, Prevacid, Aciphex, Protonix, or Nexium alone.

Each of the promotility drugs has a potential for serious side effects and should be used with caution. Metaclopramide (trade name Reglan) can cause lethargy, depression, and abnormal muscle reactions. Cisapride (trade name Propulsid) can cause potentially fatal cardiac arrhythmias when given to individuals with preexisting heart disease or those taking drugs that can interact negatively with Propulsid (for example, toenail fungus drugs like Sporonox and antibiotics like erythromycin and Biaxin). You should ask your pharmacist if any medication you are taking might interact with Propulsid. You should avoid grapefruit products while on Propulsid. In fact, Propulsid has essentially been taken off the market because of its potential to cause cardiac arrhythmias. You can get the drug only if your doctor fills out a form requesting the drug. I personally use the promotility drugs for patients who have regurgitation or nausea as a prominent feature of GERD. I also use metaclopramide (sometimes in combination with a proton pump inhibitor) in patients who have reflux symptoms aggravated by slow stomach emptying (see gastroparesis, chapter 6).

When the prescription-strength H_2 receptor antagonists (Tagamet, Zantac, Pepcid, Axid) or promotility drugs (Reglan) in combination with appropriate dietary measures fail to control your reflux symptoms, the next step is usually substituting the H_2 blocker or promotility drug with a proton pump inhibitor.

Many gastroenterologists start their patients on proton pump inhibitors since H_2 blockers work effectively in GERD patients only about 50 percent of the time. By using proton pump inhibitors right away, patients get relief more quickly and some studies have shown that this results in

overall cost savings (fewer trips to the doctor, fewer endoscopic procedures).

Proton pump inhibitors block the enzyme that pumps protons or hydrogen ions (H+) from special cells in the stomach. Hydrogen ions combine
with chloride to form hydrochloric acid. By blocking the so-called proton
pump omeprazole (brand name Prilosec), lansoprazole (brand name Prevacid), rabeprazole (brand name Aciphex), pantoprazole (brand name Protonix) and esomeprazole (brand name Nexium) can effectively shut down
acid production in the stomach. They are stronger than the H_2 blockers and
more likely to alleviate symptoms of heartburn and heal esophageal inflammation (esophagitis). A single dose of a proton pump inhibitor in the morning before breakfast is usually enough to control symptoms all day and all
night.

The proton pump inhibitors (PPI) are just about equally effective in
their ability to heal esophageal inflammation caused by acid reflux (reflux
esophagitis); however, some people find that one PPI may work better
than another to relieve their heartburn and/or other GERD symptoms.
Most of the time it is difficult to predict which PPI may work best for any
given patient. Most doctors will just prescribe their favorite PPI and see
what happens. If your GERD symptoms are not completely relieved after
two to four weeks on a PPI, there are several things you and/or your doctor can do.

PPIs work best if taken 30 to 60 minutes prior to the first meal of the
day. If you don't eat breakfast, take the PPI before lunch. Some doctors may
recommend taking the PPI 30 to 60 minutes before dinner for their patients
with nighttime heartburn who continue to have symptoms when the drug is
taken before breakfast. PPIs should not be taken at bedtime because they
work best if a meal is consumed 30 to 60 minutes later (the meal activates
the proton pumps in the stomach cell and PPIs can only knock out active
proton pumps). PPIs should not be taken during a meal. This is especially
important when taking Prevacid or Nexium since food can decrease the absorption of these drugs by one-third to one-half. Protonix and Aciphex do
not seem to be affected by food but ideally should still be given 30 to 60
minutes prior to the first meal of the day.

People with severe esophagitis may do better with a 40 mg. PPI (Protonix or Nexium), rather than a 20 mg PPI (Prilosec or Aciphex) or a 30 mg
PPI (Prevacid). Nexium has been shown to be more effective than Prevacid
in healing severe reflux esophagitis and Protonix has been shown to heal severe esophagitis as effectively as mild to moderate esophagitis by eight
weeks. In one study Protonix and Nexium had equal effectiveness in healing esophagitis.

In those individuals who take their PPI intermittently whenever their heartburn acts up, choosing a PPI that has a fast onset of action may be an advantage. (Remember antacids and combination antacid/H_2 blockers such as Pepcid Complete work much faster than PPIs) Among the PPIs Aciphex seems to work quickly with approximately 80 percent of patients reporting some relief of heartburn on the first day the drug is taken. Similar results have been reported for Protonix. Without direct head-to-head studies comparing the different PPIs, it is difficult to know for sure that one PPI is truly better than the next.

For those individuals who continue to have nighttime GERD symptoms despite treatment, Protonix may offer some advantage. After a single dose, Protonix seems to be present in the blood at higher concentrations for a longer period of time than the other PPIs. Furthermore, there is some evidence that Protonix, once bound to the proton pump, may inhibit the pump's activity for a longer period of time. This longer duration of action may help control symptoms throughout the night. For some people, giving the PPI 30 to 60 minutes before dinner rather than breakfast may improve nighttime symptoms. In some instances you may need to be given a PPI before breakfast and before dinner to control GERD symptoms.

If a morning dose of a PPI or even a morning plus an evening dose fails to control symptoms experienced in the middle of the night (2 A.M.), some doctors recommend adding a bedtime dose of an H_2 blocker (for example, Pepcid 40 mg). While the proton pump inhibitors are generally more effective than H_2 blockers, the surge in acid secretion that occurs in the middle of the night seems to be better controlled by H_2 blockers. That being said, a recent article from the Cleveland Clinic failed to show any clinical benefit in treating GERD by adding a bedtime dose of H_2 blocker. I tell my patients on a PPI not to take a daily H_2 blocker at bedtime because the effect of the H_2 blocker can wear off over time. I recommend that they take a combination antacid/H_2 blocker (Pepcid Complete) only if they develop symptoms in the middle of the night (an H_2 blocker should not be taken within 4 hours of a PPI).

The PPIs do not affect the strength of the lower esophageal sphincter and therefore do not prevent stomach contents from refluxing back into the esophagus (regurgitation). On the other hand, PPIs inhibit acid secretion and in doing so also decrease the volume of fluid secreted into the stomach. If there is less volume of fluid, there is less likelihood of regurgitation. Protonix is the only PPI approved by the FDA to prevent regurgitation, although the other PPIs also likely benefit regurgitation.

Once symptoms have been controlled and esophageal healing has taken place, the drug can be stopped (usually 8 to 12 weeks). During this period, it is very important to adhere closely to the recommendations outlined in the Self-Help Nutritional Program. If symptoms recur, a "maintenance" dose of a PPI may be necessary. The maintenance dose is either the regular dose of the PPI (e.g., Prilosec 20 mg, Prevacid 30 mg, Aciphex 20 mg, Protonix 40 mg, or Nexium 40 mg) or one-half the regular dose (there is no Aciphex 10 mg tablet). In general, the full dose works slightly better than a half dose. Switching from a PPI to an H_2 blocker for maintenance usually does not work. When symptoms recur in those individuals who experience total relief of symptoms with an H_2 blocker, the maintenance dose of the H_2 blocker is usually the same as the original dose that relieved symptoms.

Serious side effects have not been seen with long-term use of the H_2 blockers or proton pump inhibitors. There was initial concern that long-term use of the proton pump inhibitors could cause malignant carcinoid tumors of the stomach. Rats receiving high doses of omeprazole for two years developed these tumors. As far as we know, no person has ever developed a carcinoid tumor from Prilosec or any other PPI, even though some people have taken Prilosec for more than ten years. All drugs have a potential for side effects, and none is a substitute for an overall health program.

Rarely do all measures fail to relieve symptoms, but if heartburn remains severe and disabling, you may be a candidate for surgery to increase the strength of the LES. Usually this type of "anti-reflux surgery" can be performed laparoscopically. Multiple small incisions are made in the upper abdomen to permit insertion of surgical instruments. The upper part of the stomach, called the fundus, is wrapped around the end of the esophagus making it more difficult for stomach contents to reflux back up into the esophagus. The procedure requires only one or two nights in the hospital. Although this is an effective procedure, it is necessary for only a small percentage of patients and is usually performed only if the patient doesn't want to take medication for the rest of his life. Those individuals who fail medical management also do not have as good results with surgery.

A new procedure can correct acid reflux using an endoscopic suturing machine. (EndoCinch). Originated by a London gastroenterologist, the procedure can be performed in less than an hour on an outpatient basis, using conscious (twilight or low-level) sedation.

The Stretta procedure is another endoscopic method to treat GERD. In this case tiny prongs puncture the lining of the esophagus near the stomach and create a microwave-induced thermal injury to the esophagus. The scarring that occurs acts to prevent acid reflux. There also is the Enteryx procedure, in which a liquid polymer is endocsopically injected into the wall of the esophagus to tighten the lower esophageal sphincter. In addition, a new endoscopic stapling device called the NDO Plicator, which appears to be technically easier than EndoCinch, is now available.

GERD *and* H. Pylori

We now know that the bacterium *Helicobacter pylori (H. pylori)* can infect the stomach and cause inflammation (gastritis), stomach ulcer, duodenal ulcer, and even stomach cancer (see chapter 6). However, it is thought that the bacteria does not cause GERD. In fact, stomach infection with *H. pylori* seems to protect GERD sufferers from developing severe esophagitis and Barrett's esophagus. Patients with Barrett's esophagus have a lower incidence of *H. pylori* infection than the general population and GERD patients with *H. pylori* infection may get worse heartburn after being cured of *H. pylori* with antibiotics, possibly because stomach contents are less acidic in most people with *H. pylori* infection.

Currently, gastroenterologists are in a quandary whether or not to treat *H. pylori* infection in people with GERD. On the one hand, we don't want to make symptoms worse; on the other hand, the ability of *H. pylori* to cause precancerous changes in the stomach (atrophic gastritis; see chapter 6) may be hastened by using proton pump inhibitors (for example, Prilosec) for a long period of time. So, in those GERD patients who need a proton pump inhibitor to control their symptoms, it might be a good idea to eradicate *H. pylori*. For those who do not require stong heartburn medication, it may be better to leave *H. pylori* alone (most of the time *H. pylori* just causes gastritis without symptoms). Until we know for sure what to do, I recommend discussing the options with your doctor and then making the decision together. I always treat *H. pylori* when found in my patients.

Esophageal Motility Disorder (Noncardiac Chest Pain and Trouble Swallowing)

In order for the swallowing process to function smoothly, several things must happen in the correct sequence. When you place a morsel of food in your mouth, the food is moved voluntarily to the back of your throat (pharynx). Everything that happens afterward is involuntary (outside your conscious control). Pharyngeal contractions transfer the morsel through a valve or sphincter in the upper esophagus (upper esophageal sphincter or UES), which must relax for the food to pass into the body of the esophagus. As the UES closes, contractions begin in the upper esophagus and then proceed sequentially downstream along the body of the esophagus to the valve or sphincter located at the end of the esophagus where it joins the stomach (lower esophageal sphincter, or LES). This propagated sequence of contractions is called a primary persistaltic wave. When the contraction reaches the end of the esophagus, the LES must relax in order for the food to pass into the stomach. It takes about 8 seconds for food to pass from your throat to your stomach and when all goes well with esophageal contractions (esophageal motility), you should not feel a thing when you swallow.

In some individuals, the swallowing process is abnormal, and depending on the type of problem, the result can be chest pain, trouble swallowing (dysphagia), or painful swallowing (odynophagia).

Noncardiac chest pain similar to angina can be caused by the esophagus going into spasm. Patients with nutcracker esophagus (stronger-than-usual contractions which normally travel down the esophagus) or diffuse esophageal spasm (the entire esophagus contracts at the same time instead of sequentially and there may be forceful and longer-than-usual contractions as well) may develop severe chest pain below the breastbone. Occasionally food may even stick in the esophagus because of persistent spasm. Interestingly, the same drugs used to treat angina (nitrates like Isordil and calcium channel blockers like Cardizem) may help relieve the pain caused by esophageal spasm.

Dysphagia both for solids and liquids is a common symptom in patients with esophageal motility disorders. Patients with cancer of the esophagus or a peptic stricture have more trouble swallowing solids than liquids.

Dysphagia is especially prominent in disorders in which the body of the esophagus fails to contract at all (aperistalsis). Patients with scleroderma, a connective tissue disease, have little or no esophageal contractions because the muscle becomes replaced by scar tissue. The esophagus becomes a flaccid tube and the LES is wide open all the time, allowing free reflux of stomach contents. In this condition food empties into the stomach just by gravity and complications of acid reflux (see above) are common. Treatment involves use of a proton pump inhibitor and elevation of the head of the bed at night. Promotility drugs are of no use because the muscle layer of the esophagus is destroyed.

Achalsia is another motility disorder complicated by aperistalsis. But in this case, dysphagia may be very severe because the LES is very tight and does not relax with swallowing. Ingested food may sit in the esophagus for days fermenting and increasing the risk of choking (aspiration of food) when the person lies down. Early on, nitrates (e.g., Isordil), calcium channel blockers (e.g., Cardizem), and anti-cholinergic drugs (e.g., Bentyl) may relax the LES and help the person to swallow. As the disease progresses the LES must be forcefully dilated with a balloon (pneumatic dilatation) or be surgically cut (Heller myotomy). Temporary relief can often be achieved by endoscopically injecting botulinum toxin (Botox) into the LES.

Esophageal motility disorders that cause spasm (nutcracker esophagus, diffuse esophageal spasm, nonspecific motor disorder of the esophagus, and hypertensive LES) can also cause dysphagia and odynophagia. Painful swallowing can also be caused by esophageal cancer, severe peptic esophagitis, and infectious esophagitis (caused by monilia [yeast], herpes virus, or cytomegalic virus [CMV]), so endoscopic evaluation is essential in all patients with dysphagia and/or odynophagia.

Patients with noncardiac chest pain, dysphagia, or odynophagia who have a normal-appearing esophagus at the time of endoscopy likely have an esophageal motility disorder or acid reflux. A specific diagnosis can be made by having an esophageal motility study and a 24-hour pH study (see chapter 3).

6   *Peptic Ulcer Disease and Other Stomach Disorders*

*P*eptic ulcer disease is a group of disorders in which a portion of the mucous membrane that lines the stomach or the duodenum (the first portion of the small intestine) becomes inflamed and then ulcerated. Inflammation is called gastritis when it is in the stomach, and duodenitis when it is in the duodenum. Ulcers in either location are called peptic, named for the digestive enzyme pepsin, which breaks down protein.

Inflammation

Inflammation of the gastrointestinal tract has many causes: arthritis drugs, ingestion of corrosive substances, allergies, alcohol, *Helicobacter pylori (H. pylori)* infection (see below), shock, surgery, or other significant physical stress—anything that might cause the stomach to produce excessive acid or weaken the mucous membrane that lines the stomach. Gastritis and duodenitis are not usually serious conditions but can sometimes cause significant bleeding. These are both usually curable conditions, but if neglected may lead to complications.

• Gastritis

Gastritis, an inflammation of the stomach lining, usually asymptomatic, may cause epigastric (upper middle) abdominal discomfort, nausea, and vomiting. Gastritis may come on abruptly (acute) or it may be a chronic condition. Certain drugs, bacteria, viruses, and alcohol can cause gastritis. In some people, extreme physical stress or the development of liver failure can cause gastritis and ulceration, also known as stress-related mucosal damage or stress ulcer. *H. pylori* is the most frequent cause of chronic gastritis.

Correct diagnosis is made by examining the stomach lining through an endoscope, a long slender tube passed down the esophagus to the stomach. A bit of tissue can be removed through the endoscope for analysis to help determine the type of inflammation and possible cause.

Although gastritis is common and usually does not cause significant problems, your doctor may want to treat your gastritis if you have symptoms. If the inflammation is caused by alcohol, aspirin, or NSAIDs, merely avoiding these substances can be enough. If *H. pylori* is present, one of the antibiotics regimens described below should cure the gastritis but may or may not cure the pain in the epigastric area (see nonulcer dyspepsia below).

Antacids containing aluminum and magnesium may help relieve symptoms of gastritis by neutralizing gastric acids. A trial of an H_2 blocker like Pepcid (20 mg twice a day) or a proton pump inhibitor like Protonix (40 mg a day) may also be useful to heal gastritis and treat symptoms.

• Duodenitis

Inflammation of the duodenum may produce the same vague symptoms as gastritis, a burning sensation in the upper abdomen, but is often asymptomatic. Infection with *H. pylori* is the most common cause of duodenitis. Diagnosis of duodenitis is made by endoscopy at which time an area of redness of the lining of the duodenum but no visible ulcer is seen.

Like gastritis, treatment for duodenitis, when it produces symptoms, is similar to treatment for an ulcer (see below).

Peptic Ulcers

Peptic ulcer disease (PUD) is a common disorder that affects millions of individuals in the United States each year and has a major impact on health care costs. In the last two decades, major advances have been made in the understanding of the causes of PUD, particularly regarding the role of *Helicobacter pylori* infection and nonsteroidal anti-inflammatory drugs (NSAIDs). This has led to important changes in diagnostic and treatment strategies, with the potential for improving the clinical outcome and decreasing health care costs.

A peptic ulcer is a chronic sore or break in the mucosal membrane lining of the stomach (gastric ulcer), duodenum (duodenal ulcer), or less commonly, the esophagus (esophageal ulcer).

Ulcer pain (burning, gnawing, discomfort) is typically worse when the stomach is empty because acid can more readily come in contact with the irritated lining of the stomach or duodenum. Food helps set up a barrier and tends to neutralize acid. That is why ulcer pain seems to lessen after eating.

Stomach ulcers usually cause pain in the upper mid-abdomen (epigastric area) or just below your rib cage on the left side. Eating may aggravate stomach ulcers at first, especially certain foods, but then the burning sensation subsides as the food begins to buffer the stomach acid. Stomach ulcers occur more often in people over the age of forty. This higher incidence in older people may be caused by increased use of drugs such as aspirin and NSAIDs, which are often used to treat arthritis (see below).

Duodenal ulcers usually occur in younger people between the ages of twenty and forty, probably, in part, because younger people produce more acid. Burning pain from duodenal ulcers may be felt in the epigastrium or a bit to the right. Eating often relieves pain quickly because of an immediate buffering effect, but irritants in certain foods can produce more pain.

Smoking and alcohol consumption may exacerbate ulcers but probably do not cause them. Nor do spicy foods appear to be a cause. About 10 percent of Americans will develop an ulcer in their lifetime.

Ulcers occur only in the presence of stomach acid, but they are not necessarily caused by excessive quantities of acid. Even people who produce low levels of acid sometimes develop ulcers while others who produce large amounts of acid may be ulcer free. Distortion of the balance between acid and protective mucus is the likely cause. With inadequate "mucosal defense," even a small amount of acid can cause an ulcer.

Most people think stress is the cause of their ulcers and most of the time they are wrong. Many people under great stress never develop ulcers, while others who lead seemingly quiet lives do. We know there are basically three ways to get an ulcer.

• Aspirin and NSAIDs

A significant percentage of patients taking nonsteroidal anti-inflammatory drugs (NSAIDs) experience some type of adverse gastrointestinal symptoms and up to 25 percent of people may develop ulcers. Only 1 to 2 percent of people will bleed while taking NSAIDs. NSAIDs cause gastrointestinal damage by two independent mechanisms: a topical effect (the pill directly irritating the stomach) and a more important systemic effect (after absorption into the bloodstream) caused by the NSAIDs blocking the enzyme cyclooxygenase (COX) which is necessary to help the stomach lining defend itself against acid and pepsin.

Aspirin and NSAIDs, such as Motrin and Advil, can erode the stomach lining. These drugs block the production of the hormone prostaglandin (PGE) by interfering with the enzyme cyclooxygenase (COX) necessary to make PGE. If you have arthritis you want to reduce PGE because it causes joint inflammation. However, PGE also has a good side. It stimulates mucus and bicarbonate production in the stomach. The mucus acts as a protective layer between the acid and the stomach lining. Bicarbonate actually neutralizes stomach acid. By blocking the production of PGE, aspirin and NSAIDs break down the so-called mucosal defense and an ulcer may develop. The elderly, smokers, people with severe heart disease, and people taking steroids like prednisone along with aspirin are particularly prone to developing ulcers when taking arthritis medicine.

Currently there are arthritis medications that can calm inflamed joints with less chance of causing stomach trouble. There are two different COX enzymes (COX-1 and COX-2). COX-1 produces a normal level of PGE—not enough to cause joint inflammation but enough to protect the stomach. COX-2 is activated by inflammation and is responsible for the overproduction of PGE in inflammatory conditions like arthritis. Current drugs such as Celebrex, Mobic, and Bextra block COX-2 more than COX-1. These so-called COX-2 inhibitors have less potential to cause peptic ulcers than traditional arthritis medications because they allow normal amounts of PGE to be produced. When aspirin (even 81 mg baby aspirin) is taken with Celebrex the risk of bleeding ulcers increases. There is also mounting evidence that COX-2 blockers, and perhaps even COX-1 blockers (Naproxen) to a lesser extent, may increase the risk of heart attack and stroke. In fact, Vioxx, a COX-2 blocker, was recently voluntarily withdrawn from the market.

The prevalence of ulceration in NSAID users has been reported as being between 14 and 31 percent with a twofold higher frequency of gastric ulcers compared with duodenal ulcers. Among the strategies used to decrease the risk of ulcer development are: (1) the use of analgesics other than NSAIDs (e.g., acetaminophen); (2) the use of the lowest possible dosage of NSAID; (3) the use of a COX-2–selective NSAID; (4) the use of low doses of corticosteroids instead of NSAIDs; (5) avoidance of concomitant use of NSAIDs and corticosteroids; and (6) the use of preventive therapy (see below).

• Too Much Acid

Ulcers can also be caused by extreme overproduction of acid. While the mucous protection of the stomach lining can hold up against even a heavy acid load, at times secretion of acid is so great not even a normal mucosal defense is enough. Rare conditions like gastrinoma (Zollinger-Ellison syndrome), in which a tumor of the pancreas secretes the acid producing hormone gastrin, are associated with severe ulcer disease.

• *H. Pylori*

There has been a lot of talk about *H. pylori*. What is *H. pylori*? *H. pylori* is a spiral-shaped bacterium that is found in the gastric mucous layer adherent to the lining of the stomach. *H. pylori* produces a variety of proteins that appear to mediate or facilitate its damaging effects on the stomach lining. The enzyme urease produced by the bacteria helps the bacteria survive in an acidic environment. Other proteins secreted by the bacteria cause inflammatory reactions which may ultimately lead to development of an ulcer or even gastric cancer.

One of the most common causes of ulcers is bacterial infection of the stomach by *H. pylori*. The knowledge that peptic ulcer disease is often an infectious disease shocks a lot of people. Did you know that if you have *H. pylori*, your spouse has a 70 percent chance of having it as well? Your parents and children are also more likely to be infected.

The discovery by Barry Marshall and Robin Warren, Australian doctors, that most ulcers are caused by a bacterial infection of the stomach stunned the medical world. We now know that one in three adult Americans is infected with *H. pylori* and more than 80 percent of adult Japanese, Latin Americans, Asians, and Africans are infected. Once you are infected, there is a 15 to 20 percent chance of developing an ulcer in your lifetime.

H. pylori–infected individuals are also at higher risk for stomach cancers and lymphoma, but the risk is very low (less than 1 percent). The World Health Organization (WHO) has declared *H.pylori* to be a class-I carcinogen (see stomach cancer).

Acid kills most bacteria, but *H. pylori* can exist only in an acidic environment. That's because *H.pylori* produces an enzyme called urease that converts stomach urea to ammonia. Since ammonia has a high pH (basic) it neutralizes acid and permits *H. pylori* to thrive.

Infection with *H. pylori* usually occurs in childhood. That's because the bacteria is usually transmitted from person to person by the fecal-oral route. That is, stool contaminated with *H. pylori* (the bacteria can be shed from the stomach down the gastrointestinal tract) finds itself on a child's finger and into the mouth of another child. Because of improving hygienic habits as a child grows older, most infection occurs before the age of five. *H. pylori* can also be transmitted by the oral-oral routes (drooling, kissing), vomit-oral, and environmentally (water supply) in some parts of the world (e.g., Peru and Himalaya).

Contrary to the age-old belief that the best way to get an ulcer is become

CEO of a Fortune 500 company, we now know the best way to get an ulcer is to be infected with *H. pylori*. And the best way to get infected with *H. pylori* is to be poor (at least as a child). Poor hygiene and crowded living conditions as a child are major risk factors for *H. pylori* infection. Minority groups are much more likely to be infected with *H. pylori* than American Caucasians.

The older you are, the more likely you are to be infected with *H. pylori*. At first glance, this seems incongruous. I just told you *H. pylori* infection usually occurs in childhood. Why should older people be at risk?

The elderly grew up in an America far different from today's America. In the 1920s and '30s, hygiene was not dissimilar to that seen in developing nations today. Greater wealth, less crowding, and better public works allow most children today to grow up *H. pylori*–free. In fact, *H. pylori* infection seems to be dying out in the United States along with ulcers and stomach cancer.

Once infection occurs, *H. pylori* often sets up shop in your stomach for life (or until you get treatment; see below). *H. pylori* doesn't invade the lining in your stomach; it just sits in the mucous layer producing various chemicals and proteins that can damage the stomach lining. Most infected individuals develop gastritis, but nothing else, and live in relative harmony with the bacteria. Only a minority of people develop ulcers or cancer. It is not clear why some people infected with *H. pylori* get ulcers and others do not. Certain host factors (for example, genetic predisposition) and infection with virulent strains of the bacteria are probably important factors in determining the natural history of *H. pylori* infection.

There is increasing evidence that *H. pylori* infection can cause problems outside the gastrointestinal tract. Inflammation that goes on for a long time can make blood clot more easily and can make platelets, a component of your blood, "more sticky." Some studies have linked *H. pylori* to the development of atherosclerosis leading to a heart attack and stroke. Studies have linked *H. pylori* to dental plaque and causing cavities. At the present time, the association of *H. pylori* with these disorders is not well established.

***How to Find Out If You Are Infected with* H. Pylori.** *H. pylori* infection can be diagnosed by a simple blood (serological) test, stomach biopsy at the time of endoscopy, urea breath test (testing exhaled breath after drinking a chemical solution), and by detecting *H. pylori* in stool. The serological test, endoscopy, and breath test are all equally effective (about 90 percent) in detecting the presence of *H. pylori*. Young people (younger than forty-five) with ulcer symptoms will usually get the serological test, breath test, or stool antigen test. Older individuals are usually referred for endoscopy to make sure stomach cancer is not present.

Your doctor will usually want to know if you are infected with *H. pylori* if you have ulcer symptoms. If you are under the age of forty-five, I recommend the serological (blood) test to check for the presence of *H. pylori*. However, recent studies show that the stool antigen test is just as good in the detection of *H. pylori* as serology. The blood test detects the presence of antibody against the bacteria, whereas the stool antigen test detects antigen (a portion of *H. pylori* bacteria). The antibody test just determines whether you have been exposed to the bacteria and does not prove that you are currently infected. A positive stool antigen test indicates active (current) *H. pylori* infection.

If you are over the age of forty-five or have evidence of gastrointestinal bleeding (vomiting blood, black tarry bowel movements, or anemia), your doctor will recommend a diagnostic procedure—probably an endoscopy— in order to rule out stomach cancer and/or determine the site of bleeding. At the time of endoscopy, a biopsy of the stomach can be obtained for a CLO-test, which determines the presence of *H. pylori* by detecting the presence of the enzyme urease in the stomach tissue. Biopsies of the stomach can also be sent to the pathologist. Under the microscope, the bacteria can be seen in the stomach mucous layer in infected individuals.

Once you have been treated for *H. pylori,* your *H. pylori* serology test may remain positive for years even though you are no longer infected. If ulcer symptoms return after *H. pylori* treatment and you are under the age of forty-five, or if you are over the age of forty-five and already had an endoscopy, the *H. pylori* breath test and stool antigen test can determine if you are still infected. The breath test should be performed no sooner than two months after your treatment for *H. pylori*. You are asked to drink a solution of urea containing a radioactive isotope of carbon. If you are infected with *H. pylori,* the bacteria will digest the urea and release radioactive CO_2, which is absorbed into your bloodstream and exhaled through the lungs into a balloon. Radioactive CO_2 in your breath can be measured by a machine that detects radioactivity. Children can be given a similar test using a non-radioactive isotope of carbon.

Endoscopy to diagnose persistent *H. pylori* infection can be performed as an alternative to the breath test. The breath test can also be used to diagnose *H. pylori* infection in those people who have never been treated; however, I find the serologic test to be preferable due to its low cost and ease of administration.

Diagnosis of *H. pylori* may be warranted in several clinical situations (see box below).

It is not currently recommended to screen the general population for the presence of *H. pylori*. The cost of such screening would be large as it is

Reasons to Diagnose and Treat H. pylori *Infection*

Strongly Recommended	Strength of Supporting Evidence
Active peptic ulcer disease	Unequivocal
History of peptic ulcer disease	Unequivocal
Bleeding peptic ulcer	Unequivocal
MALT lymphoma (see below)	Unequivocal
Gastritis with severe abnormalities	Supportive
Following the resection of stomach cancer	Supportive

Advisable	
Nonulcer dyspepsia after full investigation	Equivocal
Family history of stomach cancer	Equivocal
Long-term treatment with proton pump inhibitor for GERD	Supportive
Planned or existing treatment with NSAIDs	Equivocal
Following stomach surgery for peptic ulcer disease	Supportive
Patient's wishes	Equivocal

Uncertain	
Prevention of stomach cancer in the absence of risk factors	Equivocal
People with no symptoms (the general population)	Equivocal

Adopted from the Maastricht consensus report on the management of *Helicobacter pylori* infection.

anticipated that millions of people would be infected and need treatment. Treatment regimens cost anywhere from $35 to $300 and more. There is also worry that widespread treatment with the few antibiotics that kill *H. pylori* may cause the bacteria to become resistant to these antibiotics and they wouldn't be available when we really need them (to treat active peptic ulcer disease, gastrointestinal bleeding, etc.) Nevertheless, some people may want to know if they are infected. Researchers are still evaluating the benefits of screening large populations of people for *H. pylori,* and recommendations for diagnosis and treatment of this disease may change in the future.

Ulcer Treatment

Drug therapy is always recommended to treat ulcers because drugs help speed healing. Untreated ulcers can bleed, perforate, or cause obstruction, and it is best to heal them as quickly as possible. Ulcers are seldom malignant, although any gastric ulcer is potentially malignant and needs to be evaluated, especially if you are over forty-five years old. Four types of drugs are used to heal ulcers: antacids to neutralize stomach acid; sulcrafate to protectively coat the ulcer; H_2 receptor antagonists to inhibit acid production; and proton pump inhibitors, which also inhibit acid production. It is rarely necessary to use more than one type of ulcer medication.

Antacids neutralize acid: two tablets or two tablespoons of an antacid, such as Maalox or Mylanta, are given one and three hours after meals and at bedtime for patients with an active ulcer. Antacids can also be given as needed to control symptoms (studies show that low doses of antacids work just as well as larger doses). Antacid therapy properly used may be as effective as some prescription drugs (see below). For many people, antacids taken regularly can ultimately relieve pain and, along with changes in the diet and lifestyle, may be enough to heal the ulcer. Nevertheless, this anti-ulcer regimen is quite cumbersome and does not treat *H. pylori*. Therefore, it is rarely if ever used today to treat peptic ulcer disease. Antacids are most frequently used on an as-needed basis when patients develop symptoms of heartburn or burning epigastric pain.

Carafate (sucralfate) can heal ulcers as well as antacids or H_2 blockers, but the drug is not used in any of the *H. pylori* drug regimens (see below). Sucralfate is occasionally used to heal an NSAID ulcer after the NSAID has been discontinued, but sucralfate cannot prevent the development of an NSAID-induced stomach ulcer. Sucralfate is sometimes given through a nasogastric tube (tube through the nose) to extremely ill patients in the intensive care unit to prevent stress ulcers from forming in the stomach. Nowadays, most ulcer patients will be prescribed an H_2 blocker or a proton pump inhibitor in the ICU setting.

Drug treatment of peptic ulcer disease today depends on the cause of the ulcer. For those patients whose ulcers are caused by asprin or nonsteroidal anti-inflammatory drugs, the preferred treatment is to discontinue the aspirin or NSAID and then treat the individual with one of the standard anti-ulcer medications (an H_2 blocker such as, Pepcid, Zantac, Tagamet, Axid; a proton pump inhibitor such as Protonix, Nexium, Prilosec, Prevacid, or Aciphex; or Carafate, which works by binding to the raw exposed surface of inflammed or ulcerated tissue forming a protective coating, allowing healing to occur).

Once healing has occurred, it is likely the person will never get an ulcer again if he stays away from aspirin or NSAIDs. If these drugs cannot be avoided, the recommendation is to give the drug Cytotec (misoprostol) along with the asprin or NSAID once the ulcer has been healed by a standard ulcer drug. Cytotec is a prostaglandin that produces mucus and bicarbonate and protects the stomach against the injurious effects of aspirin and NSAIDs. The recommended dose of Cytotec is 100 or 200 mcg four times per day. This drug may produce cramps and diarrhea. If it does, you can reduce the dose to 100 mcg three to four times per day, although studies show that only misoprostol 800 ug/day has been directly shown to reduce the risk of ulcer complications such as perforation, hemorrhage, or obstruction.

A drug called Arthrotec is a combination of Cytotec (200 ug) plus the NSAID Diclofenac (50 to 75 mg). The lower dose of Diclofenac can be given either twice or three times per day and the larger dose can be given up to two times per day. Arthrotec is convenient because you don't have to remember to take a second drug in order to protect your stomach.

If you absolutely cannot tolerate Cytotec but need stomach protection from aspirin and NSAIDs, the next best thing is a proton pump inhibitor. I usually give Prevacid 30 mg, Protonix 40 mg, or Nexium 40 mg per day along with the aspirin or NSAID. At the present time, only Prevacid is approved by the FDA for the prevention of NSAID ulcers. The advent of the COX-2 inhibitor era (see above) may circumvent the need to use ulcer drugs in many patients taking arthritis medicine; however, even COX-2 inhibitors like Celebrex and Vioxx may cause ulcers that bleed although at a lower incidence than other NSAIDs.

I believe ulcer patients taking aspirin or NSAIDs on a chronic basis need to be checked for *H. pylori* infection. If the *H. pylori* test is positive, I recommend treating the patient for *H. pylori*.

Patients that are found to have an *H. pylori*-related ulcer or need to have *H. pylori* eradicated for some other reason (see box on page 63) can be treated with one of eight FDA-approved treatment regimens (see box on page 67). I rarely use options 1 or 2 listed in the box because the effectiveness of the treatment is only 70 to 80 percent and the regimen may be more expensive than other treatments. The advantage of treatments 1 or 2 is that you only have to take four or five tablets a day. Treatment option 3 (standard triple therapy) is complicated, requiring up to eighteen tablets a day. Furthermore, many people have drug side effects following this regimen, and alcohol use is prohibited in anybody taking metronidazole. I tend to use this regimen in those people where cost is an issue, since this is the cheapest regimen. Although inexpensive, the regimen is 90 percent effective. I also tend to use standard triple therapy for patients who are allergic to penicillin. For convenience, it can be prescribed as Helidac kit where everything is prepackaged with written instructions. Helidac is more expensive than your doctor ordering each drug separately. When a proton pump inhibitor like Protonix is added to standard triple therapy, it is known as quadruple therapy and the effectiveness of the regimen is enhanced. Options 4, 5, 7, and 8 (proton pump inhibitor–based triple therapy) tend to be the preferred regimens recommended by most gastroenterologists. Because they are more expensive than option 3, I tend to use one or the other if the patient has a prescription plan. Option 4 can be prescribed as PrevPak for convenience of administration, but as with the Helidac kit, the cost is higher. Although options 4 and 5 tend to be better tolerated than option 3, some people have difficulty taking Biaxin (clarithromycin) due to gastrointestinal distress. Biaxin intolerance is more likely to occur with options 1 and 2, which use a higher dose of Biaxin. Option 6 is rarely used in the United States and is recommended only in patients who are allergic or intolerant to Biaxin or for infections of *H. pylori* that are known or suspected to be resistant to Biaxin. Option 3 is more commonly used in patients who are allergic or intolerant of Biaxin.

Some *H. pylori* infections have developed a resistance to metronidazole or Biaxin. If I fail to get rid of *H. pylori* using a Biaxin-based regimen, I will retreat, using option 3 or 6. Conversely, if option 3 doesn't work because of resistance to metronidazole, I tend to use option 4, 5, 7, or 8. Although unusual, if a person is not cured of their *H. pylori* infection after two different treatment courses, I endoscope the patient and take several biopsies for bacterial culture to determine which antibiotics are able to kill the bacteria.

Most of the time, there is no need to make sure *H. pylori* treatment has been successful. Many of the regimens are 90 percent effective and we just assume the treatment worked. In some patients who have severe complications of peptic ulcer disease, like bleeding or perforation, we do document *H. pylori* eradication by performing an endoscopy or breath test two months after finishing treatment. You can get an *H. pylori*–related ulcer to heal just by giving an H_2 blocker or proton pump inhibitor. However, if you heal the ulcer but don't get rid of *H. pylori*, there is an 80 to 90 percent chance the ulcer will return within a year.

Getting rid of *H. pylori* does not give full protection against developing another ulcer. In some studies, 40 percent of patients develop recurrent peptic ulcer disease even though they are no longer infected with *H. pylori*. Nobody knows the reason why these patients develop ulcers. When this hap-

---

FDA-Approved Treatment Options for Helicobacter pylori

1. Prilosec 40 mg once a day plus Biaxin 500 mg three times a day. If an active ulcer is present, continue Prilosec 20 mg once a day for an extra two weeks. *Or,*
2. Tritec 400 mg two times a day plus Biaxin 500 mg three times a day for two weeks. If an active ulcer is present, continue Tritec 400 mg two times a day for an extra week. *Or,*
3. Metronidazole 250 mg four times a day plus tetracycline 500 mg four times a day plus Pepto Bismol two tablespoons or tablets four times a day for two weeks. If an active ulcer is present, add a proton pump inhibitor like Protonix 40 mg a day and continue the proton pump inhibitor for an extra two weeks. *Or,*
4. Prevacid 30 mg two times a day plus amoxicillin 1 g two times a day plus Biaxin 500 mg two times a day for ten or fourteen days. If an active ulcer is present, continue Prevacid 30 mg once a day for an extra two weeks. *Or,*
5. Prilosec 20 mg twice a day plus amoxicillin 1 g two times a day plus Biaxin 500 mg two times a day for fourteen days. If an active ulcer is present, continue Prilosec 20 mg once a day for an extra two weeks. *Or,*
6. Prevacid 30 mg three times a day plus amoxicillin 1 g three times a day for two weeks.* If an active ulcer is present, continue Prevacid 30 mg once a day for an extra two weeks. *Or,*
7. Nexium 40 mg a day plus amoxicillin 1 g twice a day plus Biaxin 500 mg twice a day for ten days. If an active ulcer is present, continue Nexium 40 mg once a day for an extra two weeks. *Or,*
8. Aciphex 20 mg twice a day plus amoxicillin 1 g twice a day plus Biaxin 500 mg twice a day for seven days. If an active ulcer is present, continue Aciphex 20 mg once a day for an extra two weeks.

*Indicated for patients who are either allergic or intolerant to Biaxin or for infections with known or suspected resistance to Biaxin.

---

pens, the ulcer can usually be controlled by an eight-week course of an H_2 blocker or a six-week course of a proton pump inhibitor. If a person continues to develop peptic ulcer disease, a maintenance dose of an H_2 blocker (half the prescription strength, e.g., Zantac 150 mg at bedtime, Pepcid 20 mg at bedtime, or Axid 150 mg at bedtime) may be necessary on an indefinite basis.

Ulcer patients who are not taking NSAIDs and are not infected with *H. pylori* should have a blood test measuring their serum gastrin level. As I mentioned, a rare pancreatic tumor secreting gastrin can cause severe peptic ulcer disease. In the United States we are finding more and more people with ulcers who do not take NSAIDs, who are not infected with *H. pylori,* and have a normal gastrin level. There are obviously other causes for peptic ulcer disease. Patients with NSAID-negative, *H. pylori*–negative ulcers can be treated with a prescription-strength H_2 blocker or proton pump inhibitor. An active peptic ulcer should never be treated with an over-the-counter-strength H_2 blocker (except maximum strength Pepcid AC twice a day).

Self-Help

The Self-Help Nutritional Program, in conjunction with drug therapy, can help relieve the symptoms of peptic ulcer disease. After the condition is healed, the Self-Help Nutritional Program, which is higher in fiber, may help reduce the incidence of recurrent ulcers. This can be especially important for patients who do not take NSAIDs and who are *H. pylori* negative. However, dietary therapy cannot be relied on to prevent ulcer recurrence.

One patient of mine with peptic ulcer disease demonstrates how it often takes a combination of drug therapy, along with changes in lifestyle and diet, to heal and manage ulcers. Brendan, a forty-year-old rising star in his management consulting firm, began his day with an hour of paperwork on a commuter train and ended it the same way twelve hours later. His normal breakfast consisted of four cups of strong coffee, three cigarettes, and a Danish. He made time for lunch only when entertaining a client.

On the way home from work at night, Brendan usually nursed a Scotch on the rocks and smoked five more cigarettes. Around 8:30 P.M. he would eat a huge meal when, he said, he could finally relax and enjoy food. The foods he enjoyed most were curries, red-hot Italian tomato sauces, and any Mexican food, as long as it had plenty of salsa.

For two months prior to seeing me, Brendan had awakened with a burning, gnawing sensation in the pit of his stomach and a feeling of nausea. Eating a cracker usually helped subdue the gnawing feeling. His wife joked that he might be pregnant. His symptoms tended to return in the late afternoon. One day, when he noticed a dark tarry bowel movement, Brendan called his family physician, who referred him to me.

His physical exam was normal, except for mild tenderness when I pressed on his epigastric area (upper mid-abdomen). A complete blood count was within normal limits, so it was unlikely that Brendan had lost a lot of blood, and there was no evidence of active bleeding.

I prescribed a proton pump inhibitor that he could take once a day, which I thought was more in keeping with his lifestyle than multiple-dose drugs. I also told him to carry antacid tablets in his pocket in case his symptoms became suddenly uncomfortable during the day or night. I performed an endoscopy and found a small duodenal ulcer that had been the cause of the bleeding and pain. Endoscopic biopsies for *H. pylori* were negative and Brendan told me he had not been taking any aspirin or nonsteroidal anti-inflammatory drugs.

We discussed the stresses in his life and "taking time to smell the roses," but this advice was largely lost on Brendan. He wasn't interested in changing his charged-up lifestyle. However, he listened to the advice about dietary management. I recommended cutting back on coffee and using decaf, if possible. I also prescribed a quick high-fiber cereal for breakfast, a sandwich and decaf beverage for lunch, and eliminating alcohol and spices from his diet. I told him the importance of having three meals a day in order to avoid long periods of fasting.

I reminded him that since he is not allowed to smoke either at home or at work (thank goodness for take-charge wives, obnoxious nonsmokers, and the Clean Air Bill), he might as well give up smoking altogether. He said he would try but didn't sound as if he meant it.

One week later, he returned feeling much better. I told him to continue the proton pump inhibitor for a total of six weeks and to call if his symptoms returned. I gave him a home test to check his stool for blood. He was still smoking.

Non-ulcer Dyspepsia

Dyspepsia, which literally means "bad digestion," is a term used imprecisely by many physicians. Nonulcer dyspepsia (NUD) refers specifically to pain or discomfort centered in the upper abdomen. Heartburn or pain under the breastbone is not considered to be dyspepsia. The symptoms are usually chronic, lasting on and off or constantly for more than three months. True ulcer disease as well as gallbladder and pancreatic disease are excluded by having a normal endoscopy and ultasound and/or CT scan (see chapter 3). The discomfort may at times be relieved by antacids and food. However, dyspepsia may not respond to conventional antiulcer drugs and at times the best treatment is self-help measures.

Food. Avoid spicy sauces, coffee, tea, cola, alcoholic beverages, orange juice, tomato juice, and radishes.

Drugs.   Antacids may be taken one hour after each meal and at bedtime, or on an as-needed basis to relieve pain. You can also try an over-the-counter H_2 blocker (described in chapter 5). Do not take aspirin or aspirin-containing products, ibuprofen, or other anti-inflammatory medicines to relieve stomach pain. Stop smoking. Some people may respond to higher doses of H_2 blockers or a proton pump inhibitor. If the pain is severe, or if it persists or recurs, see your physician. Stomach pain may be caused by a gallbladder attack, inflammation of the pancreas, or ulcers. In older adults, there's even a small chance that such pain could be caused by stomach cancer. So if you experience stomach pain repeatedly, it's important to get a proper diagnosis by your physician. Although up to 50 percent of people with NUD may be infected with *H. pylori* according to some studies, there is no convincing evidence that treatment of *H. pylori* will be effective in treating the abdominal pain. Nevertheless, there are some individuals who seem to get better after treatment for *H. pylori* and most gastroenterologists would probably give it a try. The latest thinking is that some patients with NUD may have heightened sensitivity to stomach distention similar to the situation with irritable bowel syndrome (see chapter 9). Eating multiple small meals, which are less likely to cause stomach distention, and avoiding foods that slow down stomach emptying, such as greasy foods, may help. Some physicians, including myself, have had some success in treating patients with a tricyclic antidepressant drug like Elavil. Elavil may be effective in preventing sensations in the gut from reaching the brain.

If your epigastric pain is not a burning type of pain, does not improve with Prilosec, Prevacid, Aciphex, Protonix, Nexium, and you tend to fill up easily when eating, your non-ulcer dyspepsia may be caused by a condition known as gastroparesis (see below).

• Gastroparesis

Do you experience pain in the middle of the upper abdomen (epigastrum) after eating? Do you feel bloated after eating? Do you feel full after eating just a small amount of food? Are you nauseated? If the answer to these questions is yes, you may have a condition called gastroparesis (literally translated, "weak stomach") in which the stomach empties food into the intestine more slowly than normal. Gastroparesis is associated with many medical conditions. Surgical procedures, such as vagotomy (cutting nerves to the stomach) can result in poor stomach emptying. Metabolic disorders (diabetes and renal failure), arthritic conditions (scleroderma), central nervous system disease (stroke, head trauma, brain tumor), and infections (viral) may also cause slow stomach emptying.

Medications (narcotics, antispasmodics) commonly cause or worsen gastroparesis. In many patients there is no obvious cause and we call this idiopathic gastroparesis—a fancy way of saying we have no idea what is causing the problem. Symptoms related to idiopathic gastroparesis are relatively common, yet the condition is rarely diagnosed correctly by physicians.

Idiopathic gastroparesis usually affects women under the age of forty. Perhaps the sex hormone progesterone, which slows down the gut (now you know why pregnant women have nausea and constipation), makes young women more prone to gastroparesis.

If your doctor suspects you may have gastroparesis, he or she may either treat you on a strong hunch (empiric therapy) or order a test to confirm the diagnosis. The best way to diagnose gastroparesis is to have a gastric emptying scan. Although there are many variations to this test, usually a weak radioactive substance (technesium 99) is added to an egg sandwich, which is then eaten. The patient lies under a machine that measures radioactivity. The time it takes to empty half of the radioactive substance from the stomach into the intestine is calculated ($T\frac{1}{2}$ of gastric emptying). A $T\frac{1}{2}$ significantly longer than one hour suggests slow stomach emptying (the normal values may differ from institution to institution). Your doctor may also recommend that you have an endoscopy or upper GI series to make sure you do not have gastric outlet obstruction where an ulcer or tumor blocks food from leaving the stomach. Treatment of gastroparesis involves a combination of diet and drugs.

Gastroparesis Diet.   The objective of dietary therapy is to avoid foods that slow stomach emptying and to avoid overeating. Fatty, greasy foods slow stomach emptying because they cause release of the hormone cholecystokinin (CCK), which contracts the pyloric valve at the end of the stomach. Fiber-containing foods (roughage) also empty slowly. Receptors in the first portion of the small intestine that sense osmotic forces (osmoreceptors) slow down stomach emptying when activated. Sugary foods and drinks exert a strong osmotic force and should be avoided. Stomach emptying is also controlled by the caloric value of a meal. The pyloric valve can only "spit out" two calories per minute into the small intestine. The more the calories, the longer it takes for the stomach to empty. Small but more frequent meals are recommended. Instead of three squares a day, five or six small meals make more sense.

Drugs.   The goal of drug therapy is to accelerate stomach emptying. The so-called promotility drugs metaclopramide (Reglan), cisapride

(Propulsid—no longer available unless your doctor fills out a lengthy request to the manufacturer), and erythyromycin (E-mycin) are often useful in treating gastroparesis, but should be used only on a long-term basis with caution (see chapter 5 for more information on these drugs). Domperidone works very well for gastroparesis (10 to 20 mg before meals and at bedtime) but is not on the U.S market. Some of my enterprising patients get it overseas or through the Internet.

In the case of diabetic gastroparesis, drug treatment may need to be given indefinitely. Sometimes sudden symptoms of gastroparesis can be avoided by careful control of blood sugar. Idiopathic gastroparesis may improve spontaneously over months and years, especially if related to viral gastroenteritis.

If promotility drugs do not relieve nausea and vomiting, anti-nausea medications—like Compazine, Tigan, Phenergan, or in severe cases, Zofran—may be useful. Occasionally, Reglan may be combined with erythromycin in difficult cases. Zelnorm, used to treat constipation-predominant irritable bowel syndrome (see chapter 9), may also be useful in treating gastroparesis and non-ulcer dyspepsia. Recently, patients with gastroparesis were given botulinum toxin injections into the pylorus, which seemed to result in improved symptoms and gastric emptying.

One exciting new approach in the management of gastroparesis is gastric pacing, which requires the surgical placement of cardiac pacing wires onto the outer wall of the stomach. Patients activate the pacer just before meals and use the device for several hours after eating. In nine patients followed for at least one month, improved gastric emptying and significant reductions in symptoms were noted. In another study, twenty-four patients followed for a mean of thirty months had long-term symptom relief and reduced medication requirement with gastric pacing.

Stomach Cancer

Stomach cancer is caused by environmental factors such as diet and *H. pylori* infection, pernicious anemia, previous radiation, gastric surgery, chronic gastritis, as well as genetic factors that cause predisposition to the disease. *H. pylori* is now thought to be responsible for most cases of stomach cancer involving the bottom half of the stomach. Stomach cancer near the junction between the esophagus and the stomach is usually not related to *H. pylori* infection.

Stomach cancer is a very serious condition. Symptoms usually arise later due to the large capacity of the stomach and often the tumor is not curable at the time of diagnosis. For this reason, the mortality rate for patients diagnosed with stomach cancer is exceedingly high. Fortunately, the incidence of stomach cancer has been decreasing in the United States for several decades. In the Far East the incidence of stomach cancer remains high, probably due to the high rate of infection with *H. pylori,* as well as certain dietary factors.

Nobody knows for sure why the incidence of stomach cancer is decreasing in the United States. Lower infection rates with *H. pylori,* a known carcinogen and cause of stomach cancer, may be a partial explanation. However, other factors are probably also important.

Because the incidence of stomach cancer is relatively low in the United States, the American Cancer Society does not recommend routine endoscopic screening for the tumor as they do for colon cancer (see chapter 16). Early diagnosis can occasionally be achieved if warning signals such as internal bleeding are immediately investigated. Many people over the age of fifty are having their stool checked for blood on an annual basis. If blood is found, it is generally recommended that the patient have a colonoscopy or at least a sigmoidoscopy plus barium enema. If these studies are negative, however, an upper endoscopy examining the esophagus, stomach, and duodenum may clinch the diagnosis. While most of the patients will have esophagitis, gastritis, or peptic ulcer disease, occasionally an unsuspected stomach cancer is found. Not infrequently, precancerous changes in the stomach lining are found at the time of endoscopy.

Chronic infection with *H. pylori* in some susceptible individuals causes a change in the lining of the stomach to resemble the small intestines (intestinal metaplasia). As with Barrett's esophagus (see chapter 5) this type of change in the stomach lining increases the risk of developing cancer. The risk of stomach cancer after acquiring intestinal metaplasia in the stomach is not nearly as great as that seen with Barrett's esophagus causing esophageal cancer. Therefore, it is currently not recommended that patients with this precancerous change in the stomach be endoscoped on a regular basis. Nevertheless, I recommend to my patients that they have an endoscopy every five to ten years after discovering intestinal metaplasia.

Anyone experiencing early satiety (see gastroparesis, above) should have an upper GI series or endoscopy to rule out stomach cancer, especially if they are over the age of forty-five. Anyone who has multiple family members with stomach cancer should be checked for *H. pylori* infection, and some gastroenterologists recommend a screening endoscopy in this situation. Stomach cancer may run in families, either because the members of the family are genetically susceptible to the disease or because the members of the family have infected each other with *H. pylori.*

Although screening of the general population for *H. pylori* and treating those who are infected would be expected to reduce the incidence of stomach cancer, it is not felt to be cost effective in the United States at this time. Furthermore, no one has proven that eradicating *H. pylori* after twenty to forty years of infection would prevent the development of cancer.

Avoidance of stomach cancer may also be possible by proper diet and vitamin supplementation. Smoked foods, pickled vegetables, salted fish, excessive dietary salt, foods with nitrates such as lunch meats and hot dogs as well as charcoal-broiled foods, produce nitrosamines that cause cancer. Vitamin C can prevent nitrosamine formation and therefore fresh fruits should be substituted in the diet for foods that produce nitrosamine. Recent studies in animals show high-dose folic acid may play an important role in prevetion of gastric cancer. *H. pylori* may increase the formation of nitrosamine by preventing Vitamin C secretion in the stomach. The Self-Help Program outlined in this book is relatively low in carcinogenic-producing foods, but I advise taking supplemental vitamin C (250 to 500 mg per day) for those with a family history of stomach cancer and those who have been infected with *H. pylori.*

Once the diagnosis of stomach cancer is made, surgery is the treatment of choice. If it has spread to the lymph nodes or to the liver you may also need chemotherapy. When stomach cancer is diagnosed early and thought to be cured by surgery, a careful search for *H. pylori* should be made. When the bacteria is not found in the stomach by biopsy, a serological blood test should also be obtained. If evidence *of H. pylori* infection is found, one of the antibiotic regimens outlined in this chapter should be given and treatment success proved by endoscopy or breath test. A Japanese study of stomach cancer patients surgically treated and cured demonstrated that getting rid of *H. pylori* prevented another stomach cancer from forming. In individuals who did not receive treatment for *H. pylori,* a substantial percentage developed a second stomach cancer within a few years.

H. pylori can also cause other forms of stomach cancer. Non-Hodgkin's lymphoma of the stomach is probably related to *H. pylori* most of the time and MALT lymphoma of the stomach (a low-grade lymphoma) is always caused by *H. pylori.* Patients with severe gastritis should have biopsies taken looking for MALT lymphoma. In cases of early MALT lymphoma, treatment of *H. pylori* may completely cure the patient. In more advanced cases surgery, radiation, or chemotherapy may be necessary. Non-Hodgkin's lymphoma of the stomach can often be treated with radiation alone. Occasionally chemotherapy with or without surgery is also necessary.

7 *Pancreatis*

*B*urning pain in the upper abdomen can also be caused by an inflamed pancreas, the oblong organ that lies within the curvature of the duodenum and extends toward the spleen, which puts it in close proximity to several vital structures (see figure in chapter 2).

The pancreas is divided into two independent sections: the endocrine section secretes many important hormones, including insulin, directly into the bloodstream; the exocrine section produces a wide variety of digestive enzymes that process food into a form that can be absorbed by the small intestine. The exocrine section also secretes a bicarbonate-rich fluid that is important in neutralizing stomach acid. Pancreatitis primarily affects the exocrine pancreas.

Pancreatitis may be acute or chronic. In acute pancreatitis the gland usually returns to normal after a single attack. In chronic pancreatitis there is permanent damage to the gland and its function is impaired.

Acute Pancreatitis

• Symptoms and Causes

The most important symptom of acute pancreatitis is steady pain in the upper abdomen (epigastrium), sometimes boring straight through to the back. The pain is usually severe, although sometimes it can be mild. The pain is usually worse when you move around or lie down, but eases when you sit up and lean forward. Pain may be associated with vomiting, fever, and shock (low blood pressure).

On ultrasound or CT scan the pancreas may appear enlarged, but an accurate diagnosis of acute pancreatitis is usually confirmed by laboratory tests that measure a rise in serum amylase, a pancreatic enzyme released into the blood during an attack.

The principal cause of acute pancreatitis in men is alcohol abuse; in women it is gallstones. Other less common causes include an ulcer on the portion of the duodenum next to the pancreas, injury (such as surgery on the biliary tract or a blow to the abdomen), high levels of calcium or triglycerides in the blood, and certain drugs (sulfa drugs, thiazide diuretics, steroids, and birth control pills).

• Treatment

Acute pancreatitis usually requires hospitalization and intravenous fluids. No solid food should be consumed during an acute episode. As the pain and inflammation subsides, a low-fat diet should be followed. Unfortunately, drugs do not help. If a gallstone in the bile duct is the cause of an acute episode, it can be removed by a special endoscopic procedure called endoscopic sphincterotomy. Initially, a catheter is inserted in the bile duct, dye injected and X-rays are taken (endoscopic retrograde cholangiography or ERC; see chapter 3). If stones are found in the bile duct, a small cut is made at the junction between the bile duct and the small intestine by an electric current passed through a wire (endoscopic sphincterotomy). The stones can then be pulled from the bile duct into the small intestine by a special balloon or basket. Since the bile duct and pancreatic duct join together in most people (see figure, chapter 2), removing bile duct stones can relieve obstruction of the pancreatic duct and allow the pancreas to heal.

It may take several days, or even several weeks, for an acute episode to pass and for the pancreas to return to normal functioning. Some scarring may remain. If the cause of the attack is removed—if the gallstones are removed or, if alcohol was the precipitating factor, if the individual stops drinking—a recurrence is less likely.

Chronic Pancreatitis

• Symptoms and Causes

Chronic pancreatitis is a progressive disease that over a period of months and years slowly destroys the cells of the exocrine pancreas and eventually the endocrine pancreas as well. Symptoms may be the same as in the acute form, with attacks becoming more frequent as they continue.

Rarely, there may be no pain at all. The later signs of the disease may be weight loss and elevated blood sugars.

Chronic pancreatitis seems to result from a cascade of events, often beginning with alcohol abuse. Recurrent acute episodes lead to a chronic condition, especially when alcohol is involved. Those individuals with chronic pancreatitis who do not abuse alcohol may have one of the two abnormal genes necessary to develop cystic fibrosis (heterozygote for cystic fibrosis).

As chronic pancreatitis progresses, the endocrine pancreas may also be destroyed, and diabetes is the result. Digestion continues normally until about 90 percent of the pancreas is destroyed. When production finally shuts down, food can no longer be processed and therefore cannot be absorbed by the small intestine.

People with chronic pancreatitis may lose weight and have large bulky stools. They may be ravenously hungry, often consuming enough extra food to maintain body weight. The extra food intake often puts a strain on the damaged pancreas and causes pain. Some people with severe pain cannot compensate for their inefficient digestion by eating more food and will lose a significant amount of weight. As chronic pancreatitis progresses, the endocrine pancreas may also be destroyed, and diabetes is the result.

Measuring pancreatic enzymes in the blood is usually not helpful in making the diagnosis because serum amylase levels often are not elevated in the chronic form of pancreatitis. Abdominal X-rays or scans may be ordered, along with a special endoscopic procedure called endoscopic retrograde cholangiopancreatography (ERCP), which allows the physician to view the extent of tissue damage.

• Treatment

Elevated blood sugar levels can be controlled by giving insulin. Pancreatic extract can be given to correct greasy stools and weight loss resulting from underproduction of digestive enzymes. Pain management is a critical part of treatment. At this time, except for addicting painkillers, no drugs consistently help the pain of chronic pancreatitis. Certain drugs that block pancreatic secretion (e.g., high doses of pancreatic enzymes) may help rest the pancreas and thus provide some relief, but often this therapy is not sufficient to control pain, especially in alcoholics. Nevertheless, I often give patients with chronic pancreatitis eight tablets of Viokase or Cotazyme*

---

*Enteric-coated preparations like Pancrease and Creon should not be used to treat the pain of chronic pancreatitis, but are effective treatment for greasy stools caused by a poorly functioning pancreas.

four times a day along with an H$_2$ blocker or proton pump inhibitor (see chapter 6) to prevent stomach acid from destroying the enzymes.

New drugs are in development that may be effective in treating the pain of chronic pancreatitis. Sandostatin (octreotide acetate), a synthetic form of the hormone somatistatin that inhibits pancreatic secretion, is currently marketed for treatment of severe diarrhea, but some studies suggest that it may help some patients with chronic pancreatitis.

Although most doctors are not aware of it, there have been promising results using antioxidants for the pain of chronic pancreatitis. A group in Manchester, England, has been using a combination of antioxidant vitamins (beta-carotene, vitamin C, and vitamin E) along with the trace metal selenium and the amino acid methionine. I reviewed their findings, which were presented at the 1998 World Congress of Gastroenterology in Vienna, Austria, and was so impressed I tried the regimen on my patients with only mixed results. In England, the combination product is already available in pill form. If you and your doctor want to try it in America you'll have to visit your pharmacy or health-food store and purchase each item separately (see box for specific dose recommendations). It apparently is of no use to just take vitamins or just take the methionine. It only works if you take everything. The Manchester group recommends following vitamin and selenium levels as well as blood glutathione (a by-product of methionine) to make sure the levels do not get too high. When selenium levels are too high (selenosis) you may experience hypothyroidism and hair and nail loss. Too much methionine can precipitate psychological problems in susceptible individuals.

Because management of the pain of chronic pancreatitis has been so unrewarding, patients with persistent pain are often treated surgically—either by removing most of the pancreas or, if possible, draining the pancreatic duct. Even with the best type of operation (lateral pancreaticojejunostomy or Puestow procedure) only up to three-fourths of patients experience a reduction of pain. Obviously, before resorting to surgery, every effort should be made to control pancreatitis with dietary management (a low-fat diet), drug and possibly antioxidant therapy. Narcotic painkillers should be avoided because of the likelihood of addiction.

Another type of surgery that is easier and less risky is bilateral thoracoscopic splanchnectomy. A rigid viewing tube is placed through a small incision on each side of the chest or thorax. The splanchnic nerve, which carries pain fibers from the pancreas, is located and cut on each side. Even less risky is something called a celiac plexus block, where parts of the splanchnic nerve in the upper abdomen near the pancreas are located and then destroyed by an injection of pure alcohol through a long needle passed

Antioxidant Treatment for Chronic Pancreatitis

Antioxidant	Daily Dose
Beta-Carotene	15–30 mg
Vitamin C	500 mg
Vitamin E	200 units
Selenium	600 micrograms
Methionine	1 gram twice a day

through the abdominal wall by CT scan guidance. Celiac plexus block can also be performed by endoscopic ultrasound-guided injection.

Self-Help

Gabriel, a forty-two-year-old computer salesman, had a burning pain in the pit of his stomach that felt as if it was boring straight through to his back. The pain was unremitting. It became worse when he ate and seemed unbearable whenever he lay down. He tried antacids, which did not help. His family physician ordered an upper GI series, but nothing showed up. An ultrasound of his gallbladder showed no evidence of gallstones. Blood tests were normal, although on one occasion the serum amylase was slightly elevated.

When Gabriel was referred to me, we talked about his life. He told me that he had separated from his wife three years before. He had always entertained clients with three-martini lunches, but over the last few years his alcohol consumption had gradually increased. He now drank a fifth of vodka a day and had several glasses of wine with meals. His sales performance had worsened and he had received a few warnings from his boss regarding his working hours and sales quota.

I felt Gabriel had the classic signs and symptoms of chronic pancreatitis related to alcoholism. I performed endoscopic retrograde cholangiopancreatography (ERCP) on Gabriel, passing a flexible tube with a light down his esophagus, through the stomach, and into the duodenum, to locate the opening of the pancreatic duct. (The tube is similar to an endoscope except that the light and optics are on the side rather than the tip.) Dye was then injected to fill the duct, and X-ray pictures were taken to show any abnormalities. In this case, the X-rays revealed a dilated duct with several narrowed areas.

The immediate treatment for Gabriel was to get him off alcohol to stop further destruction of his pancreas. I arranged for a three-week inpatient detoxification and a referral to Alcoholics Anonymous. At the same time, I started him on a low-fat, high-carbohydrate diet, identical to the Two-Week Master Program. The pain that usually occurred when he ate was reduced. We added high does of pancreatic extract, and that further reduced pain. Although he was not completely pain-free, he was able to get by without narcotics and without surgery.

If you asked Gabriel what helped him the most, he would tell you that the low-fat diet brought the greatest pain relief. The Self-Help Nutritional Program is enormously helpful in managing chronic pancreatitis because it helps reduce stimulation of the pancreas. Smaller meals throughout the day may produce less pain than larger meals. People suffering from pancreatic failure can also get some additional nutritional help by taking prescription pancreatic extracts to replace digestive enzymes and insulin if diabetes ensues. Alcohol should be strictly avoided.

8   *Gallbladder Problems*

*T*he gallbladder is a pear-shaped sac with thin, smooth walls lying just underneath the liver and attached to it by fibrous tissue. The liver produces quantities of yellowish-green bile; a system of bile ducts carries the bile from the liver into the gallbladder, where it is stored. When you eat fatty foods, the gallbladder contracts and pushes the bile back through the ducts into the small intestine, where it helps digest the fat. Normally the gallbladder and bile duct do their work unnoticed. When gallstones form, the gallbladder often becomes diseased and a fatty meal that makes the gallbladder contract may result in a chronic nagging "grungy" feeling in the right upper quadrant of the abdomen. This is a very common condition.

Although more than 20 million Americans have gallstones, the stones do not always cause problems. About 80 percent of people who have them never notice them at all; even if the stones are discovered by a physician they will be left untreated unless they begin to cause symptoms.

Gallstone Types and Symptoms

There are two main types of gallstones: cholesterol stones and pigmented (calcium bilirubinate) stones. In America, most gallstones are cholesterol gallstones, and women are affected four times as often as men. In Asia, gallstones are more often pigmented.

Bile is mainly composed of cholesterol, bile salts, and phospholipids made by the liver. Cholesterol, like most fats, is insoluble in water. Bile salts and phospholipids have special chemical properties that allow them to keep cholesterol in solution. If the liver overproduces cholesterol (for example, obesity, pregnancy) or if there is a deficiency of bile salts in bile (for example, Crohn's disease, use of bile salt binders like cholestyramine to treat high blood cholesterol) then cholesterol crystals can precipitate out of solution and begin to form cholesterol stones. The process can accelerate if the gallbladder does not contract well (for example, very low-fat diet or fasting, use of the drug Sandostatin, see chapter 12 on diarrhea). The concentration of cholesterol in bile has very little to do with blood cholesterol levels. So even if your serum cholesterol is normal, you can still have gallstones.

Pigmented or calcium bilirubinate stones are composed of the bile pigment bilirubin combined with calcium. Old red blood cells when removed from the bloodstream by the spleen release the red pigment hemoglobin. Hemoglobin is converted to the yellow pigment bilirubin, which is then picked up by the liver and released into bile. If the body destroys too many red cells (a condition called hemolysis), excess bilirubin is produced and pigment stones can form in the gallbladder. Sickle-cell anemia causes early destruction of red cells and almost everyone with this condition has had a gallbladder operation by the age of twenty.

If a gallstone blocks the outflow of bile from the gallbladder, it can be the source of considerable pain. This so-called biliary colic is a sharp pain or a painful spasm on the right side, just under the rib cage. Sometimes you can feel the pain radiate to your back under the right shoulder blade. Symptoms often flare after meals because the gallbladder normally contracts after you eat fatty or greasy foods.

Occasionally when a stone blocks the outflow of bile, the gallbladder becomes inflamed, a condition called cholecystitis. Gallbladder inflammation without stones present, called acalculous cholecystitis, may be brought on by prolonged fasting, severe illness, or for no obvious reason at all.

Sometimes stones leave the gallbladder and stick in the common bile duct (the connection between the liver and the small intestine). Bile can back up into the bloodstream and cause jaundice (yellow tinge to the skin). Fever due to infection in the bile duct (cholangitis), severe right upper abdominal pain traveling to the upper back, and the pain of pancreatitis are common. Symptoms will continue unless the stone passes into the small intestine on its own or is removed by ERCP with sphincterotomy (see chapter 7, Pancreatitis).

Treatment

On three separate occasions, Bernadette experienced severe pain on her right side, just under the rib cage, about three hours after eating fatty food.

Once the pain was so severe that it traveled to her back and she developed nausea and vomiting. Bernadette had all the risk factors for gallstones: she was a woman, she was over forty years of age, and she was overweight. Ultrasound confirmed that she had a single stone measuring 1.5 centimeters or five-eighths of an inch across.

Because she was reluctant to have surgery, we attempted to dissolve the stone with Actigall (ursodeoxycholic acid) and recommended a low-fat diet similar to the Two-Week Master Program. Bernadette did well on the diet and her symptoms completely disappeared—until one afternoon when she indulged in a couple of slices of pizza. She immediately experienced pain on her right side. This convinced her of the importance of diet therapy.

The Self-Help Nutritional Program is ideal for people with gallbladder problems of all kinds because it is naturally low in fats, which means that fewer demands are placed on the gallbladder and it contracts less forcefully. Although the dietary program cannot actually dissolve gallstones, it may reduce the frequency and severity of painful attacks. Because dietary fiber reduces the amount of cholesterol in bile, the tendency to form gallstones is also reduced. By changing the chemical composition of the bile through diet, it is possible to halt the growth of stones or in rare cases, even cause the stones to shrink.

Gallstones can sometimes be dissolved medically, leaving the gallbladder intact. Patients who have small, uncalcified stones and a functioning gallbladder can try dissolving the stones with Actigall. Actigall is a bile salt so it helps dissolve cholesterol in bile. Actigall is given two or three times a day depending on body weight and is continued for several months after the stones disappear on ultrasound. The drug does not work in everyone and stones could reform once the drug is stopped. For these reasons dissolving gallstones with Actigall is not very popular.

Most cases of symptomatic gallstones are treated by surgically removing the gallbladder. The gallbladder usually can be removed by laparoscopic surgery (using multiple small incisions) with a one night stay in the hospital and relatively quick recovery at home. For technical reasons a large incision is necessary, on occasion, to remove the gallbladder.

Irving, a fifty-five-year-old, overweight trial attorney, developed a severe attack of biliary colic associated with fever right in the middle of a trial. At the time of surgery, his gallbladder was so inflamed it could not be safely removed by laparoscopic surgery. He required a large incision, five days in the hospital, and a month to recover. To make matters worse the jury's verdict favored the other side. Well, you can't win them all.

Most people do well after gallbladder removal. The body works just fine without a gallbladder. Digestion proceeds normally. Rarely a patient will develop diarrhea immediately following a cholecystectomy. This usually can be treated with Imodium AD or Questran (cholestyramine). Occasionally, abdominal pain is wrongly attributed to gallstones and therefore surgery does not relieve the symptoms. Pain after eating fatty foods can also be caused by irritable bowel syndrome, GERD, or a tight valve at the junction between the common bile duct and small intestine (sphincter of Oddi dysfunction). Removal of the gallbladder will not relieve pain caused by these conditions.

Obesity, Dieting, and Gallstones

There has been controversy over whether dieting to lose weight causes gallstones. It is well known that obesity itself causes cholesterol gallstones to form. In fact, the heavier you are, the greater your risk for gallstones. A fifty-year-old adult of normal weight without symptoms of gallbladder disease has about a 9 percent risk of having gallstones. That risk increases twofold for mild obesity (20 to 30 percent above ideal body weight) and up to sixfold for morbid obesity (more than 100 percent above ideal body weight).

Some studies suggest that the risk of developing gallstones may increase transiently during active weight loss. These studies were all done using either stomach bypass surgery or very low-calorie diets (about 500 calories a day). In the studies using very low-calorie diets, ultrasound of the gallbladder was performed before and after losing weight. About 25 percent of obese subjects who did not have gallstones detectable by ultrasound before dieting had detectable stones after losing weight.

If very low-calorie diets do on occasion cause gallstones, it may be related to poor stimulation of the gallbladder—with less fat (1 to 2 grams a day) there is less gallbladder contraction. Stagnant bile loaded with cholesterol is the setting for gallstone formation.

At this time, there is no evidence that diets of higher calorie and fat value (750 calories or above) cause gallstones. However, high calorie intake (greater than 3,000 calories per day) or high cholesterol intake (greater than 1,000 milligrams of cholesterol per day) are associated with gallstone formation.

The good news is that after you have lost your excess weight, your risk of developing gallstones goes back to normal. Considering the health risks of remaining obese (such as heart disease, diabetes, cancer, stroke, and infertility), I feel it is imperative to try to lose weight with an appropriate combination of diet and exercise (see chapters 28 and 29) despite the small risk of developing gallbladder disease.

Ursodeoxycholic acid (Actigall or Urso) can prevent the development of cholesterol gallstones while a person is on a very low-fat diet or after anti-obesity surgery. Aspirin may offer some protection against gallstone formation but does not work as well as Actigall.

9

Irritable Bowel Syndrome (IBS)

*I*rritable bowel syndrome (IBS) is really a constellation of symptoms, usually involving a change in bowel habits and abdominal pain. IBS is one of the most common health problems in the Western hemisphere. For some reason, young women tend to be much more susceptible to IBS than men. IBS is sometimes called colitis, but in fact this is a misnomer because no "itis", or inflammation, is present. It also goes by the names of spastic colon, spastic colitis, and mucous colitis. All of this nomenclature means the same thing—irritable bowel syndrome.

Symptoms of IBS

Many people have gastrointestinal complaints several times a year, including abdominal pain, constipation, and diarrhea. They should visit a physician for a diagnosis. These symptoms may be caused by a potentially serious disorder, such as inflammation of the bowel (colitis) or cancer. In the case of colitis or cancer, specific structural abnormalities are seen on diagnostic tests. In IBS, which can cause identical symptoms, no such structural abnormality exists. In fact, the diagnosis often depends on having normal results from diagnostic tests, including a barium enema, sigmoidoscopy, an upper GI series and small bowel follow through, stool culture, and analysis of stool for white cells and parasites.

When all of these test results are normal but symptoms persist, it is likely the person has IBS. In a young person with the classical IBS symptoms of lower abdominal cramps, diarrhea alternating with constipation, abdominal bloating or distension, and mucus coating the surface of the stool, we often make the diagnosis on symptoms alone and avoid tests. Those patients who mainly suffer from diarrhea and abdominal pain have diarrhea-predominant

IBS. Those who have mainly constipation and pain have constipation-predominate IBS.

Make no mistake, this is a real physiological disorder, not a psychosomatic ailment as was originally thought. IBS usually means that the bowel does not contract properly. It may contract forcefully after eating, causing severe cramps or spasm. Diarrhea may occur from hypermotility of the bowel. Normal contractions of the bowel may decrease in frequency or become weaker, leading to constipation.

Many IBS sufferers do not have any detectable colon motor function abnormality. They seem to have a heightened sensitivity to pain perception when the colon is stretched or distended. In one study a special balloon was inserted into the rectum of IBS sufferers as well as normal subjects. As air was slowly added to the balloon, the people were asked to note when they could first feel the balloon and when it caused pain. Across the board people with IBS sensed the balloon and had pain with a lower volume of air than normal subjects.

Normally, an urge to defecate occurs about 15 to 30 minutes after a meal. Stomach distension by the meal and release of various gastrointestinal hormones activate the nerves to the colon, which in turn stimulate the muscle of the bowel wall to contract. This so-called gastrocolic reflex can be exaggerated in IBS sufferers and they may find themselves rushing to the toilet suffering cramps and diarrhea even before the meal is over. Fatty foods and large meals seem to aggravate this problem.

Many people with IBS notice that their abdominal pain subsides after a bowel movement. By contrast, pain tends to increase when more frequent loose bowel movements occur. Some people feel they have had an incomplete bowel movement and need to go again. While this symptom, called tenesmus, is associated with IBS, it can also be caused by a tumor in the colon. For this reason, anyone who has tenesmus as a symptom should have a diagnostic workup that includes sigmoidoscopy and a barium enema or colonoscopy to rule out the possibility of a more serious ailment. The consensus definition and criteria for IBS have been formalized (see table).

It's interesting that even when IBS symptoms are severe they rarely disturb a person's sleep. If symptoms do arise in the night, it usually suggests that some organic problem, such as inflammatory bowel disease or long standing diabetes, is the cause.

IBS may be present from infancy, but tends to begin in young adulthood. A young person with IBS symptoms and no other manifestations of organic disease—no fever, rectal bleeding, or weight loss—usually doesn't require diagnostic studies. Adults past the age of forty or fifty who begin to

Criteria for IBS

Manning Criteria	Rome II Criteria
Pain relieved by defecation More frequent stools at the onset of pain Looser stools at the onset of pain Visible abdominal distension Passage of mucus Sensation of incomplete evacuation	At least 12 weeks or more, which need not be consecutive, in the previous 12 months of abdominal pain or discomfort that has 2 of 3 features: Relief with defecation Onset associated with a change in the frequency of stool Onset associated with a change in form (appearance) of stool

suffer from IBS symptoms can usually recall having had similar episodes in the past. Even so, when an older person begins to have these symptoms, he or she should be evaluated with a full diagnostic workup to rule out potentially serious gastrointestinal disease.

Some women with IBS notice they are constipated during most of their menstrual cycle but when they begin their period they develop diarrhea. Some normal women also notice more fluid stools during their menstrual flow probably because levels of progesterone, which inhibits bowel function, drop precipitously just before menstruation begins. Again, IBS patients have an exaggerated response to a normal or physiological process.

It has been reported that women with IBS are more likely to have experienced sexual or physical abuse than the general population and these individuals may benefit from recognizing the association and receiving psychotherapy. IBS may begin after an episode of food poisoning or other intestinal infection.

In some individuals IBS is part of a more global gastrointestinal tract motility problem. Some people have non-cardiac chest pain, GERD, gastroparesis, and/or non-ulcer dyspepsia as well as IBS.

Occasionally, patients with chronic diarrhea and abdominal pain who have a normal-appearing colon actually have a condition called microscopic colitis rather than IBS. Biopsy of the normal looking colon will show inflammation similar to patients with ulcerative colitis. (See chapter 15 for more information on microscopic colitis.)

Treatment

Melissa is a twenty-three-year-old secretary who complained of abdominal cramps. She had had this problem since her early teens. It would become especially severe before exams and during dates in high school. The pain was in the left and right lower abdomen. It was worse just before moving her bowels, and improved after a bowel movement.

Melissa also had frequent episodes of diarrhea, containing mucus but no visible blood. Then she would go for days without moving her bowels. Her symptoms of diarrhea seemed to get worse around the time of her period. She had recently seen her gynecologist for a pelvic exam, which proved to be normal. Because Melissa is sexually active the gynecologist cultured her cervix for chlamydia and gonococcus. Both tests were negative.

Melissa had none of the symptoms more characteristic of inflammatory bowel disease (rectal bleeding, fever). But at times her symptoms were so severe she would hunch over and clutch her abdomen, and then have to run to the bathroom. Since most of her symptoms occurred during working hours, especially when she was under specific deadlines set by her unsympathetic boss, Melissa spent a good part of the day in the ladies' room.

Except for the usual childhood diseases, Melissa had no past history of illness. She did not smoke cigarettes and had stopped drinking alcohol because it "gave her the runs." No one in her family had ever had colon cancer or inflammatory bowel disease.

Melissa's physical examination was entirely within normal limits except for some mild discomfort in the lower abdomen. I felt she had the classic symptoms of IBS and did not need any further diagnostic evaluation. That was the good news. The bad news was that although IBS is not considered a serious medical disorder, it is usually impossible to control all of the symptoms all of the time.

IBS may stay the same or worsen over time; it is usually an intermittent, lifelong condition that may require lifetime management. One of the important goals of treatment is to instill a positive attitude. For that reason, I believe it's important to avoid negative labels when speaking of IBS. I use the word "condition" or "disorder" to describe IBS rather than the word "disease." Reassurance that symptoms are not serious goes a long way in helping individuals deal with IBS. I tell my patients there are no strict rules about what is a normal bowel movement, and some abdominal discomfort associated with colonic spasm is normal for some people. It also comforts my female patients to know they are not alone. Since some of the symptoms of IBS are personal, women tend not to tell their friends about it. One of my more adventurous patients came back to see me after taking a quick poll of her friends, family, and fellow office workers: 30 percent suffered from IBS.

On the other hand, I have found that once people start talking about their bowels they may go on and on with whoever will politely listen. I try to discourage this type of obsessive talking in order to encourage taking one's mind off the disorder and getting on with a productive life. I once told Mrs. Frawly, an elderly patient of mine, that I have a great interest in hearing about her bowel complaints, but that her neighbors and Mr. Frawley (who had called me the week before) would prefer that she and I dealt with this problem alone. The result was that my visits with her now last one hour instead of 30 minutes, and she still seeks "outside help" with her delicate complaints.

I am not a therapeutic nihilist when it comes to IBS treatment. At times, antispasmodic drugs can alleviate the painful lower abdominal cramps. Fiber products, stool softeners, and laxatives can help treat constipation; fiber products, antispasmodics, and other antidiarrheal products can help treat diarrhea. However, as with any kind of medical therapy, you have to consider the cost and risk-to-benefit ratio. Many of the drugs used to treat IBS have side effects. For example, antispasmodics such as Bentyl (dicyclomine), Pro-Banthine (propantheline bromide) and Levsin (hyoscamine) can cause grogginess, dry mouth, difficulty urinating, constipation, and a fast heart rate. Harsh laxatives can lead over time to a flaccid colon that doesn't function properly.

*I*n addition to their potential side effects, many of these drugs are expensive and are usually only modestly effective over the long term. The long term is the real issue. IBS is a lifelong condition and by nature is relatively innocuous. It is difficult to recommend using strong drugs on a regular basis. However, symptoms can come on quite suddenly at times and can be severe. At times like these, intermittent drug therapy may be the best help.

By far the best approach for the long-term management of IBS symptoms is diet. A high-fiber diet significantly affects the colon, or large intestine, throughout its entire course. Fiber, with little help from the friendly bacteria residing in the colon, supplies the cells lining the colon with their primary fuel—short-chain fatty acids. With its spongelike action of holding on to water, fiber also increases the bulk of stool and helps absorb excess fluid. These properties make fiber useful in treating symptoms of both constipation and diarrhea. Extra bulk moves the stool through the colon faster, which relieves constipation without producing diarrhea.

A high-fiber diet is not a cure-all for IBS, but it seems to help most patients, especially those with constipation. In some people, a high-fiber diet may make symptoms of diarrhea or bloating worse, however, this does not usually happen if vegetables and grains naturally high in fiber are gradually introduced into the diet. But a few people with IBS continue to have such symptoms and should discontinue a high-fiber program.

Anyone who suffers from the symptoms of IBS should have a medical evaluation. Many physicians prescribe an antispasmodic agent such as Donnatal (belladonna alkaloids combined with phenobarbital), Bentyl (dicyclomine), Levsin or Nu-Lev (hyoscamine), or Pamine for their IBS patients to have on hand in case of sudden lower abdominal cramps. A drug called Zelnorm (tegaserod) has shown to be effective in treating women with constipation-predominant IBS, helping to reduce symptoms of bloating, pain, and increase frequency of bowel movements. Zelnorm is a serotonin-like drug that stimulates fluid secretion and motility in the intestines. It is taken twice a day (every day) even when symptoms are under control. It is best not to take the drug with food. When Zelnorm is stopped, symptoms usually return within a few days.

Lotronex (alosetron), a drug that blocks the chemical serotonin, has been recently re-approved by the FDA for treating female patients with severe diarrhea-predominant IBS. Lotronex has been shown to cause ischemic colitis (damage to the colon caused by inadequate blood supply) in approximately 1 in 700 people using the drug. Therefore, the FDA has imposed several restrictions on its use. Only doctors who have completed a brief information course can prescribe the drug using a special sticker. It should only be used to treat women with severe symptoms not responding to standard anti-diarrheal products (Imodium, Lomotil). Some IBS patients benefit from low dose (10–25 mg at bedtime) Elavil (amitriptylline) an antidepressant that seems to work by filtering out painful stimuli from the gut to the brain. Elavil also has some antispasmotic properties. For some of my patients it has truly been a "magic bullet."

Warm compresses to the lower abdomen may also ease the discomfort of cramps. Stress management can also play an important part in reducing the frequency and intensity of symptoms. Stress plays an important role in causing acute attacks of IBS, and reducing stress can help relieve the attack. The problem is that the attack may not occur until several hours after stress has passed. Stress has a residual action in the body, almost a reverberation. Taut muscles set up a chain reaction through the gut (see chapter 18).

In the long run, close adherence to the Self-Help Nutritional Program can help prevent IBS attacks and minimize those that do occur. And a little tender loving care and reassurance by a physician can go a long way in helping individuals suffering from IBS deal in a positive way with their symptoms.

10 *Gastrointestinal Gas*

Gas can affect the GI tract from the esophagus to the anus. Eructation (belching), bloating, distension, cramps, and flatulence are familiar and common symptoms related to the presence of gas in the GI tract. The type of symptom depends on where the excess gas is located. Gas in the stomach is different from gas in the colon, or large bowel.

We don't usually think of these symptoms as pathological; however, when they occur on a frequent basis they may be caused by specific gastrointestinal disorders. Some people feel gas pains or cramps even if they don't produce large amounts of gas. People with IBS, for example, have a lower threshold for pain caused by a distended colon (see chapter 9).

Gas in the Upper GI Tract—Eructation

Eructation, or belching, is the most common symptom of gas in the upper GI tract. The composition of belched gas is similar to that of air (mostly nitrogen), which gives us a good clue to its origin. Belching is due to large amounts of air in the stomach, usually caused by excessive swallowing of air. Swallowing air is often a nervous habit related to stress and anxiety. Gulping food also tends to cause accumulation of air in the stomach. Chewing gum, sucking on a pipe or cigar for a long time, or taking long drags on a cigarette can also cause excessive stomach gas. Patients with severe lung disease such as emphysema tend to swallow extra air. And some people huff and puff during exercise to such an extent that some air gets swallowed.

The fate of excess swallowed air varies according to the individual and may differ at times in the same person. When you are standing up, stomach air is always in the upper part of the stomach, near the opening of the esophagus. It is normal for the LES valve between the stomach and the esophagus to relax when you swallow; if excess air is present in the stomach, a belch could follow. If this one-way valve is weak, the path of least resistance may be for the air to reflux back up into the esophagus and pass out through the mouth, leading to chronic belching.

If the air doesn't escape through belching it can get temporarily trapped in the stomach and cause bloating and a full feeling in the upper abdomen. Some people may even get painful abdominal distension. Eventually, the air will pass into the small intestine and beyond and can add to the "gas load" normally present in the bowel.

The major treatment for upper GI tract gas is to avoid excessive air swallowing. Relaxation techniques for stress management may be helpful. Giving up gum chewing, smoking, and carbonated beverages, and learning to eat and drink slowly can also reduce air swallowing.

The Self-Help Nutritional Program is useful for this condition because it avoids or minimizes foods that cause the LES valve to relax. Since the Self-Help Nutritional Program is also low in fat, the stomach will tend to empty faster and there should be less bloating in the upper abdomen. If gas is trapped in the stomach, however, you may want to encourage belching. In that case, sucking on a peppermint candy may help relax the LES, allowing you to belch and ease gas buildup in the stomach. The same action tends to cause heartburn, though—always a trade-off!

Over-the-counter medications such as Mylicon (simethicone) help break up gas bubbles and can promote belching to relieve stomach gas pains (see Part Three). If simethicone itself, or products like Mylanta, which contain simethicone, do not work, you will probably have to ride out your attack of gas pain. Fortunately, most episodes are not severe and resolve on their own within a few minutes to a few hours. You may be able to help things along by pressing on your abdomen to help move the gas out of the stomach.

Lower Intestinal Gas—Flatulence

Although swallowed air can pass into the intestines and lead to a distended, bloated abdomen and flatulence, most flatulence is caused by gas produced in the colon by bacteria.

Gas buildup in the lower GI tract usually consists of oxygen (O_2) and nitrogen (N_2) from swallowed air, carbon dioxide (CO_2) formed by the combination of stomach acid and bicarbonate from the pancreas and CO_2, methane (CH_4) and hydrogen (H_2) formed by bacterial fermentation of ingested food. All of these gases are odorless. Less than 1 percent of intestinal gas is odiferous but the human nose is sensitive enough to detect hydrogen sulfide and other sulfur gases present in trace amounts.

Different foods produce different gases, and individuals have varying responses. About 30 percent of the population have bacteria in their colon that produce excessive amounts of methane. Certain plant foods—cabbage, broccoli, brussels sprouts, cauliflower, dried apricots, and beans—are more likely to have sulfur-containing proteins or amino acids and can produce gas that has a fairly potent odor. Beans and other legumes are major hydrogen gas producers because they contain a special type of carbohydrate that is poorly absorbed but quickly digested by bacteria in your intestines. But they are important sources of nutrients and you may not want to eliminate them from your diet. If you suffer from intestinal gas, you may want to take an enzyme that will help your body digest the carbohydrate in beans and legumes. Beano contains an enzyme that the body lacks, capable of digesting the carbohydrate in beans and many vegetables. Take three to ten drops just before eating and you may find you have less gas after eating beans, but Beano will not help you with gas formed by consuming lactose or fiber products.

Fiber can also cause problems. Some otherwise indigestible fiber is quite digestible by certain strains of intestinal bacteria, leading to flatulence. Milk also creates gas in many people. Lacking the enzyme to digest the lactose in milk, their intestinal bacteria have a field day and produce distension and flatus (hydrogen gas) in abundance. For people who can fully digest milk, milk may cause no flatus at all (see below).

Everyone passes gas every day of their lives. The average person passes gas approximately thirteen times a day. But when it gets out of control or if passing even normal amounts of gas is intolerable to you, there are several things that may help.

The high-fiber Self-Help Nutritional Program, which recommends that you *slowly incorporate fiber into your diet,* decreases flatulence by moving newly made feces rapidly through the large intestine. When some people get enthusiastic about the Self-Help Nutritional Program they suddenly increase their fiber intake from their customary 10 grams daily to 50 grams or more. The bacteria in their intestines run amok, often creating diarrhea and embarrassing quantities of gas. The amount of fiber in the recipes in this book—between 20 and 30 grams a day—should not be a major problem for most people.

By carefully checking their Flag Foods (see chapter 26) and making some recorded observations, most people can determine which foods are most likely to produce excessive flatus for them. If you find that you still have excessive flatulence, there are several antiflatus products available over the counter (see Part Three), but for most people these are unnecessary.

Some people don't want to eliminate gas-forming foods from their diet, and some people continue to pass gas no matter what they eat. Their primary concern is the noise and the odor. You can't eliminate the noise, but if odor is a problem for you, try activated charcoal capsules. Because activated charcoal is an absorbent, it can reduce the volume of intestinal gas by about 75 percent and deodorize the gas as well. People who have had a colostomy can also use charcoal capsules to reduce odor.

Activated charcoal is a natural product. It has enormous internal surface area, which makes it very absorbent and adsorbent, meaning that it attracts other particles to its surface. For this reason, it should be taken at least two hours before or one hour after any medication or hormones that you might be taking for other reasons. The usual dose is two to four charcoal tablets (Charcocaps) taken just before eating and one hour after meals. Charcoal tablets or capsules are available without a prescription at pharmacies and health food stores.

Charcoal-filtered underwear has been shown to be effective in removing the odor from flatus. Mylicon (simethicone) may help, although it often isn't as effective for flatulence as it is for belching.

Lactose (Milk) Intolerance

One common and little recognized cause of gas or flatulence is lactose intolerance, or lactase deficiency. *Lactase* is an enzyme produced in the intestine to digest *lactose,* the sugar in milk. Lactose is a combination of two sugar molecules, glucose and galactose. Before the intestines can absorb lactose, the double molecule must be split by the lactase enzyme present in the lining of the small intestines. Without this splitting action, the double molecule travels intact through the GI tract to the large intestine. There, bacteria cause the sugar to ferment, thus releasing hydrogen gas and drawing fluid osmotically through the intestinal walls into the bowel. The result is bloating, cramps, gas or flatulence, loose stools, or diarrhea. This problem is called either lactase deficiency or lactose intolerance, but it is not an allergy to milk and has nothing to do with fat content of milk—skim milk can cause as many problems as whole milk.

Except in rare instances, almost all babies are born with high levels of lactase in their intestines to digest milk. Lactase remains high throughout the first year or two of life, and then begins to drop off. In some people, usually as adults, lactase nearly disappears. It is very common for the body to lose its ability to manufacture lactase, and lactase deficiency eventually occurs in the majority of the world's population, particularly among African Americans, Native Americans, Jews, and Asians, groups that have a 70 to 80 percent incidence. On occasion, lactase deficiency may be caused by a disease of the small intestine like sprue or Crohn's disease. Even though people with lactose intolerance experience uncomfortable symptoms, they are still able to derive some nutritional benefits from the fat and protein in milk products.

Not every adult becomes lactose intolerant. Northern Europeans and their American descendants and a few African populations seem to retain their ability to digest lactose even as they grow older. But it's also possible to have a lactase deficiency and not realize it. It sometimes sneaks up on people as they grow older. Symptoms of bloating and gas develop gradually and people therefore get used to them.

Roger Moore, a thirty-eight-year-old executive, was one of those people who had always had excessive flatulence, but for the last several years the condition had gotten progressively worse. When he came to see me he was at the point where he was afraid to go to a board meeting because of embarrassment about his noticeable symptoms. Roger avoided beans and other legumes like the plague, but his flatulence continued unabated. He occasionally had cramps in his lower abdomen and loose stools. His family doctor ordered X-rays of the upper and lower GI tract, which proved to be completely normal. Roger had recently traveled outside the United States, so a stool analysis for parasites was carried out, and that also proved to be negative. Roger's father also had excessive gas, but it never seemed to bother him. The family just joked about it.

Roger was an African American, and this and his family history made me suspect he might be lactose intolerant. He said he never drank milk, but after a little prodding he admitted he did use milk in his cereal and cream in his coffee. He was also an avid fan of ice cream. I was almost certain that he was lactose intolerant, but to prove it I performed a hydrogen breath test, in which a small tube is placed in the nostril and a quantity of exhaled air extracted. Air can be tested just as blood or urine can be analyzed. In this case, a gas chromatograph is used to analyze the breath for excess hydrogen, which a lactose-intolerant person will exhale after taking a dose of lactose.

Roger's test was distinctly abnormal. He was delighted to learn that simply avoiding milk products would cause a drastic reduction in his episodes of flatulence. He now uses lactase-added milk, and he can even eat ice cream if he swallows two tablets of lactase enzyme along with it. His father has started using lactase products too.

You can test yourself for lactose intolerance simply by drinking four glasses of milk on an empty stomach and waiting to see if any symptoms develop. Symptoms should appear within two to four hours. More sophisticated scientific tests are available to measure the increase in serum glucose after ingesting lactose by mouth (lactose tolerance test) or to measure the hydrogen content in your breath after ingesting lactose (breath hydrogen test), the test used for Roger.

For most people, lactose intolerance is not an all-or-nothing phenomenon. Many people can consume small amounts of milk or milk products and have no noticeable reaction. Most people with lactase deficiency have no trouble with the amount of milk that might be added to a cup of coffee, and they can often handle dairy products like yogurt, some cheeses, and butter. However, some people are so lactose intolerant that they must avoid all sources of lactose.

Lactose is in all forms of milk, including skim and low-fat milk products. People who need to consume low-lactose products can try lactase-added milk, acidophilus milk, and lactase drops and tablets (see chapter 21).

11   *Constipation*

Constipation is a disorder in which there is difficulty moving one's bowels. It is a common problem, particularly for those living in the Western hemisphere, and for some people it can be chronic and worrisome.

What is considered a "normal" bowel movement varies with the individual and geography. In the West, where diet tends to be low in roughage and fiber, stools tend to be low in weight; the normal number of bowel movements ranges from one movement twice a week to one or two movements a day. In rural Africa and other countries where grain is a dietary staple, movements are bulkier and much more frequent, as often as six or seven times a day.

Not everyone can or needs to have a bowel movement every day. Most people miss a day now and then and don't even notice it. However, for those who have chronic difficulty, who must strain to produce a dry, hard bowel movement, constipation can be uncomfortable and painful. Constipation often produces a bloated feeling because the bowel distends with gas and liquid, as well as large amounts of stool in the colon.

Causes

The most common cause of constipation is insufficient fiber in the diet, but many other causes contribute to chronic constipation. People with IBS may have constipation because the colon doesn't always contract properly. In others, the anal sphincter pressure is too high (anismus). Some medication may also cause constipation: iron supplements, antidepressant medications, painkillers, and some medications for hypertension. People suffering from low thyroid (hypothyroidism) or an excess of calcium in the blood tend to suffer from constipation. So do pregnant women and people who are sedentary or confined to bed rest. Depression at times can cause constipation. Travelers almost universally complain of constipation on the first few days of a trip, although it is difficult to say just why this is so. It may be a change in sleeping or eating habits or water intake, or sitting long hours while traveling. Some people have a cathartic colon, or "lazy bowel," decreased bowel contractions often caused by excessive use of laxatives.

Some people develop constipation because they are too busy to move their bowels when they get the urge to defecate. Others may ignore the urge whenever they are outside their home. The longer the stool remains in the colon, the more water the colon reabsorbs. The stool gets smaller, firmer, and thus more difficult to evacuate. Over time, this disregard for the urge to have a bowel movement can interfere with the normal pattern of bowel habits and require relearning of the conditioned defecatory reflex.

Less commonly, constipation can occur when nerves to the bowel are severed during surgery. This can occur with some types of back surgery and after a hysterectomy. Bladder function may also be affected.

A word of caution about constipation: if you suffer from chronic constipation it's important to have a checkup to make sure no serious disease is present and that no underlying hormonal or electrolyte imbalance is causing the constipation. A *recent change* in bowel habits, especially a narrowing of stools, may signify colon cancer and also requires a thorough evaluation. This is especially true when rectal bleeding is present. Any new onset of constipation, especially for those over age forty, should be evaluated by a physician.

Treatment

Mildred Rosenberg is a seventy-two-year-old woman who had always had some degree of constipation. Recently, however, she noticed that her bowel movements were even less frequent, only once a week. It required a lot of effort to produce a few small, firm pieces of stool. The only way Mildred could have a larger bowel movement was to take Correctol.

When we talked about her lifestyle, Mildred said that her usual arthritis had been getting worse, which had considerably slowed down her usual activities. At times she took aspirin with codeine for pain, but usually she took ibuprofen. She did not take any other medication. Her diet was noticeably deficient in fiber. There was no evidence of blood in her stool, weight loss, or any family history of colon cancer.

My impression was that Mildred had the same constipation she had all her life, but that it was being made worse by inactivity and occasional codeine. To be certain no other problem existed, I ordered a barium enema and also examined her colon by flexible sigmoidoscopy. Both studies were normal.

The obvious treatment for Mildred was a change in diet. Because her diet was so low in fiber, I recommended one tablespoon of Metamucil and one glass of prune juice each day. She also began to add small servings of cereal, whole wheat bread, raw fruit, and vegetables to her daily diet, until after two weeks she was up to 25 grams of fiber a day. With this regimen she was able to have two to three well-formed bowel movements each week, without straining. This was a significant improvement for her (not everyone needs to have a bowel movement every day) and she did not require enemas, laxatives, or even a stool softener.

Treatment of constipation depends on what's causing the problem to begin with. A change in drug therapy may be the answer for people who are on treatment regimens that produce constipation as a side effect. For most people, however, the answer will come from a change in diet, just as it did for Mildred.

Increasing fiber in the diet, in the form of fruits, vegetables, and grains, adds bulk and also increases the amount of water in the stool, which aids in its passage.

In most cases the Self-Help Nutritional Program, which recommends between 25 and 30 grams of fiber a day, is all that is necessary to treat constipation. Drinking plenty of water and getting regular exercise is also important. Runners often notice that they have a strong urge to defecate after a strenuous workout. For a quick fix, try that old standby prune juice. It works and it's good for you.

Bowel Retraining.   People who tend to ignore their body signals may over time have lost the ability to recognize when it's time to move their bowels. In this situation, it may help to go to the bathroom at the same time every day when a bowel movement is most likely to occur, usually about thirty minutes after breakfast or after a cup of caffeinated coffee (caffeine is a stimulant to the GI tract). Remember, however, that caffeine is a Flag Food for heartburn—again, what helps one GI problem may exacerbate another. (Nicotine, while a recognized colonic stimulant, is not recommended as a treatment for constipation or anything else.)

When you attempt to "retrain" your bowel, remember to take your time. Your mother may have told you to "do your business" quickly and get off the toilet, possibly to avoid hemorrhoids but probably because most of us grew up in a house with one bathroom. Today, even small houses usually have 2.5 bathrooms for the average 2.5-member family, so take your time.

If breakfast time finds you at work, any large meal will do for bowel retraining. When food enters your stomach it encourages the colon to contract. This impulse is transmitted by nerves that innervate the colon; certain hormones may also be involved. This reaction is called the gastrocolic reflex. Some people, especially those with IBS, have an exaggerated gastrocolic reflex. As soon as they eat they have to run to the bathroom. In bowel retraining the gastrocolic reflex works in your favor.

Drugs.   Scores of laxatives on the market can provide a quick fix to relieve constipation. They fall into several different categories according to their mechanism of action.

Bulk laxatives add volume and fluid to the stool. Metamucil, Effersyllium, and Perdiem are psyllium seed laxatives that add nonirritating bulk and promote normal elimination. FiberCon, which has a similar bulking action, contains the fiber calcium polycarbophil. You may notice an increase in wind (flatulence) and stomach bloating when you start taking fiber supplements. This is normal and tends to settle down after a few months as the gut becomes used to the increase in fiber. Calcium polycarbophil may cause less bloating and gas.

Stool softeners like Colace (docusate sodium) are not laxatives but contain surface-active agents that help keep stools soft for easy, natural passage.

Magnesium salts like Phillips Milk of Magnesia and Haley's M-O work by increasing the fluid in the GI tract. Dulcolax (bisacodyl) is a stimulant laxative that acts directly on the colon to make it contract.

Miralax is a prescription drug that contains the same ingredient found in Golytely, the colonoscopy prep. Miralax works very well for some individuals. Visicol tablets (prescription drug) or Fleet's phospho soda (OTC), also used as colonoscopy preparations, can be used in cases of severe constipation with a physician's supervision. Zelnorm, a new drug that acts on serotonin receptors in the intestines to increase the motility of the colon and stimulate secretion of fluid, has been successfully used in constipation associated with irritable bowel syndrome (see chapter 9). Zelnorm can also be used to treat garden variety constipation not related to irritable bowel syndrome. Lactulose is another prescription drug to treat constipation. Since it is a nonabsordable carbohydrate it can cause excessive bloating and flatulence.

Phenolphthalein-containing laxatives have been taken off the market because they may cause cancer. Avoid any laxative that you may have kept in your medicine cabinet that contains the chemical phenolphthalein.

In general, it is always best to try the gentlest agents first. Over time, harsh laxatives can damage the bowel and ultimately make you dependent on laxatives to move your bowels. For most people I recommend starting with a bulk laxative and/or stool softener and, if necessary, adding a magnesium salt (milk of magnesia, citrate of magnesium). Only in very difficult cases would a stimulant laxative or prescription drug be the treatment of choice.

Enemas.   Enemas, while not popular with most people, are safe and quite effective in treating constipation. A simple tap water enema can distend the rectum, creating the normal stimulus that initiates defecation. For your convenience a Fleet's enema can also be used.

Management of Severe Constipation

Even after taking stool softeners, fiber-bulking agents, Zelnorm, and other laxatives, some individuals still are unable to move their bowels. If a sigmoidoscopy, barium enema, or colonoscopy rules out a bowel obstruction, then other diagnostic tests and treatment modalities may be necessary. In this situation we will often perform a Sitzmarker study. A capsule containing markers that will show up on an X-ray is swallowed by the patient. Two and five days later an X-ray is taken. If none of the radiopaque markers appear on the X-ray, then the patient does not have a severe bowel motility problem. If the markers are found hung up on the right side of the colon, a likely diagnosis is colonic inertia or slow transit constipation, which means the entire colon is sluggish. In severe cases of colonic inertia that have been unresponsive to all medical measures, surgery may be necessary. The entire colon, excluding the rectum, can be removed and the small intestine attached to the rectum. This obviously should be undertaken only in patients with the most severe problems.

If the Sizmarkers pool at the very end of the colon in the rectum, the patient may have an anorectal motility problem (dysfunctional anal sphincter) or obstructed defecation. In this case, a special barium enema study, called a defecogram or defecography, and anorectal manometry (measuring pressures at the anal sphincter) are often recommended. With defecography, a barium paste is injected into the rectum. The patient sits in a special chair and is asked to try to evacuate his or her bowels. A videotape of the procedure is taken and analyzed by a radiologist.

Measuring the pressures in the anal sphincter and rectum may also shed light on what's causing the problem with defecation. In some cases, behavioral modification techniques can be employed with positive results. In severe cases, a diverting colostomy, where the large intestine is brought out to the skin, may be necessary.

12   *Diarrhea*

Diarrhea is defined as stool output in excess of 300 grams (about three-quarters of a pound) a day and an increase in the fluidity of stool.

Causes

Diarrhea may be due to a disturbance in osmosis, secretion, or motility of the bowel; sometimes it is caused by a combination of two or more problems.

• Osmotic Diarrhea

The small and large intestines are lined with a semipermeable membrane. Fluid normally diffuses through the membrane and an equal osmotic pressure is maintained on either side. Food particles that cannot be absorbed by the intestine exert osmotic pressure and cause fluid from the bloodstream to cross the lining to try to balance the fluid concentration on either side. This excess of fluid in the intestine produces diarrhea.

People who frequently consume magnesium-containing antacids, such as Mylanta or Maalox, or laxatives, such as milk of magnesia, may have an osmotic diarrhea because magnesium cannot be absorbed by the intestine and will exert a strong osmotic force.

People who have lactase deficiency (milk intolerance) also have problems with diarrhea. In this case, the milk sugar lactose cannot be absorbed by the small intestine. Bacteria in the colon break the lactose into simple sugars, which then exert an osmotic force in the colon, resulting in loose stools.

Fasting will generally improve osmotic diarrhea since the osmotically active agent will be eliminated.

• Secretory Diarrhea

As food passes through the GI tract, the cells lining the inside of the tube absorb fluid and nutrients and pass them into the bloodstream. These same cells also secrete fluid from the bloodstream into the interior of the GI tract.

Normally, intestinal cells absorb more fluid than they secrete, and there is a "net absorption." However, sometimes things can go awry and the cells secrete excessive fluid, causing a "net secretion" and diarrhea. In this case, even fasting will not stop the diarrhea.

Certain bacteria such as the cholera bacteria, *Vibrio cholerae, Salmonella,* and *Escherichia coli* (the cause of traveler's diarrhea) give off toxins that can stick to the intestinal lining. Although these toxins do not damage the intestinal lining, they do cause the cells to secrete massive amounts of fluid, which results in voluminous watery diarrhea typical of food poisoning. This is a common cause of acute severe diarrhea.

Some rare endocrine tumors give off hormones (for example, vipoma) or the chemical serotonin (carcinoid tumors), which cause intestinal secretion. In this case, diarrhea doesn't improve and requires specialized treatments. An injectable drug Sandostatin is particularly effective in these difficult cases.

Any disease that damages the lining of the intestine, such as Crohn's disease, a common form of inflammatory bowel disease, tends to impair absorption and leads to net secretion and diarrhea.

Motility Disorders

The normal contractions, or motility, of the small intestine act like a cleansing wave to prevent stagnation of fluid and overgrowth of bacteria. Certain diseases such as longstanding diabetes and scleroderma can affect the nerves and muscles of the intestine, so that bowel contents move sluggishly along the gastrointestinal tract, giving bacteria the opportunity to multiply. As bacteria compete for food they impair absorption of nutrients and can cause weight loss and diarrhea.

Some people with irritable bowel syndrome (see chapter 9) have a colonic motility problem, which may lead to diarrhea, although many people with irritable bowel syndrome have normal colonic motility. In developed countries, irritable bowel syndrome remains the most common cause of chronic diarrhea in women.

Complex Causes

In certain instances, diarrhea may be caused by all of these problems working in unhappy concert. In patients with Crohn's disease, for example, the last portion of the small intestine, the ileum, is often inflamed (ileitis). This means that bile from the liver cannot be absorbed normally and travels instead into the large intestine, where it stimulates secretion of fluid and leads to secretory diarrhea. Because the small intestine is inflamed, lactase production is impaired, which results in milk intolerance and loose stools (osmotic diarrhea). Prolonged inflammation can lead to scarring and the bowel can become obstructed, interfering with normal motility. (For such complex causes, treatment must also be diverse. In this particular case, drug therapy may be needed to decrease inflammation, bind bile salts, and/or suppress bacterial growth.)

Acute Diarrhea

Diarrhea that has been present for less than two weeks is usually referred to as acute diarrhea. Most infectious causes of diarrhea (viral or bacteria) are self-limited infections and, even without treatment, resolve within days.

Most cases of diarrhea are not too serious. Sudden onset of diarrhea associated with fever, vomiting, and cramping pains in the stomach is often caused by flu or other viruses (viral gastroenteritis).

Food poisoning, another common cause of diarrhea, is caused by bacteria, or toxins produced by bacteria, that have overgrown in food and find their way into the GI tract. Foods with high protein content such as meat, chicken, fish, and eggs more readily support overgrowth of bacteria than do carbohydrates. Dry foods are also less likely to cause food poisoning. One important key to prevention is refrigeration: food should never be allowed to sit without refrigeration for more than three hours.

Just how severe these sudden attacks of diarrhea can be was illustrated by the famous airplane incident in the 1970s when a commercial

Common Causes of Bacterial Food Poisoning

Bacteria	Typical Source of Infection*	Clinical Presentation
Salmonella	Uncooked eggs, Chicken	Fever, "pea soup" diarrhea
Shigella	Contaminated food or water	Bloody diarrhea
Campylobacter jejuni	Uncooked chicken	Bloody diarrhea
E. coli 0157:H7	Uncooked beef	Bloody diarrhea
Vibrio cholerae (cholera)	Contaminated water	Severe dehydration; "rice water" diarrhea
Staphylococcus	Unrefrigerated food (e.g., mayonnaise)	Nausea, vomiting
Enterotoxigenic E. coli (traveler's diarrhea)	Contaminated water	Severe diarrhea beginning during or after a trip to a tropical locale

*Many of these bacteria are also transmitted person to person by the fecal-oral route.

airliner nearly crashed into the sea because everyone aboard, including the pilot, had eaten food overrun with salmonella bacteria. The pilot had to overcome severe diarrhea and cramps to maneuver the plane onto the runway.

Acute diarrhea can also be caused by parasites. Amebic dysentery caused by the parasite *Entamoeba histolytica* is a common cause of diarrhea, especially in developing nations, where the water supply may be contaminated. Most often amebic dysentery is a self-limited disease. Occasionally, if it is not treated with metronidazole (Flagyl), patients can develop severe complications, including a liver abscess. Another common water supply contaminant is *Giardia lamblia*. Individuals who drink water from mountain streams or use well water are prone to develop giardiasis. Although in most cases giardiasis is a self-limited acute disease, some individuals, especially those with impaired immune systems, may go on to chronic infection and present with symptoms similar to malabsorption with weight loss. We are beginning to see many individuals infected with

Blastocystis hominis. Although some physicians feel this is not a patho-
genic (disease-causing) organism, most physicians now believe that patients infested with a large amount of Blastocystis may develop a diarrheal
illness. Most parasitic diarrheal diseases are treated with metronidazole
with good results. Alinia (nitazoxanide) is another drug used to treat parasitic disease. Its advantage over metronidazole is that it can treat cryp-
tosporidiosis as well as giardia.

Chronic Diarrhea

When diarrhea persists beyond two to four weeks, it is referred to as
chronic diarrhea. Since most of the common infectious causes of diarrhea
are self-limited and last only a few days, diarrhea that continues beyond
two weeks often is caused by other diseases. Most of the time your doctor
will start by ordering stool tests, including routine culture, examination
for ova and parasites, and assay for *Clostridium difficile,* the cause of
antibiotic-related diarrhea (see below). If you have lost weight and have
diarrhea, your doctor will probably check your stool for the presence of
fat, which would indicate you are either not absorbing your food (disease
of the small intestines) or not digesting your food (your pancreas is not
making digestive enzymes: see chapter 7). If these stool tests are negative,
in all likelihood your doctor will recommend either a sigmoidoscopy or a
colonoscopy to rule out inflammatory bowel disease. An upper GI series,
including an X-ray of your small intestine, may also be ordered. Examples of disorders that lead to chronic diarrhea include irritable bowel syndrome, inflammatory bowel disease (ulcerative colitis and Crohn's
disease), and certain bowel infections (giardiasis, amoebiasis, *Clostridium difficile*–related colitis).

Occasionally people will develop diarrhea after they have their gallbladder removed. Although nonspecific antidiarrhea medication like Imodium may help, the drug that seems to work the best is cholestyramine
(Questran), which binds bile salts. Remember: you should always see your
doctor if you develop severe diarrhea or the diarrhea persists beyond two
weeks.

• Treatment

With mild diarrhea of short duration there is usually no need for treatment. More significant diarrhea, especially when associated with lighthead-
edness and thirst from dehydration, does require treatment.

Fluids.   The most important action to take if you have an attack of diarrhea is to drink plenty of fluids to avoid dehydration. Gatorade is useful to replenish lost electrolytes such as sodium and potassium. Pedialyte is a good fluid and electrolyte replacement for infants.

Diet.   A clear-liquid diet will sustain you until the bout of flu or food poisoning is over: bouillon, soup broth, carbonated beverages, fruit juices, and gelatin. Avoid milk and dairy products since the milk sugar (lactose) may be poorly absorbed even in people who normally tolerate it well and thus may worsen the diarrhea. Start with foods light in carbohydrates such as bread or pasta.

Drugs.   For the occasional bout, especially if you have IBS, over-the-counter remedies such as Pepto-Bismol, Kaopectate, and Imodium A-D may give symptomatic relief but should not be used for more than three days without the advice of your physician. Diarrhea associated with IBS may be relieved by Donnagel, an antispasmodic and antidiarrhea agent. Lotronex, a drug that blocks serotonin receptors in the intestines, has been successfully used for severe diarrhea associated with irritable bowel syndrome but has some restriction to its use in the United States. Lotronex should be used only for severe chronic diarrhea associated with the irritable bowel syndrome (see chapter 9) when other remedies have not worked. The prescription drug Lomotil (diphenoxylate/atropine) should be tried if there is no response to Imodium. Antidiarrhea drugs are not recommended for people with food poisoning and people with moderate to severe inflammatory bowel disease.

Extreme Measures.   If a severe acute episode doesn't resolve itself within 24 to 48 hours, seek medical attention. People with high fever or bloody diarrhea should consult their physician immediately.

Malabsorption.   Patients with loose, greasy stools and weight loss may have a disease of the small intestine causing malabsorption. Diseases such as celiac disease or sprue (see chapter 17), immunoglobin deficiency, and Whipple's disease damage the small intestine and impair the absorption of food. If your doctor analyzes your stool and finds fats, you may be referred for a biopsy of the small intestine (usually done by endoscopy) to make a specific diagnosis. Treatment will depend on the cause of the malabsorption (e.g., gluten-free diet for sprue, antibiotics for Whipple's disease).

Traveler's Diarrhea

The warmer and sunnier the climate of the country you are visiting, the more likely it is that you will develop traveler's diarrhea, the so-called Montezuma's Revenge so common in Mexico and Central America. Travelers to the Middle East, Asia, and Africa are also vulnerable to traveler's diarrhea.

Symptoms are abrupt and include watery diarrhea, sometimes accompanied by disabling stomach pains and cramps. Fever, dehydration, nausea, vomiting, and prostration may all be part of the picture.

Whether you develop traveler's diarrhea does not necessarily depend on a roll of the dice. The illness is caused by ingesting toxigenic bacteria in contaminated water and food.

Food.   The best prevention is careful eating habits when traveling to endemic areas. Always drink bottled water, soft drinks, or fruit juices. Boiling water for five to ten minutes will kill the bacteria. But freezing water won't harm the bacteria, so forgo ice cubes in your drinks.

The most common contaminated foods are vegetables and fruits. It may seem absurd to go to a tropical paradise like Mexico and pass up the beautiful fruits and vegetables. Washing fruit in local water obviously will not help. So, if you can't peel it, don't eat it. That means that lettuce is out, and avocados are in.

Hand to Hand.   Like the bugs that cause the common cold, harmful bacteria can be passed from hand to hand or from money to hand. Wash your hands frequently when traveling and carry antiseptic towelettes to dry off.

Drugs.   If you follow these basic precautions you may be able to avoid traveler's diarrhea, or if you do pick it up your symptoms are likely to be mild. If it catches you, however, the best quick fix is Pepto-Bismol (see Part Three), and to a lesser extent Kaopectate or Donnagel. Certain prescription antibiotics (for example, Bactrim, Cipro) can also help. Make sure you follow the directions given on the labels and do not exceed recommended dosages.

Some travelers are not willing to risk coming down with traveler's diarrhea, which in its worst instances can be severely incapacitating. The attacks have ruined many expensive, long-planned vacations. One man I know had to be helicoptered off the beach in Acapulco and brought back to the United States for treatment. There are some prescription and OTC medicines you can take *before traveling* that will offer some protection against diarrhea. A word of caution: even with preventive medication, you should still follow the precautions given above.

One of the most effective drugs is doxycycline. Like many antibiotics, doxycycline can cause photosensitivity, which means that you are more likely to get sunburned. Since you are probably traveling in a sunny country, excess sun exposure can be a problem. Make sure you wear a high-rated sunscreen (30 or above) and skip lying on the beach.

Trimethoprim sulfa (Bactrim DS), another effective antibiotic, produces a lesser degree of photosensitivity. The newest antibiotic and arguably the treatment of choice for traveler's diarrhea is Xifaxan (rifaximin). Ask your doctor for a prescription before you leave for the tropics.

Pepto-Bismol is the best OTC drug to prevent traveler's diarrhea. The bismuth in the product can suppress growth of bacteria, but a lot of Pepto-Bismol is required to be effective as preventive treatment. A reasonable regimen is two tablets four times a days starting 24 hours before you leave and continuing for two days after you return from your trip (as long as your overall use doesn't last longer than twenty-one days).

Pepto-Bismol contains salicylate, which, like aspirin, can cause ringing in your ears at high doses. If you experience this side effect, cut back on the dose until there is no more ringing.

Diarrhea Associated with AIDS

Patients with acquired immune deficiency syndrome (AIDS) are prone to develop diarrhea. The diarrhea is usually caused by an infectious agent—either a bacteria parasite, or virus. Certain bowel infections are only present in those AIDS patients with very poor immune function (low CD4 count). Diarrheal diseases in AIDS patients such as those caused by cytomegalovirus (CMV), Mycobacterium Avium (MAI), cyclospora, isopora, and microspora infection of the small intestine can sometimes be diagnosed by taking a biopsy of the colon or small intestines at the time of endoscopy. At times no infectious agent can be found in AIDS patients with severe chronic diarrhea and the diarrhea is just attributed to AIDS-induced bowel dysfunction. In individuals where a specific infectious agent cannot be found, diarrhea refractory to Imodium A-D or Lomotil may often respond to Sandostatin injections.

Diarrhea Caused by Drugs

Just about any drug can cause diarrhea. If you are taking medication, ask your doctor if it could be causing your diarrhea.

Antibiotics may cause diarrhea because they change the normal flora of the colon, permitting overgrowth of certain toxic bacteria. Mild diarrhea caused by antibiotics may be helped by Lactinex, a combination of *Lactobacillus acidophilus* and *Lactobacillus bulgaricus*. Usually the diarrhea improves by itself after stopping the antibiotic, but if it is severe or persists, consult your doctor. You may need a prescription for another antibiotic (vancomycin or metronidazole) to destroy the bacteria causing the problem.

The cause of antibiotic-related diarrhea and antibiotic-related colitis is the bacterium *Clostridium difficile.* This bacterium is usually not detectable in the stool of normal individuals, but when normal bacteria are suppressed by antibiotics this bacterium may grow and cause problems. *C. difficile* gives off a toxin that damages the lining of the colon and can cause fever, lower abdominal cramps, and severe diarrhea. If not treated the patient could go on to require surgery for a bowel perforation. If you have diarrhea and have taken antibiotics in the recent past or are currently on antibiotics, your doctor will probably order a stool test for the bacterium *Clostridium difficile.* Test results may not be available for up to three days, so if you are very ill your doctor may start either metronidazole or vacomycin before the results of the test are known. *C. difficile*–related diarrhea has now become the most common cause of diarrhea in hospitalized patients. Although usually associated with a course of antibiotics, the organism can also be transmitted from patient to patient. Therefore, health-care personnel, including doctors and nurses, should wash their hands carefully after examining a patient with antibiotic diarrhea. Hospital epidemics of *Clostridium difficile* diarrhea are well documented.

It may take up to four or five days for the diarrhea to resolve after starting metronidazole or vacomycin. Usually the fever will improve before that. It is important to know that up to 25 percent of people with antibiotic-related diarrhea will develop recurrent diarrhea once the metronidazole or vacomycin has been stopped. *Clostridium difficile* multiplies by forming spores. Although metronidazole and vacomycin kill the bacteria, they do not touch the spores. After treatment for *Clostridum difficile* has been stopped, the spores may hatch and new bacteria can cause disease. Once you have a relapse of *Clostridium difficile*–related diarrhea you are more likely to have more relapses. The world record holder, I am told, is a woman who had more than forty relapses before her problem subsided. Each gastroenterologist has his or her own formula for how to get rid of recurrent antibiotic-related diarrhea, but there is no one proven way to get rid of the problem. If the diarrhea recurs, you just need to restart the same antibiotic that relieved the diarrhea the first time. In other words, the recurrent diarrhea is not related to *Clostridium difficile* being resistant to metronidazole or vacomycin; the drug will still work just as well the next time around.

13 *Diverticulosis and Its Complications*

Definition

Normally stool is pushed along as muscles in the colon wall contract in waves. Over the years little pouches may form along the outer surface of the colon wall. These pouches, called diverticula (singular diverticulum), usually form at weak spots where blood vessels poke through the wall of the bowel. They most commonly develop in the section of the colon heading toward the rectum where stool is becoming more solid. Diverticulosis—which simply means having diverticula—is very common, especially among older people. About 30 percent of Americans over age 60 have some degree of diverticulosis.

Cause

It is thought that a diet poor in fiber tends to generate stools that are drier, smaller, and more difficult to move, which makes the muscles in the colon wall work harder. This leads to a higher pressure, which in turn may push the inner lining of a small area of the colon through the muscle wall to form a diverticulum.

Symptoms

Diverticula usually cause no harm or symptoms. In some cases, pain and spasm in the abdomen and/or bloating can occur in painful diverticulosis along with diarrhea or constipation. However, it is not clear whether diverticula actually cause these symptoms. They may be due to other conditions such as irritable bowel syndrome in people who just have diverticula.

Complications

Complications of diverticulosis are not common but when they occur can be serious, and in some cases life-threatening and need immediate attention.

• Diverticulitis

Diverticulitis occurs when a diverticulum becomes inflamed and infected. It results from dry, hard stool or food matter getting stuck in the mouth or opening of the diverticulum. Bacteria in the trapped stool may then multiply and cause infection. Symptoms of diverticulitis include a constant pain, usually in the lower left side of the abdomen (where diverticula commonly develop), fever, constipation or diarrhea, nausea and vomiting, and rarely a small amount of blood mixed in the stool. In some cases urinary symptoms such as burning and/or hesitancy can occur when the bowel inflammation is close enough to the bladder to irritate its wall. If the infection is severe, an abscess (collection of pus) may develop.

In the acute situation, a CT scan (see chapter 3) may show a thickened colon wall or abscess cavity. The white blood count is often elevated. After the infection is treated and resolves, your physician may recommend a barium enema or a colonoscopy to confirm the diagnosis.

Treatment of severe diverticulitis usually means hospitalization. Antibiotics and fluids are given intravenously while the patient fasts in order to rest the bowel. Milder cases can usually be treated with a clear-liquid diet (see appendix I) at home and oral antibiotics (usually Bactrim or Cipro along with metronidazole). After a day or two, if symptoms improve, the diet can be advanced to a low-residue diet (see appendix II). After a week or so, when the attack has fully subsided, a more healthy high-fiber diet (as outlined in the Self-Help Nutritional Program) can be followed. Chronic, recurrent attacks are usually treated surgically to avoid serious complications.

Infected diverticula occasionally cause a blockage (obstruction) of the gut, or form a channel (fistula) to other organs such as the bladder or the skin. In the former case, stool and gas are mixed with the urine. A diverticulum may rarely burst and cause infection inside the abdomen (peritonitis). Surgery is usually needed to treat these serious but uncommon complications.

• Diverticular Bleeding

Diverticulosis is a common cause of bleeding from the GI tract. Symptoms include passing blood with or without stools. The amount of blood varies with the severity of the bleeding and can be large enough to warrant blood transfusion. In most cases, there is no abdominal pain associated with this condition (as opposed to diverticulitis). When the bleeding is heavy, management may involve hospitalization and blood transfusion and in some cases surgery to resect the part of the bowel involved in the bleeding. Bleeding from diverticulosis can be recurrent, and in this case surgery also is recommended.

Prevention of Diverticulosis and Its Complications

In most cases of diverticulosis, the disease doesn't cause symptoms and no drug is needed. A high-fiber diet is considered an effective preventive treatment since it increases fecal bulk and softens stool; it also decreases the pressure inside the colon, thus preventing formation of diverticula. A low-fiber diet can result in constipation. Straining to produce a bowel movement increases pressure in the colon and may cause weak spots of the colon to bulge and become diverticula.

If you already have diverticulosis, the Self-Help Nutritional Program can help keep existing diverticula free of obstruction, which can lead to infection (diverticulitis). Even a mild increase in fiber intake can significantly improve stool bulk and softness and speed the transit of stool through the colon.

14   *Hemorrhoids and Fissures*

Hemorrhoids

Hemorrhoids are dilated, engorged veins in the rectum, which can protrude through the anus. Hemorrhoids are caused by increased pressure around the anus, often from chronic constipation, with straining to defecate, over months and years. Hemorrhoids are also common during pregnancy and often accompany obesity. Some people simply have a natural predisposition to them.

Hemorrhoids may bleed, but often this appears as fresh, red blood on the toilet tissue, rather than as darker blood mixed with stool. See your doctor in either case. About half of people over age fifty have hemorrhoids. An examination of the rectum through a sigmoidoscope or colonoscope is usually performed to exclude cancer. Mild cases of hemorrhoids, where the person is only experiencing anal itching and/or mild bleeding, can often be controlled by drinking plenty of fluids and eating a high-fiber diet. More severe cases can be very uncomfortable, and a wide variety of topical analgesics are used to soothe inflammation and relieve itching (see Part Three). Stool softeners and laxatives are also used for relief. Sometimes hemorrhoids may be banded (rubber bands applied around them). When this is performed, the hemorrhoid will eventually slough off. This is especially effective for large hemorrhoids that bleed. Some doctors use a laser to treat hemorrhoids. Sometimes surgery is required, in which case the hemorrhoids are cut out and sutured over. Hemorrhoidal surgery can be very painful and I usually advise it only for patients with severe symptoms.

Fissures

A fissure is a crack or tear in the skin of the anus, usually caused by constipation and straining to defecate. Sometimes fissures occur following anal surgery or in association with proctitis or other diseases. Since the surface of the skin at the anus has been broken, defecation irritates the fissure and may cause the sphincter muscle around the anus to go into spasm, resulting in intense pain.

Topical creams, stool softeners, and warm baths are used to ease symptoms. Some people resort to laxatives. And in severe cases, surgery may be required.

• Treatment

The Self-Help Nutritional Program can go a long way to helping anorectal problems like hemorrhoids and fissures. The high-fiber program can prevent hemorrhoids and encourages hemorrhoid healing by improving stool bulk and intestinal transit time. It also softens stool and helps relieve constipation, prevent bleeding, lessen pain, and heal fissures.

Adding a bulking agent (for example, Metamucil) or stool softener (for example, Colace) to the diet twice a day is also helpful. Creams, foams, lotions, suppositories, or ointments can be soothing and promote healing when hemorrhoids or fissures cause pain and itching.

Sitz baths (soaking your bottom in warm water) are often effective. The best results are obtained if you take a sitz bath for ten minutes several times a day.

Here is a brief run-down on common OTC medications that can help hemorrhoids:

• Anusol HC-1 suppositories, like most hemorrhoid remedies, work by lubricating the swollen, irritated hemorrhoidal tissue. They also contain a mild analgesic. The dosage is given in the morning and at bedtime, and after each bowel movement. Anusol HC-1 should be taken no more than three to four times a day.

• Preparation H is available as suppository, ointment, or cream. This popular drug contains a live yeast cell derivative that supposedly helps build collagen and increases the ability of the tissue to absorb oxygen. Preparation H contains no anesthetic, but it does contain shark liver oil, which acts as a lubricant. Preparation H is applied whenever symptoms occur, but should not be used more than four times a day.

• Nupercainal (dibucaine) works primarily as a topical painkiller to relieve pain and itching. Nupercainal cream, ointment, or suppositories can be used whenever symptoms occur, up to four times a day for cream or ointment and six times a day for suppositories.

- Cortaid cream, ointment, or lotion contains 0.5 percent hydrocortisone to decrease inflammation of the tissues and relieve itching. It should not be used more than three or four times a day.

- Tucks pads, ointment, or cream contains witch hazel, which is soothing to inflamed tissues. It can be applied three to four times a day.

- A bulking agent such as Metamucil or Citrucel may also be helpful in keeping the stool soft, making bowel movements less painful.

15   *Inflammatory Bowel Disease*

Crohn's disease and ulcerative colitis are potentially serious inflammatory conditions that usually involve the lower small intestine (Crohn's disease) and parts of the large intestine. Symptoms of Crohn's disease and ulcerative colitis are similar—diarrhea, bloody stool, weight loss, and fever, and it is sometimes difficult to distinguish between the two diseases (see indeterminate colitis below). Lower abdominal cramps—usually on the right side with Crohn's, on the left with ulcerative colitis—are common.

Crohn's Disease

It is estimated that as many as half a million Americans have Crohn's disease and males and females are equally affected. It is primarily a disease of adolescents and young adults affecting mainly those between 15 and 35 years of age. In another much smaller group of patients, the disease develops between the ages of 50 and 70, a so-called "second wave". However, the disease may occur in people of all ages. Crohn's Disease can involve the gastrointestinal tract anywhere from the mouth to the perianal area. About 30 percent of people who suffer with Crohn's disease have inflammation only in the ileum (the last portion of the small intestine), about 55 percent have both ileal and colon involvement (ileocolitis), and 15 percent have only colon inflammation (Crohn's colitis). With Crohn's disease, inflammation extends through the entire wall of the bowel and there can be normal healed areas in between patches of diseased bowel. The inflammation may cause the intestinal wall to thicken, and the inside diameter may narrow so much that an intestinal obstruction occurs.

About 30 percent of patients with Crohn's disease develop a fistula, an abnormal passage between two organs, or from an internal organ to the surface of the body. Internal fistulas often form between loops of intestine but can also connect to other intra-abdominal organs such as the bladder or vagina. External fistulas to the skin's surface—either the abdomen or the anal area—may be caused by the rupture of an abscess (a collection of pus). Abscesses form in about 20 percent of patients. Often, they occur around the anus, but some occur within the abdomen. Complications in other parts of the body (so-called extracolonic manifestations of inflammatory bowel disease) may include liver disease, inflammation of the eye, arthritis affecting various joints of the body including the spine, and skin disorders.

The cause of Crohn's disease is unknown. Some theories involve bacteria similar to tuberculosis bacteria, viruses, and immunological problems. Foreign substances (antigens) in the environment may stimulate the body's defenses (the immune system) to produce an inflammation that continues without control, damaging the intestine and causing the various symptoms of Crohn's disease described above. Crohn's disease is not infectious, but it does appear to have a strong genetic tendency: in one study, about 40 percent of first-degree relatives (parents, siblings, and children) of Crohn's patients developed inflammatory bowel disease. The genetic predisposition is not as great with ulcerative colitis. But interestingly, relatives of patients with Crohn's disease have a higher likelihood of developing not only Crohn's disease but also ulcerative colitis.

Symptoms of Crohn's disease depend upon the part of the bowel affected. Patients with disease of the last portion of the small intestines (ileitis) tend to have diarrhea, weight loss, right lower quadrant pain, and possibly fever. Patients with predominantly colonic involvement may have loose stools with blood and mucus similar to the symptoms in patients with ulcerative colitis. Nutritional deficiencies and weight loss are more profound in patients with small bowel disease compared to patients with primarily colonic disease. Patients with Crohn's disease who develop narrowing of the small intestines or the large intestines due to formation of a stricture may have symptoms of nausea, vomiting, abdominal distention, and constipation rather than diarrhea. Symptoms of Crohn's disease may worsen in patients who smoke cigarettes.

Diagnosis of Crohn's disease usually involves stool studies to rule out infection followed by a colonoscopy looking for the typical endoscopic findings of the disease. Patients with mild Crohn's disease of the colon may just have superficial ulcers. With more severe disease, deeper linear ulcers appear, giving the colon a cobblestone appearance. In Crohn's disease, the endoscopic abnormalities may be patchy with some areas of the colon appearing normal (skip areas). At the time of colonoscopy, an attempt should be made to enter the small intestine through the ileocecal valve in order to determine whether the person has ileitis as well as colitis. If the small intestine is not seen at the time of the colonoscopy, an X-ray called an upper GI series with small bowel follow-through or small bowel study can be ordered. Narrowing and inflammation in the terminal ileum (the last portion of the small intestines) is usually indicative of Crohn's disease (ileitis). It is important to determine whether a patient with Crohn's disease has small bowel involvement in addition to colonic involvement since treatment for small bowel Crohn's disease may be different than treatment for disease just involving the colon.

• Treatment

Treatment of Crohn's disease (including nutritional therapy) depends on two things: severity of disease and location of disease. The goal of medical treatment is to suppress the inflammatory response allowing the intestinal tissue to heal thus relieving symptoms. Once symptoms are under control, medical therapy is used to maintain remission and decrease the frequency of disease flares.

Mild Crohn's Disease. Patients with mild disease activity usually do not appear to be acutely ill. They may have mild diarrhea, mild discomfort, no fever, and minimal colonoscopic findings. Most physicians recommend one of the 5-aminosalicylic acid (5-ASA) anti-inflammatory drugs. If the disease just involves the colon, sulfasalazine (Azulfidine) can be used as long as the patient does not have a sulfa allergy and can tolerate the medication. Some people find that Azulfidine gives them headaches and nausea so I recommend starting it slowly and gradually working up to the prescribed dose (usually 1,000 mg four times a day) over a period of several days. If you're allergic or intolerant to sulfasalazine, olsalazine (Dipentum) and balsalazide (Colazaal) are alternative 5-ASA drugs. The usual dose of Dipentum is 500 mg (two tablets) twice a day. Some people find that Dipentum causes diarrhea, which can limit its use.

If Crohn's disease involves the small intestine as well as the large intestine, then mesalamine (Asacol, 800–1200 mg three times a day, or Pentasa, 1,000 mg four times a day) is the preferred 5-ASA drug. Mesalamine will start to release in the small intestine, whereas Azulfidine, Dipentum, and Colazaal are only active in the colon.

If the 5-ASA drug does not completely control symptoms then budesonide (Entocort) 9 mg once a day may be useful. Budesonide, a steroid in pill form that has more rapid clearance from the bloodstream after absorption (as opposed to prednisone), was approved by the FDA in 2001 for the treatment of mild to moderate Crohn's disease involving the right side of the colon. Studies showed that it is more effective than 5-ASA drugs and almost as effective as prednisone, but with fewer unpleasant steroid side effects.

For patients with mild Crohn's disease, a high-fiber diet such as the Self-Help Nutritional Program found in this book and possibly even a stool-bulking agent such as Metamucil or Citrucel may improve diarrhea by absorbing the water in the stool. The 5-ASA drug can be supplemented by an over-the-counter anti-diarrheal drug such as Imodium A.D., if necessary. Anti-diarrheal agents are useful in mild inflammatory bowel disease, but extreme caution should be used with these medications. They generally should be avoided in patients with moderate or severe disease because of the risk of precipitating toxic megacolon (see below). It is prudent to consult your physician prior to starting anti-diarrheal drugs such as Imodium A.D.

Moderate to Severe Crohn's Disease.   Patients with moderate to severe Crohn's disease may have fever, more intense right lower quadrant pain or generalized lower abdominal pain, and weight loss. They may also have blood in their stool. Five percent of patients with moderate to severe Crohn's disease develop significant lower gastrointestinal bleeding, which can be life threatening. Most people with more severe disease will require a steroid medication such as prednisone to control inflammation. Often a dose as high as 40 mg a day or more may be given, usually in the morning. When symptoms finally are under control, the dose of prednisone can be tapered over a period of weeks until the patient is no longer on medication. Most of the time a 5-ASA drug such as Asacol will also be started and the patient will continue taking Asacol after the prednisone has been discontinued.

If the patient relapses after being taken off prednisone or if the patient is unable to stop prednisone, I will often add an immunosuppressant drug such as azathioprine (Imuran), which may allow the person to be weaned from prednisone or at least remain on a lower dose of the drug. However, azathioprine may take three to four months to start working. Although azathioprine does have side effects such as bone marrow suppression, pancreatitis, and liver damage, I believe it is a safer drug to take than prednisone. Prednisone can cause osteoporosis, diabetes, hypertension, damage to hip joints and a host of cosmetic side effects including rounding of the face, acne, facial hair growth, obesity of the upper torso, and purplish stretch marks on the abdomen, buttocks, and thighs. I always try to keep my patients on as low a dose of prednisone as possible.

Some doctors do not use high enough doses of the 5-ASA and immunosuppressant drugs and the patient is not able to be weaned from prednisone. Although the standard dose of Asacol is 2.4 g per day in three doses (two tablets, three times a day), higher doses such as three tablets, three times a day may give better results. These drugs have limited side effects so higher doses can be used safely in the majority of patients. Likewise using Imuran at 1.5 to 2.0 mg per kilogram per day (e.g., 150 mg for a 150-pound person) may permit the patient to finally stop prednisone.

If necessary, 5-ASA drugs such Asacol, Pentasa, Colazaal, Dipentum, or Sulfasalazine can be taken for the rest of your life. There is a theoretical concern that long-term use of azathioprine, since it is an immunosuppressant, could increase the person's risk of developing a tumor in the future. In actuality, this rarely, if ever, happens and many physicians have given Imuran to their patients for several years. Patients will usually relapse when taken off Imuran.

Some physicians use a drug called 6-mercaptopurine instead of Imuran. The two drugs are almost identical and can be used interchangeably. For those individuals who are intolerant or allergic to Imuran another immunosuppressant drug, methotrexate, can be given as a weekly injection.

For those individuals who do not respond to prednisone and immunosuppressant drugs like azathioprine, 6-mercaptopurine, or methotrexate, Remicade will usually bring the disease under control. Remicade works by inhibiting the activity of tumor necrosis factor alpha (TNF), which stimulates an inflammatory response in the colon. Remicade is given intravenously over two hours as a one-time dose. The drug is very expensive and should only be used in those individuals who are truly resistant to standard treatment and those individuals who have fistulae. Those individuals receiving Remicade to treat fistulae usually receive repeat doses of Remicade at two and six weeks after the initial dose. In one study 46 percent of Remicade treated patients had complete healing of fistulae compared to only 13 percent in the placebo group. Once Remicade brings Crohn's disease under control, standard therapy is used in an attempt to maintain remission. About 40 percent of patients will relapse after going into remission with Remicade. This drug was recently approved by the FDA for maintaining remission, both in fistulizing disease and in moderate to severe disease. Remicade infusions at a dose of 5 mg per kg body weight are usually given every eight weeks. Side effects of Remicade include infusion reactions such as flushing and shortness of breath. The vast majority of these reactions can be controlled with medications such as Tylenol or Benadryl. They usually occur at the second infusion or later. Some patients have developed delayed reactions, usually about a week after the infusion, characterized by joint or muscle aches and pains. Treatment of these reactions can include a short course of prednisone. Remicade is also associated with an increased risk of infections. Although the majority of these infections are not serious (e.g., upper respiratory infection), occasionally serious infections such as pneumonia or tuberculosis can occur. A skin test for tuberculosis (PPD) should be administered to patients before they are started on the medication. Another potential problem that can be encountered with Remicade is the development of antibodies against the drug, which limits its effectiveness on subsequent injections. Some physicians think that using immunosuppressant drugs such as Imuran concomitantly with Remicade may prevent the phenomenon from happening.

Some antibiotics are effective in treating Crohn's disease. Metronidazole (Flagyl) is helpful in patients with Crohn's disease confined to the colon and in patients with perianal Crohn's disease. The usual dose is 1 to 1.5 grams per day in divided doses. The higher the dose, the more likely the patient will experience side effects including nausea, metallic taste, and numbness and tingling in the extremities caused by nerve damage. The nerve damage is usually reversible when the drug dose is lowered or stopped. Patients on metronidazole are not allowed to drink alcohol because the combination of alcohol and metronidazole can make them feel ill. Metronidazole does not seem to help patients with ileitis. Metronidazole may also be useful in preventing or delaying recurrences after surgical resection of bowel affected by Crohn's disease. Ciprofloxacin (Cipro) is often used in patients with Crohn's disease with good results, although its usefulness is not as well established as that for metronidazole. Some studies show the combination of metronidazole and Cipro works better than either antibiotic given by itself.

Thus, a patient with moderate to severe Crohn's disease affecting the colon as well as the small intestines may be treated with several drugs simultaneously. It is not unusual for one of my patients to be on prednisone, azathioprine, metronidazole, and Asacol, all at the same time.

It may be necessary for the very ill to be admitted to the hospital and receive intravenous steroids (for example, methylprednisolone). If the patient does not respond to high doses of intravenous steroids, Remicade or cyclosporine (a drug used in transplant patients to suppress the immune system) may be effective. I try to avoid cyclosporine since it is not as effective in treating Crohn's disease as it is in treating ulcerative colitis. Furthermore it can cause kidney and nerve damage and hypertension.

Nutritional management of patients with moderate to severe Crohn's disease of the small intestine may require some type of nutritional supplementation. The most severe cases may require total parenteral (intravenous) nutrition, however, usually the patient is able to tolerate nutritional supplements via the gastrointestinal tract. A nasogastric tube can be placed and the patient fed with an elemental diet. Instead of giving the patient macronutrients (carbohydrates, fats, and protein), the patient is given micronutrients (amino acids and glucose), which are easier to absorb (see chapter 31). In less severe cases of small intestine disease, I recommend a diet low in lactose, fat, and residue. A low-residue diet avoids foods rich in fiber (see chapter 19 for fiber-containing foods and Appendix II).

• Surgery

Surgery cannot cure patients with Crohn's disease. Therefore, surgery is usually only performed on patients with a bowel obstruction, abdominal abscess, or a troublesome fistula. We usually recommend giving Asacol or Pentasa after surgery in an attempt to prevent disease relapse. Occasionally, azathioprine may also be used for this purpose. The goal of surgery is to remove the least amount of small bowel as possible in order to avoid diarrhea and malabsorption caused by a so-called "short gut."

Ulcerative Colitis

Ulcerative colitis is an inflammatory disease of the colon and rectum. As with Crohn's disease, the symptoms usually start in childhood or early adulthood. On rare occasions, the disease may begin in the seventh decade or even later. Although ulcerative colitis can go into remission for long periods of time, once you have ulcerative colitis it is generally a lifelong illness. Unlike Crohn's disease, which affects the entire wall of the intestine, the inflammation associated with ulcerative colitis involves only the superficial lining of the colon called the mucosa. Ulcerative colitis almost always involves the rectum (proctitis), but can also extend beyond the rectum and at times involve the entire colon (pancolitis). Patients with ulcerative colitis do not develop perianal disease. Fistulae do not form in ulcerative colitis because the inflammation does not extend through the entire thickness of the bowel wall. While Crohn's disease often causes a patchy distribution of disease in the colon (skip areas), inflammation caused by ulcerative colitis tends to extend in a continuous fashion from the rectum. As with Crohn's disease, patients with ulcerative colitis may develop complications in other parts of the body, including arthritis of the spine and joints, skin ulcers and nodules, inflammation of the inner eyelids and whites of the eye, and liver and biliary tract disease (extracolonic manifestations of inflammatory bowel disease). The cause of ulcerative colitis is unknown but, like Crohn's disease, it is thought that the inflammation is caused by a complex interaction of genes, immunity, and environment. Diagnosis of this complex disease requires a full evaluation including stool cultures and colon biopsy. A barium enema can often give clues to diagnosis, but the "gold standard" remains a full colonoscopic exam with biopsies.

Patients with ulcerative colitis commonly complain of diarrhea, which is often bloody and lower abdominal pain, especially in the left lower quadrant. A condition called toxic megacolon or toxic dilatation of the colon may occur in patients with severe ulcerative colitis. The abdomen may become distended and abdominal tenderness may increase. Often the patient has a high fever. X-ray of the abdomen will demonstrate a markedly dilated colon. This is a medical emergency and needs to be treated promptly (see below).

Patients with long standing ulcerative colitis and Crohn's disease, especially those patients who have moderate to severe disease involving the entire colon, have an increased risk of developing colon cancer. If you have had pancolitis for at least eight years, your doctor may recommend a colonoscopy to screen for colorectal cancer. Even if no tumor is seen, your doctor will probably take biopsies throughout the colon looking for dysplasia (precancerous changes in the colon). When dysplasia is found on a biopsy specimen, the pathologist tries to determine whether the atypical cells are caused by inflammation or are true precancerous cells. A colonoscopsy is often repeated after an attempt to maximize treatment for a few months. If dysplasia persists, surgery is usually recommended (see below). We previously thought patients with Crohn's disease of the colon did not have as great a risk for colon cancer as those patients with ulcerative colitis. We now believe that patients with Crohn's disease may have an even higher risk of cancer than patients with ulcerative colitis. (See chapter 16 for recommendations on colorectal cancer screening in inflammatory bowel disease.)

• Treatment

Similar to Crohn's disease, treatment of ulcerative colitis depends on the severity and the extent of the disease.

Proctitis. Patients who have disease involving the rectum only (proctitis) usually do not have diarrhea but complain of a bloody mucus discharge and, occasionally, lower abdominal cramps. For mild proctitis, a mesalamine suppository at bedtime may be all that is necessary. If the disease extends above 15 cm from the anus at the time of sigmoidoscopy, your doctor may prescribe Rowasa enemas, which can heal inflammation of the colon up to 60 cm (about 25 inches) from the anus. Steroid enemas such as

Cortenema can be used instead of Rowasa enemas; however, there is some steroid absorption into the body through the rectum and steroid side effects can develop over time (see above). If the proctitis is more severe, your doctor may give you an oral 5-ASA drug like sulfasalazine, Asacol, or Colazaal or even a steroid like prednisone in the most severe cases.

Mild Ulcerative Colitis. Patients with mild ulcerative colitis involving the entire colon (pancolitis) usually have up to four bowel movements a day, scant blood in the stool, and a normal temperature. We usually use the combination of an oral 5-ASA drug such as Azulfidine or Colazaal along with a Rowasa enema at bedtime in patients with mild colitis. Occasionally the Rowasa enema can be avoided if the disease on the left side of the colon is mild. If you are intolerant or allergic to sulfasalazine or sulfa drugs and get diarrhea from Dipentum, Asacol or Pentasa can also be used to treat ulcerative colitis. With mild ulcerative colitis, the high fiber content of the Self-Help Nutritional Program is recommended for most patients. Occasionally a high fiber diet will aggravate even mild inflammatory bowel disease and in this case you should switch to a low-residue diet (see chapter 19 and Appendix II).

Moderately Severe Ulcerative Colitis. I frequently use a Rowasa enema along with an oral 5-ASA drug and prednisone when treating patients with moderate to severe ulcerative colitis. If the rectal inflammation is intense, the patient initially may not be able to tolerate the Rowasa enema. A mesalamine suppository (e.g., Canasa) can be given for a week or two until the patient is able to tolerate the Rowasa enema.

After symptoms have subsided, I try to gradually lower the dose of prednisone while leaving the patient on a full dose of an oral 5-ASA drug and, at times, a Rowasa enema. If the colitis flares as the prednisone dose is lowered, it may be necessary to give an immunosuppressant drug like azathioprine (Imuran) along with prednisone and the 5-ASA drug. Prednisone usually needs to be continued after starting azathioprine since the drug usually does not begin to work for three to six months. After an appropriate period of time, prednisone can be slowly tapered and many individuals can be maintained in remission with just azathioprine and one of the 5-ASA drugs.

A patient who has been in remission for more than a year may wonder whether he or she can stop oral 5-ASA medication. Occasionally people can stop their 5-ASA drug and remain in remission for years; however, if they relapse off medication I recommend they take the medication indefinitely either at the full prescription dose or half the usual dose. The issue of how long to keep someone on azathioprine is not as clear. Some doctors continue the drug indefinitely (while checking blood tests periodically). Others stop the drug after one to three years. However, when azathioprine is stopped, most patients will relapse within a few months.

Severe Ulcerative Colitis.   In patients with severe ulcerative colitis who have more than six bloody movements a day, fever, rapid pulse, and tender abdomen, hospitalization may be necessary. In this situation, a patient is usually fasted and given intravenous steroids and nutrition. If the patient does not respond to the above measures, the drug cyclosporine can be given intravenously. Most people will respond to cyclosporine within two weeks and the drug can then be switched to an oral form. Although oral azathioprine can take up three months or longer to work, intravenous azathioprine can produce a more rapid response in patients with difficult ulcerative colitis. Several small studies of Remicade have indicated a potential treatment benefit in ulcerative colitis, although definitive studies to prove benefit have not yet been completed. In patients with severe colitis, antidiarrheal drugs like Lomotil and Imodium A.D. and narcotics are generally avoided since they can precipitate the development of toxic magacolon (see below). Patients with moderate to severe active colitis should adhere to a low-residue diet (see chapter 19 and Appendix II) until their symptoms are under control. The Self-Help Nutritional Program outlined in this book is not recommended for patients with moderate to severe inflammatory bowel disease.

Toxic Megacolon.   Patients with toxic megacolon are in danger of colonic perforation. In order to decompress the bowel, a tube is put through the nose into the stomach and air and stomach contents aspirated on a continuous basis. A rectal tube may also be placed to decompress the colon. The patient is fasted and given intravenous fluids and nutrition. A high dose of steroids (methylprednisolone) is given along with antibiotics. If the patient does not respond to treatment in the first twenty-four to forty-eight hours, surgery is often performed (see below). Cyclosporine may be used in this condition. In a small trial this therapy was able to stabilize the majority of patients. However, over half still required surgery within six months.

Indeterminate Colitis.   Occasionally, it may be difficult to distinguish ulcerative colitis from Crohn's disease. Prometheus Laboratories of San Diego offers a battery of blood tests (ANCA, pANCA, ASCA) that can help distinguish ulcerative colitis from Crohn's disease. It is of particular importance to be certain you have ulcerative colitis and not Crohn's disease before undergoing surgery (see below). The Prometheus blood tests may also predict those individuals with ulcerative colitis who go on to develop inflammation of the ileal pouch (pouchitis) after ileal pouch-anal anastomosis. (Your doctor can order these tests called the IBD system when indicated by calling 1-888-423-5227.)

• Microscopic Colitis

Patients with symptoms of diarrhea and lower abdominal pain who have a normal appearing colon at the time of sigmoidoscopy or colonoscopy are often diagnosed as having irritable bowel syndrome (IBS). Usually the diagnosis is correct but in some individuals, even though the colon grossly looks normal, there can be significant inflammation seen microscopically. So-called microscopic colitis, also known as lymphocytic colitis, and a variant called collagenous colitis can cause mild to severe abdominal pain and diarrhea. When performing a colonoscopy on a patient with chronic diarrhea, I generally take random biopsies of a normal colon looking for microscopic inflammation. Microscopic colitis usually responds to the same drugs used to treat mild ulcerative colitis (5-ASA drugs). Rarely prednisone is given to patients with severe symptoms that do not respond to the 5-ASA drugs.

• Future Treatments

Interleukin-10 (IL-10) blocks the formation of proteins that cause inflammation by special white cells called monocytes. IL-10 has been shown to be effective in treating Crohn's disease, with up to 50 percent of patients experiencing a complete remission.

Some patients with inflammatory bowel disease have started to use fish oil supplements. By giving large doses of fish oils that contain omega-3 fatty acids, some studies have shown improvement in patients with inflammatory bowel disease—especially Crohn's disease. Omega-3 fatty acids produce a prostaglandin (PGE3), which has anti-inflammatory properties.

Short-chain fatty acid such as butyrate, propionate, and acetate may also heal colitis. Butyrate is the major food source for cells lining the large intestine. Giving extra short-chain fatty acids in the form of a butyrate enema has been shown to be effective in treating colitis.

Recent interest has been generated in "probiotic" therapy. This is the use of beneficial bacteria ingested in pill form to restore balance to the intestinal environment, thereby reducing intestinal inflammation. Some studies showed benefit with this approach especially in patients with pouchitis who underwent J-pouch ileoanal anastomosis (see below and see Part Four).

Ulcerative colitis may flare when an individual gives up smoking cigarettes. Of course, no doctor is going to recommend going back to smoking. However, there may be another option. Some studies show that the nicotine patch may help induce remission or at least reduce symptoms in approximately 40 percent of the patients who use the patch for more than four weeks. Other studies however, have not shown such a positive effect of the nicotine patch. Remember, only patients with ulcerative colitis benefit from nicotine. Smoking actually makes Crohn's disease worse (see above).

• Surgery

For patients who fail medical management of ulcerative colitis, or for those who develop dysplasia or cancer of the colon, total removal of the colon (colectomy) may be necessary. With ulcerative colitis colectomy can be curative if the entire colon, including the rectum, is removed. These days a permanent ileostomy (the end of the ileum is sewn to the abdominal wall and liquid stool empties into a plastic bag) is not usually required. A special operation called total colectomy with J-pouch ileoanal anastomosis can be performed. Here the surgeon creates a new rectum out of the small intestine and sutures it to the anus. This is a two-step operation requiring a temporary ileostomy.

More About Nutrition

The management and treatment of Crohn's disease and ulcerative colitis requires careful medical supervision over the long term. Dietary management may require a low-fiber, low-residue diet, especially when these diseases are in their acute phases. Patients are instructed to avoid fruits and vegetables, bran cereals and whole grain breads, seed, and nuts. A lactose-free and low-fat diet may also be important in patients with ileitis.

Once either disease is under control, the Self-Help Nutritional Program (a high-fiber diet) may help prevent the typical symptoms of these diseases including diarrhea, cramps, and perianal disease. However, all dietary management for patients with inflammatory bowel disease should be carefully supervised by a physician.

Patients with ileitis may require iron and calcium supplements: if the inflammation is severe, trace metals (zinc, cadmium, chromium) must also be replaced. Patients with ileitis may need monthly shots of vitamins B12.

Ileitis sufferers tend to form kidney stones because of excessive absorption of oxalate. Dietary management includes a low-fat, low-oxalate diet (avoid spinach, rhubarb and tea) plus calcium supplements (1 gram of calcium gluconate a day). This is one instance where extra calcium prevents kidney stone formation.

By individualizing drug and nutritional therapy most patients with inflammatory bowel disease can live long productive lives free of symptoms. Key to success is the use of multiple drugs at doses high enough to do their job and tailoring drugs and diet to disease activity and location.

For more information on inflammatory bowel disease contact the National Foundation for Ileitis and Colitis (NFIC).

16   *Cancer of the Colon and Rectum*

*C*ancer of the colon and rectum, also known as colorectal cancer, is the second leading cause of death from cancer in the United States. Only lung and prostate cancer in men, and lung and breast cancer in women, occur more frequently. In 2001, there were approximately 135,000 new cases of colorectal cancer in the United States, and an estimated 57,000 Americans died from the disease. The highest rates of this disease are seen in North America, Australia, and New Zealand, with the northeast and central states in the U.S. demonstrating more cases than the national average. The good news about colorectal cancer is that almost all cancers arise from polyps, which are benign tumors of the colon. Colon polyps are present for many years before they turn to cancer. Thus, if you develop colon polyps and they are removed, it is unlikely you will ever develop colon cancer. Even when colon cancer is at its early stages, it is definitely curable. Over 90 percent of people who have an operation to remove an early cancer survive. Unfortunately, as the cancer progresses and invades deeper into the bowel wall, the chance for survival decreases. But even when the tumor has extended through the bowel wall and invaded regional lymph nodes, there is still a 50 percent chance of cure as long as chemotherapy follows surgery. Unfortunately, once colorectal cancer has spread to the liver, it is incurable and people often succumb within a few years.

There are tried and true ways to avoid the development of colorectal cancer but most people never take advantage of them. If you adhere to the principles I outline in this chapter, you will markedly reduce your risk of developing colon cancer in the future. Just as mammography has revolutionized the early diagnosis of breast cancer, and the prostate-specific antigen (PSA) blood test in concert with a digital rectal exam has revolutionized the early diagnosis of prostate cancer, appropriate screening tests have been documented to significantly decrease the risk of death from colorectal cancer. Furthermore, we now know that by altering diet and by taking calcium and/or aspirin (see below), we may reduce our chances of developing colon cancer in the first place.

Symptoms of Colon Cancer

Most people with colorectal cancer have no symptoms at all. Symptoms, when present, often depend on where the tumor is located. The most common symptom of right-sided (ascending colon) cancers is weakness from iron deficiency anemia. These tumors may bleed chronically and a low hemoglobin may be found on routine blood testing. Tumors on the left side of the colon (descending colon, sigmoid, and rectum) are more common and may produce some obstructive symptoms since stool is firmer there and the diameter of the bowel is smaller on the left side. Abdominal distention, difficulty in having a bowel movement, constantly feeling like you haven't completely evacuated your bowels (tenesmus), and bright red rectal bleeding are more likely to be present with left-sided tumors. People may also notice a change in the caliber of the stool (pencil-thin stools).

Risk Factors for the Development of Colorectal Cancer

The older you are the higher the risk of developing colorectal cancer. Although we occasionally see colorectal cancer in people in their thirties and their early forties, most of the time this tumor arises in people over the age of fifty. When colorectal cancer is seen in individuals under forty-five years of age, there is a higher chance they have a genetic cause and family members should be screened (see below).

• Hereditary Factors

Several genetic defects have now been identified that predispose an individual to develop colorectal cancer. The adenomatous polyposis coli (APC) gene helps the body to defend against colon cancer. When the APC gene is defective, an individual has an increased risk of developing polyps and eventually colon cancer. Some Ashkenazi Jews (of Eastern European ancestry) have a particular defect in the APC gene that markedly increases their risk of getting colorectal cancer. When the APC gene is truly disabled, familial adenomatous polyposis (FAP) may be the result. The individual develops thousands of polyps throughout the colon and unless the colon is removed the person will almost without question develop colorectal cancer early in life. The average age of presentation with symptoms is 36 years, and two-thirds of these patients already have colon cancer. Even when there is no history of FAP in the family, individuals who develop colorectal cancer have some defect on the APC gene. Thus, you can either inherit the APC gene abnormality at birth or it can be caused by a spontaneous mutation in your DNA after birth.

A defect of the APC gene is not the only cause of colorectal cancer. About 5 percent of colorectal cancers are caused by another gene defect that causes hereditary nonpolyposis colorectal cancer (HNPCC). Patients with HNPCC not only develop colorectal cancer, but may also develop breast, uterine, ovarian and prostate cancer. HNPCC more commonly affects the right side of the colon, thus, when a tumor is found on the right side of the colon, the person should be carefully screened for other tumors and their family history be carefully taken. Some of you may remember when President Reagan developed colon cancer. His cancer developed on the right side of his colon, and, within a year, his brother also came down with a right-sided colon cancer. There is a tumor marker blood test for suspicion of HNPCC that detects a defect in the DNA repair process called MSI (micro-satellite instability). MSI is present in more than 90 percent of colon cancers in HNPCC. People who should be tested for HNPCC are those that fulfill the so-called Amsterdam criteria (see below).

Ideally, anyone whose family history is suggestive of a hereditary syndrome should seek out a cancer risk-counseling program, which can evaluate their family and help them make appropriate decisions about testing.

Even though approximately one-third of all colon cancer cases arise from inherited susceptibility, the known syndromes (e.g., FAP, HNPCC,

---

Amsterdam I Criteria for the Diagnosis of Hereditary Nonpolyposis Colorectal Cancer

There should be at least 3 relatives with colorectal cancer; all of the following should be present

- One should be a first-degree relative of the other two (a parent, child, or sibling)
- At least two successive generations are affected
- At least 1 colorectal cancer should be diagnosed before age 50
- FAP should be excluded

etc.) only account for the minority of cases. At the present time, there are not reliable genetic markers to screen most families who have relatives affected with colon cancer.

• Diet and Nutritional Factors

Colorectal cancer can also be caused by environmental factors, such as diet and lifestyle. When people move from low-incidence places such as Japan or Africa, to a high-incidence country such as the United States, the occurrence of this disease in their offspring increases to that of the adopted country. There is a body of medical literature that demonstrates an increased risk of colorectal cancer with high intake of red meat. It was previously felt that the high fat content of meat was responsible, but more recent interest has focused on compounds such as heterocyclic amines and polyaromatic hydrocarbons that are produced when food is "charbroiled." These compounds may be carcinogenic, and there are individual differences in the ability to metabolize such compounds. Laboratory studies have demonstrated that these compounds can cause colorectal cancer in animals. Eventually, we may be able to make specific dietary recommendations on red meat but the jury is still out for the time being.

Obesity is a risk factor for colorectal cancer, especially when body fat is predominately around the waist (android or male pattern of obesity). Research indicates that the amount of food, rather than the type, may be important. Recent studies have shown that obese women were 50 percent more likely, and obese men 80 percent more likely to develop colorectal cancer.

A high-fat diet seems to predispose to colorectal cancer. On the contrary, a high-fiber diet and a diet rich in vegetables and fruit seems to lower the risk of developing colorectal cancer. The fiber hypothesis has been popular for almost 40 years. Recent studies indicate that is probably not correct. A recent large study found no protective effect of fiber from any source (cereals, fruits, or vegetables). Also, two randomized trials of fiber did not show that it can prevent early cancers of the colon. However, the fact that fiber, per se, is not protective does not mean that fiber-containing foods, such as vegetables, are not protective. In fact, most of the studies have found a moderate protective effect of high vegetable intake against colorectal cancer.

Alcohol and smoking may also increase the risk of developing colon cancer. The majority of studies that have looked at smoking and colorectal cancer have found an effect. Large recent studies of health professionals have demonstrated significantly increased risks among smokers who had been smoking for at least 35 years. The majority of studies support an association between alcohol and cancer. The risk is increased for both men and women, and included moderate drinkers (e.g., one drink per day). The science behind this research centers on the effects of alcohol on the metabolism of methyl groups and the low levels of folate seen in these individuals.

• Inflammatory Bowel Disease

Patients with both ulcerative colitis and Crohn's disease of the colon have an increased risk of colorectal cancer. The risk is even higher in those individuals who have had colitis for more than eight years, severe colitis, and colitis involving the entire colon. Promising research has demonstrated that the use of ursodeoxycholic acid may decrease the risk of cancer in patients with ulcerative colitis, but this has not yet become standard preventative treatment. The 5-ASA drugs (see chapter 9) may also have a protective action against colon cancer.

Screening Techniques

The goal of screening is to discover early cancers that have a greater than 90 percent chance of cure and to discover polyps that have the potential to develop into colon cancer. When a person comes to my office, the first thing I do is take a history. I inquire about any symptoms that could possibly be related to colon cancer (see above). I also take a family history asking the person if anyone in their family has ever had colon polyps or colon cancer. Finally, a complete physical examination always includes a digital rectal examination where a doctor's gloved finger is inserted through the anus into the rectum. A low-lying rectal cancer can be palpated (felt). The prostate can be checked for evidence of tumor and a sample of stool is extracted and tested for occult blood (see below).

Individuals with a Higher Than Normal Risk of Developing Colorectal Cancer

- Family history of individuals with colon polyps and colon cancer (especially if parents or siblings develop cancer under the age of sixty)
- Family history of FAP or HNPCC
- Long-standing inflammatory bowel disease
- Individuals who have already had a polyp or colon cancer

The American Cancer Society has specific recommendations on how to screen individuals for colorectal cancer. After my initial exam, I stratify individuals into normal risk for colon cancer or high risk for colon cancer. Normal-risk individuals are those who have no symptoms, no disease that can predispose to the development of colon cancer, and no close relatives with colon cancer. Most individuals will fall into this category. For them, I recommend an annual digital rectal exam starting at age 40, at which time a stool sample can be tested for the presence of blood. A colonoscopy should also be performed starting at age fifty and repeated every ten years, if the colon appears normal. A barium enema and a sigmoidoscopy can be substituted for a colonoscopy, but these two tests have their limitations. It is well known that less than 50 percent of all colorectal cancers are within reach of the sigmoidoscope. Therefore, cancers could easily be missed using this test. Barium enema exams may miss up to 50 percent of polyps less than 1 cm in size, and have a high degree of reader variability in their interpretation. In the National Polyp Study, the incidence of cancer was reduced by 76–90 percent in patients that had regular colonoscopies according to the newly established guidelines.

Those individuals who are at greater risk for developing colorectal cancer (see box, above) require a colonoscopy when screening for colorectal cancer. Asymptomatic individuals who have one or more family members (parents, siblings) with colorectal cancer should have their first colonoscopy at age forty or ten years before they reach the age their family member was when his or her colon cancer was discovered, whichever is earlier. Annual digital rectal exam and stool for occult blood testing should commence starting at age 40. If normal, the colonoscopy should be repeated at five-year intervals. If polyps are found at the time of colonoscopy, the test is usually repeated in one to three years, depending on the number and size of the polyps and whether or not they are on a stalk (pedunculated) or flat against the wall of the bowel (sessile). When a cancer is found and removed, a colonoscopy is usually repeated one year later. (Some advise a colonoscopy at six months and then annually for four more years after diagnosis.)

Those individuals who have an extraordinarily high risk of developing colorectal cancer, for example, those patients with a family history of FAP, should have a sigmoidoscopy beginning at age 12. If polyps are found, a complete colonoscopy is necessary. Those individuals with an HNPCC family history should be screened by colonoscopy at age 20. If no polyps are found at the time of colonoscopy, the colonoscopy is repeated every three years—repeated every year if polyps are present. Blood tests are available that can test the individual to determine if they have inherited the gene for FAP or HNPCC. Another can detect the presence of the abnormal APC gene found in Jews of Eastern European ancestry. However, many physicians would still recommend intensive screening for colorectal cancer even if those tests are negative.

Patients with ulcerative colitis who have had the disease for 12 years or greater for left sided colitis or eight years for colitis involving the entire colon should be screened by colonoscopy annually or at least every two years. Patients with Crohn's disease who have had the disease for 10 years or greater should have a colonoscopy every two years. The ileum must be examined as well in patients with long standing ileitis. Inflammatory bowel disease poses a difficult problem in diagnosing colorectal cancer since this is one instance where the cancer arises directly on the wall of the colon rather than in a polyp. Since the colon is already inflamed, it may be difficult to differentiate colon cancer from inflammatory bowel disease. When a colonoscopy is performed in patients with inflammatory bowel disease, multiple random biopsies are taken along the colon. Pathologists will look for precancerous changes (severe dysplasia) and, if found, we recommend that the colon be surgically removed.

If you have symptoms that could be attributed to colorectal cancer (tenesmus, rectal bleeding, new constipation, pencil-thin stools, iron deficiency anemia), a colonoscopic evaluation is essential.

Currently, there are no tumor markers that will accurately screen for colorectal cancer like the one for prostate cancer. Carcinoembryonic antigen (CEA) is a tumor marker for colorectal cancer, but it is not sensitive enough to pick up early cancers. Furthermore, it can be elevated in smokers and in other conditions so it should not be used to screen the general population for the presence of colorectal cancer. If, however, a colon cancer is found, a CEA level is recommended before surgery. If elevated, the test can be repeated after surgery to see if the entire tumor has been removed. Furthermore, the blood test can be used in follow-up screening for cancer recurrence. A special test called a CEA-scan is available at some hospitals. This test may be more sensitive than CT-scan in diagnosing colon cancer.

Over the past few years some new technologies have been developed. People often ask about the "virtual colonoscopy" test. This test is a special CT scan that takes "slices" of a person's body and then reconstructs them into a three-dimensional view of the colon. This test still requires a bowel cleansing preparation and is limited by its inability to remove any lesions that it may detect. The "virtual colonoscopy" is also dependent on the expertise of the radiologist reading the study and has been recently shown to miss small polyps. If a polyp is found, the patient still has to have a conventional colonoscopy to remove it. That being said, virtual colonoscopy may still develop into an important diagnostic tool, especially for normal risk individuals. Another new test that is discussed is the video capsule endoscopy test. During this test, the patient swallows a small pill that has a camera on the end. This camera takes thousands of pictures of the intestines. This test is only designed to examine the small intestine and is not an appropriate tool for screening colorectal cancer. There have been developments in stool tests, looking for specific proteins and antigens that are associated with colorectal cancers. At this point in time, the stool antigen tests are not yet sensitive or specific enough to be used for cancer screening and are still considered somewhat investigational.

When the above guidelines are followed, an individual's risk of dying from colon cancer is markedly decreased. Unfortunately, only 25–40 percent of adult Americans are screened appropriately for colorectal cancer. It is distressing to see individuals diagnosed with advanced colorectal cancer who have never been screened even though they visit their primary care physician regularly. Even when patients are offered colorectal cancer screening they often refuse fearing that the test will be uncomfortable or too embarrassing. I try to work my patients through these fears, and when they come back to my office after having undergone a colonoscopy or sigmoidoscopy, they almost uniformly say, "That wasn't bad at all. I'm sorry I waited so long to have it." It is only through better public education of patients, as well as of doctors, that we will be able to make a large dent in preventing and treating this very common cancer.

How to Lower Your Risk of Developing Colorectal Cancer

Since colon cancer is more common in obese individuals and in people who consume a high-fat, low-fiber diet, it makes sense to maintain a normal body weight and eat a low-fat, high-fiber diet to avoid colon cancer. It has been shown that increasing fruits and vegetables in your diet will lower your risk as well. A high-fiber diet increases the bulk of your stool. This decreases the concentration of carcinogens in the stool and speeds waste through the colon so that the carcinogens have less contact with the wall of the colon. Fiber is fermented by bacteria in the colon to form short-chain fatty acids such as butyrate, propionate, and acetate, which may confer some protection against colon cancer. Several studies have now shown that individuals who take calcium supplements have a lower rate of developing polyps once a polyp has been diagnosed and removed. In fact, some studies even suggest that the size of existing polyps can shrink in those individuals who are taking calcium supplements (e.g., 1 g of calcium carbonate a day). Likewise, similar research suggests that folic acid supplements (1 mg per day) may be helpful as well.

A breakthrough in the prevention of colorectal cancer is the discovery that aspirin and nonsteroidal anti-inflammatory drugs (NSAID) confer significant protection against the development of colorectal cancer. This has been shown in a variety of studies. At this point in time, it is unclear what the optimal dose of aspirin should be in order to aid in cancer prevention. Unfortunately, low-dose aspirin used to prevent the development of coronary artery disease may not be sufficient to protect against colon cancer. A full prescription dose NSAID or at least one regular aspirin a day is probably necessary. The risk of taking such medication (e.g., gastrointestinal bleeding) has to be weighed against the risk of developing colon cancer in any individual.

In general, I recommend to all of my patients who are at higher than normal risk of developing colorectal cancer to adhere to a sensible diet, low in fat and high in fiber and fruits and vegetables. Red meat should be limited to less than two servings per week. Regular exercise should be encouraged (30 minutes per day of moderate activity) and obesity should be avoided. I advise them to take a calcium supplement (e.g. Caltrate) and I make a decision about treating them with an NSAID such as Sulindac or aspirin on an individual basis. Sensible modifications in diet and lifestyle may decrease your risk of colorectal cancer by as much as 70 percent. The most important strategy to decrease your chances of getting cancer is screening (see above).

• Treatment

Colorectal cancer can only be cured if it is removed from the body before it has spread to other organs. Occasionally the cancer may be confined to a polyp, and when the polyp is removed the person is cured without surgery. Most of the time, however, the affected part of the colon needs to be removed. If the cancer arises in the lower rectum, it may be necessary to remove the entire rectum and the person will be left with a permanent colostomy. If the tumor has invaded through the entire wall of the bowel, or has reached adjacent lymph nodes, a course of chemotherapy is usually given after the person has recovered from surgery (usually 5-fluorouracil with leucovorin or levamisole). Research involving new chemotherapy agents such as interferon, irinotecan, topotecan, oxaliplatin and others appears promising. Targeted therapy with radiolabeled antibodies, which directs treatment to the tumor is currently being investigated. Radiation is only given to patients with rectal cancer in order to shrink the tumor before surgery and to prevent a local recurrence after the tumor has been removed. More extensive chemotherapy may be offered to those individuals whose tumor has spread to distant organs like the liver; however, the success rate is extremely low.

If you are fifty years of age or older, call your doctor today to schedule a colonoscopy. It could be the smartest thing you have ever done.

17 *Food Allergies*

An allergy is an exaggerated reaction to a substance that in most people causes no response. The response is mainly to otherwise harmless substances: chemicals that come in contact with the skin, particles of dust or pollen that affect the respiratory passages or the surface of the eye, foods that affect the stomach and intestines.

Allergies are caused by a reaction of the immune system; they occur only on second or subsequent exposure to the offending agent, after the first contact has sensitized the body. Many common illnesses, such as asthma and hay fever, are caused by allergic reactions.

Many of my patients feel their GI symptoms may be caused by a food allergy. Symptoms of food allergies include nausea, vomiting, diarrhea, abdominal pain, indigestion, belching, rash, headache, runny nose, hives, asthma, and swelling of the face or throat. True food allergies are relatively rare in adults, however. Food allergies in infants and young children are much more common, possibly related to the introduction of solid food at too early an age, before the small intestine has had a chance to mature. Some allergies in children are caused by a protein in formula or cow's milk. Many of us know of babies who require a soy-based milk because of milk allergy.

In adults, the symptoms that we loosely ascribe to food allergy may actually be related to disorders of the GI tract, such as IBS, peptic ulcer disease, gastroesophageal reflux disease, or inflammatory bowel disease.

Food Intolerance vs. Allergy

Sometimes what we think of as a food allergy is really a specific food intolerance. That may sound like splitting hairs, but a true allergy is a reaction to food mediated by your body's immune system. It tends to recur quite predictably each time you are exposed to the food, and symptoms usually begin soon after exposure, not several hours later.

A food intolerance, on the other hand, simply means that a particular food causes you some sort of distress. For instance, many people develop diarrhea, cramps, and flatulence after drinking milk. This is not an allergy, but rather an intolerance to milk because of a lack in the body of the enzyme needed to digest the milk sugar lactose. (When these symptoms occur in an infant, however, especially if a rash is also present, a true milk allergy is probably the cause because all infants have plenty of lactase to digest the milk sugar.)

Some patients say they are "allergic" to fatty foods because they have pain after eating foods that contain butter or cream. Most likely, they are suffering from gastroesophageal reflux or possibly from gallstones. Fatty foods tend to relax the LES (lower esophageal sphincter) valve between the stomach and esophagus, creating heartburn. Fatty foods also cause the gallbladder to contract, and if stones are present, pain is the result.

Certain chemicals in foods can also cause reactions similar to allergic responses. Histamine, a chemical released by specialized white cells in the body in response to an allergic reaction, can cause the flushing, itching, and hives characteristic of an allergic reaction. Certain foods, such as fermented cheese, pork sausage, canned tuna, and sardines, also contain histamine, and, for some people, may produce flushing, headaches, and a drop in blood pressure. Phenylethylamine, found in chocolate, aged cheese, and red wine, causes migraine headaches in some people.

Food additives can also cause problems. One common offender is monosodium glutamate, or MSG. A Chinese meal may have up to 2.5 grams of MSG, which can make susceptible individuals dizzy or short of breath. Some people have an asthmatic reaction to sulfites, which are often added to salads and vegetables to preserve a fresh appearance. Tartrazine in yellow food dye No. 5, often added to desserts, snacks, and drinks, can cause asthma, hives, and a runny nose. Nitrates found in smoked meat and cheese can cause GI upset, headache, and hives.

All of these are intolerances; none is a true food allergy. Those foods most likely to cause a true allergic reaction in adults are milk, eggs, peanuts, fish (especially shellfish), and wheat.

Diagnosis of Allergies

Unless the offending food causes a severe and immediate reaction, diagnosis of food allergy can be difficult. It may require a detailed list of foods consumed up to seventy-two hours prior to the reaction, as well as a detailed food record kept for at least two weeks correlating food eaten with symptoms.

If this fails to yield an answer, skin testing can be tried. This is the most reliable way of diagnosing food allergy, but it is by no means perfect. An extract of the food is injected under the skin; development of a red weal and flare means you are allergic to that food. Unfortunately, the test is not always accurate. Not only are there false-positives, but also false-negatives (you have a food allergy, but the skin test is negative).

Sometimes the only way to accurately diagnose a suspected food allergy is to go on an elimination diet. You begin with a diet least likely to cause an allergic reaction—usually devoid of milk, eggs, peanuts, and wheat products. If all goes well, you add specific foods to the diet, one at a time, with wide intervals between each addition, remaining alert for allergic reactions until the culprit is spotted.

Gluten-Sensitive Enteropathy

One food allergy that has been well studied involves gluten, a protein found in wheat. For those who are allergic to it, gluten can cause damage to the cell lining of the small intestine. The result is poor absorption of nutrients, greasy stools, weight loss, and diarrhea. Gluten-sensitive enteropathy is also known as sprue, nontropical sprue, or celiac disease.

Removing gluten from the diet usually leads to prompt healing of the intestinal lining. Symptoms disappear, and the individual gains back the lost weight. Lactose may also need to be temporarily eliminated because the damaged cells temporarily lose their lactase enzyme activity.

Wheat is found in many products including bread, cake, and pasta; gluten is also present in rye and barley and, to a lesser extent, oats. As you can imagine, a gluten-free diet is quite restrictive (see box). Fortunately, sprue is relatively rare, although in some areas of the world, especially Ireland and England, it is more common.

Food List for Gluten-Sensitive Enteropathy

The following is from the Thomas Jefferson University Diet Manual.

	Foods Allowed	*Foods Not Allowed*
Fruits	Plain fresh, frozen, or canned fruits	Fruits prepared with wheat, rye, barley, or oat products
Vegetables and Rice	Plain fresh, frozen, or canned vegetables and rice; homemade creamed vegetables if made with allowed thickeners	Vegetables prepared with wheat, rye, barley, or oats; commercially creamed vegetables
Soups	All soups prepared with allowed ingredients	Soups prepared with wheat, rye, barley, or oats; canned soups (except clear broths); soup mixes; bouillon
Fats	Butter, margarine, lard, vegetable oils, shortenings (with no cereal starch added), cream, bacon fat, pure mayonnaise, homemade salad dressing, gravy, and cream sauces prepared with allowed ingredients	Fats or salad dressings prepared with wheat, rye, barley, or oat products; salad dressing prepared from dry mixes; some brands of commercial mayonnaise
Desserts	Gelatin, homemade cakes, pies, cookies, if prepared with allowed flours; homemade cornstarch, rice, or tapioca puddings prepared with allowed ingredients	Commercial cakes, cookies, pies; certain brands of puddings, ice creams, sherbets, dessert mixes, custard mixes, and icing

	Foods Allowed	*Foods Not Allowed*
Sweets	Jellies; jam; honey; brown and white sugar; molasses; pure fruit syrup; some candy; chocolate; cocoa; coconut	Some commercial cakes
Beverages	Fresh brewed coffee, pure instant coffee or tea, Sanka, herb teas; Kool-Aid, carbonated drinks, fresh or frozen fruit juices, pure wine, brandy, rum, sake, tequila, vodka which does not have grain alcohol added (some "pop" type wines have grain alcohol added)	Postum; instant tea or coffee containing grains; fruit punch powders; beer; alcoholic beverages made from malt or grain, including blended whiskey and liqueurs, such as after-dinner drinks
Miscellaneous	Salt, pure ground peppers, herbs, cloves, ginger, nutmeg, cinnamon, chili powder, dry mustard, A-1 Steak Sauce, cornstarch, food coloring, bicarbonate of soda, cream of tartar, tomato puree, tomato paste, olives, pickles, cider vinegar, wine vinegar, rice vinegar, nuts, peanut butter made without additives	Some curry powders; chili seasoning mix; chutney; gravy extracts; meat sauces; certain brands of mustard, catsup, and horseradish; soy sauce; Worcestershire sauce; chip and dip mixes; apple cider "flavored" vinegar; brewer's yeast; certain brands of peanut butter; products which contain monosodium glutamate (MSG), hydrolyzed vegetable protein, emulsifiers, starch, stabilizers, cereal fillers or thickeners, malt, or vegetable gum

18 *Stress: The Great GI Aggravator*

*T*ake my word for it, if you have a chronic digestive problem, stress is probably playing an active role in making your symptoms worse. Over the years there has been much controversy about whether stress actually causes GI problems. Many dozens of studies have been carried out trying to track down the origins of irritable bowel syndrome (IBS), for example. Some findings support the idea that IBS is psychological in origin. Others find that IBS is a functional disorder aggravated by stress. If you have IBS, or any other digestive disorder, the important thing to know is that excessive stress increases your risk of an attack and is likely to make your symptoms worse. Tension, anxiety, worry, fear—all affect the GI tract. "I feel it in my gut" is one of the most common expressions in the American language, and we aren't joking when we say it. That's exactly where we feel it.

Our awareness of the effects of stress on the digestive tract began some 150 years ago when an American army surgeon was able to observe the stomach of a patient who had been wounded by a gunshot. The wound left a permanently opened passage between the stomach and the surface of the abdomen and gave the surgeon a clear view of the interior of the stomach. For many years afterward the physician made systematic experiments and observations of the digestive process in the stomach. He noted that when the patient was upset the mucosa, the coating that protects the stomach lining, changed color. The secretion of acids also increased and normal stomach contractions slowed down, so there was slower gastric emptying.

In the following decades many studies on both humans and animals were carried out, with similar findings. One famous observation was made by two physicians who were able to closely observe a man named Tom who lived most of his life with a gastrostomy, an artificial passage created between stomach and abdominal surface. For almost twenty years the physicians observed Tom and recorded their findings. When Tom was angry, they could see the stomach mucosa turn red, and acid secretions increased. If the disturbance was prolonged, severe pain was the result. When the patient was frightened, overwhelmed, or depressed, the mucosa turned pale, and the stomach contractions and secretions decreased.

These are only some of the ways our emotions affect our bodies. Our minds and our bodies interact at every level of our existence. Acknowledging the reality of the mind/body connection is essential to understanding overstress, which all of us experience at times, and to managing it, which few of us do very well.

As an example, a neighbor of ours who was plagued with irritable bowel syndrome had been receiving nutrition counseling from Cheryl Clifford Marco, R.D., for several months. She was enormously gratified with the results of changing her diet and took an interest in developing new recipes within the program's guidelines. Alice was one of our biggest success stories. Then one day she came in to see me with a full-blown attack of cramps and diarrhea. "I can't do the diet now," she told me. "I'm in the middle of getting ready for my daughter's wedding. We're expanding the office at work and I've got a big move scheduled. It's all just too much. Can you give me something just to get me through the next few weeks? I'm dying."

Alice was making herself sick. She was so busy at work that she felt anxious whenever she took time to meet with the photographer, the minister, and the caterer for the wedding. She needed to get her house cleaned before her relatives came to stay for the wedding weekend. Her daughter called her every five minutes with questions and new ideas. Alice was waking up several times a night with her mind racing and her heart pounding. At this point, she was having severe attacks of cramps and diarrhea several times a day. As a result, she was too harried to eat regular meals, let alone consider her diet.

Even if she had been sticking to the Self-Help Nutritional Program, however, it's likely that her IBS problems would have intensified. Alice's digestive upsets had always been aggravated by stress. She did not cause her own GI problem; the problem was probably the result of a number of factors, some of which may have been inherited. What Alice was not aware of, though, was how much she could help herself by understanding her body's individual response to stress. Learning to work with stress is a task for everyone, but it's especially important for people with GI problems.

Stress is produced by everyday events as well as by major life crises. It is experienced by everyone, but handled in different ways. Any event that requires us to adapt or change is a "stressor." We all feel best when dealing with just the right number of stressors in our lives. Too few and we become lethargic and bored; too many and we feel overwhelmed.

Stress that is managed well contributes to enhanced thinking and creativity, high energy level, endurance, and improved physical performance. Interest and productivity rise as stressors in our lives increase, up to a certain "just right" level. That perfect level is different for each of us.

Above that level, prolonged or frequent stressors begin to overtax our physical and mental resources, and our effectiveness decreases. Normal stress that continues without intervals for recovery develops into a state of overstress, and major body systems start to show signs of strain.

Overstress contributes to most of the major health problems in our culture, including heart disease, high blood pressure, arthritis, respiratory problems, cancer, and GI disorders. Stress tends to be most dangerous when it is cumulative, although for people with GI problems, even one significant stress event can trigger a reaction within twenty-four hours, if not immediately. When people are constantly faced with unrelenting stress over which they have little control, they simply may not have the biological resources to cope with it. If enough stressful changes are clustered together at one time, they leave people especially vulnerable to illness.

The Fight/Flight Response and GI Disorders

The "fight/flight response" is the body's reaction to any event that seems to demand some immediate action. It is a total psychophysiological response, involving body and mind, in which multiple body systems respond rapidly to the mind's perception of some demand or danger.

Our bodies are primed to take immediate action, to either fight off the threat or to flee it. Changes in the brain, nerves, heart, circulation, muscles, and GI tract are swift and effective. Following such an overwhelming response, recovery time may bring a sense of depletion or weakness ("Let me sit down and catch my breath"). If the body is not allowed adequate recovery time, the bodily systems suffer from overwork.

The GI tract responds at every level and in complex ways during the fight/flight response. Your mouth may become dry during a time of strain. Or your stomach may turn over from sudden anxiety. Or you may have the urge to defecate when facing a fearful event. Emotional states may change the acid balance in the stomach, or alter the normal contractions of the small and large intestines. Diarrhea results when contractions are too fast, and constipation when they are too slow. These stress-related changes can intensify existing GI imbalances, increasing discomfort and triggering attacks of cramps, diarrhea, constipation, or nausea. Perhaps worse is the slow, unseen damage done to the intestines by prolonged stress. When you are tense and unknowingly clench your jaw, your gut clenches, too. Some people sit for hours working under pressure with teeth tightly clenched, never realizing the pressure they're putting on internal organs.

The Three Sources of Stress

Stress overload is not usually the result of a single event, but of an accumulation of events. The degree of stress you feel stems from three different but interrelated sources.

• The Vagaries of Life

Pure external circumstances or life events cause stress. In any large group of people, more health problems are likely to occur for those who have recently experienced the greatest number of significant life events.

In their classic assessment of stress risks, Drs. Thomas H. Holmes and Richard H. Rake, psychiatrists at the University of Washington Medical School, interviewed nearly 400 people of various ages and backgrounds, asking each one to rank a series of life events on a scale of 1 to 100. At the top of everyone's list, with the highest impact of 100 points, was death of a spouse. Divorce ranked second in the line of stress. At the bottom of the list, but still considered stressful, were the Christmas holiday and traffic tickets.

In a later analysis of health statistics the researchers discovered that many widows and widowers died soon after losing the spouse. And divorced people immediately after their divorce were twelve times as likely to become ill as married or single people. A later study of 88 patients with major illnesses found that *93 percent* had suffered an accumulation of stressful life changes.

The critical finding of these investigators was that not only negative events were stress-provoking—all life changes, whether good or bad, created stress. From this work, stress came to be defined not as an event in itself, but as the product of change.

Life events have different stress "weight" for different people, but even welcomed, happy events, like a new and better job, are considered stressors. At any given time in your life, the more changes, challenges, losses, or additions you experience together, the more likely you are to develop stress-related problems. After such an accumulation, an interval of stability is needed for relief and to prevent illness.

Alice, for example, planned to sell her house and find another job right after her daughter's wedding. She would be wiser to put off these plans for a few months to give herself some recovery time from stress overload.

The daily little hassles of life can also be a potent source of stress: the car that won't start, the long line at the supermarket or the bank, the co-worker who interrupts constantly, the irate customer, the repair person who doesn't show up, the delivery van that never arrives.

Little hassles loom large on the stress front because you have so little control over them. They seem to attack in hassle squads, and some days you can handle them better than other days. This lack of control is significant, because frequent hassles define the most stressful jobs—jobs that combine a high degree of pressure with little control over decision-making. The person who works on the assembly line may have more stress than the CEO of a major corporation. Similarly, the average waiter (high pressure, low control) is under more stress than the average bank officer (high pressure, high control), the average forest ranger (low pressure, high control), or the average janitor (low pressure, low control).

In home life as well, the more control you have over your own life events, the less stress you feel. Furthermore, believing that you have control, even when you don't, can relieve stress.

• Your Personality

The second major source of stress is your own personality, including your natural temperament, your outlook on life, and your learned way of responding to events. Some people seem more "stress prone" than others, which may be partly a matter of innate biology. We know now that infants seem to come prepackaged with their own special temperament virtually intact. From birth, infants differ widely in how low-key or active they are, how bold or fearful, how irritable or placid. Life experiences interact with these innate differences to form more or less stable personality traits that persist throughout life.

Dr. Meyer Friedman, co-author with Dr. Ray Rosenman of *Type A Behavior and Your Heart,* first theorized that high-strung, anxious, "stressed out" people were more vulnerable to heart disease and elevated cholesterol levels than more relaxed individuals. In one well-known study, it was found that cholesterol levels of accountants rose significantly during the stressful weeks preceding April 15, and dropped back down to normal after the income tax due date passed. If your personality is bad for your health, however, you can often do something about it by changing your approach to life.

Overstress is often a product of our minds, of what we believe and how we imagine things to be. We live our lives by the rules of our perceptions and beliefs. Feeling overwhelmed, anxious, outraged, dejected, or hopeless is often a result of our reactions to our life circumstances, rather than the circumstance itself. And our reactions may be based on irrational beliefs that can trap us much more completely than external circumstances ever could. We actually have a great deal of power over our lives, because while we cannot always, or even often, control external circumstance, we do have a large measure of control over our own attitudes.

Alice, for instance, believed that it was entirely up to her to plan and carry off a perfect wedding for her daughter. She believed that it was a sign of weakness and incompetence to ask for help. She thought she was more comfortable if she had complete control of everything. No one told her this, but she believed it. It was up to her to please and satisfy everyone. She measured her success by the feedback she got from others. If she did not receive some sign of appreciation for her efforts every day, she felt dejected. The result of all this was that every detail of the wedding exposed Alice to the risk of feeling incompetent, guilty, a failure. Stress reverberated through her whole body, and her digestive system reacted to this emergency situation with alarm.

I have another patient who gets a similar kind of GI reaction, even though his personality is almost the direct opposite of Alice's. By his own admission, Harry is a fairly typical Type A personality—the person with "hurry sickness," a guy who first builds a pressure cooker and then lives in it. Harry runs his own mail order business, strives to achieve higher and higher levels of productivity every day, and tends to measure his worth in the number of sales he can make. Harry is outraged when other people fail to meet his own high standards; his blood pressure rises and his stomach churns with every delay in delivery, every clerical error, and any sign of slackening in his sales force. In fact, Harry is outraged all day long. He gets mad at trains that are late, cash machines that break down, and cars that don't jump forward the second the light turns green. Riding in the backseat of a taxi crawling through a traffic jam, Harry hyperventilated and had to get out and sit on the curb before he could get his breath back. He thought he was having a heart attack. Small wonder that Harry gulps antacids after meals, which he eats at his desk in between phone calls.

Given exactly the same stressful circumstance, Harry and Alice have different emotional responses. When Alice's train is late, she feels anxious and is afraid that she will fail to live up to someone else's expectations. When Harry's train is late, he feels angry and resentful, thinking he has been abused by someone else's incompetence. Alice holds some very harsh and rigid expectations for herself; Harry holds them for others. Both suffer unnecessary levels of stress without ever increasing their own effectiveness. And both experience that stress in their bodies.

These quick-trigger stress responses appear to be relics of childhood, when we first learned that it felt good if our parents approved of us, and bad if they didn't. Or when we thought other people were good if they fulfilled our wishes, and bad if they didn't. Often the response is based on false premises and negative thinking. We learn to react in preprogrammed ways. But just because these are old, old responses, which we have practiced faithfully for years, doesn't mean that we are stuck with them forever. Stress relief means recognizing not only the circumstances that cause us stress, but the *attitudes* that exacerbate them.

• Your Physical Self

The third component that determines how susceptible each of us is to stress overload is our individual physiology. Physiological differences influence how much privacy and quiet we need, how much stimulation, and how much predictability we need in our lives. For instance, some people are bored and depressed if they know exactly what's going to happen every day. Others must have routine to function at their best. Some people function best in a quiet environment; others thrive on having other people around. Each of us has a different pressure/performance curve. Some people can tolerate very high degrees of pressure before reaching peak performance. Others function best under mild or moderate pressure.

I think of one patient of mine, Nancy, who had just received a big promotion that should have pleased her very much. For years she had been in charge of planning and producing print materials for a large corporation. Even though she coordinated her work with that of other divisions in the company, she was largely autonomous in her job. A promotion to the customer service division; a job well within her abilities, brought her more prestige and money, but in the new position she had to supervise ten employees who handled customer complaints. Both employees and customers were often stressed out, presenting Nancy with one "people problem" after another. She began to have frequent attacks of heartburn and burning in the pit of her stomach. She woke up every morning dreading the day ahead. She longed to return to her solitary job in publications, and was convinced that she was weak because she couldn't tolerate the pressure of her new job. "You can't get anywhere in life if you can't take the pressure," she would say to me.

The fact is that stress is often the result of a mismatch between our temperament and the circumstances in which we find ourselves. For many reasons, some of which stem from her basic physiological temperament,

Nancy is someone who does her best in a situation where she functions independently. I don't believe, as she does, that this is weakness of character on her part. In her previous job she had plenty of responsibility and plenty of other kinds of pressure that she handled well. The answer for Nancy may be to aim for a career move that allows her to function at her own personal peak performance.

A person's basic physiology also influences the way the body expresses stress overload. Some people have tension headaches; others have ulcer attacks. Some can't sleep at night; others have stomach cramps. Different people express stress in different ways. Nausea, heartburn, diarrhea, cramping, or constipation can all be responses to stressful situations.

An emotional response to overstress may also be rooted in physiology. You may have observed some people become very cool when stress seems overwhelming. Whether we become keyed up or detached, combative or timid, passive or hyperactive under stress may be tendencies built into our basic temperaments.

For example, people who often feel anxious or depressed may be victims of their biochemistry as well as their outlook on the world. When anxiety and depression appear to be important components of GI problems, psychotherapy may help. In a study of two groups of patients with irritable bowel syndrome, those who received psychotherapy improved both psychologically and physically, while the symptoms of those who received routine medical treatment either stayed the same or got worse. Because of the powerful link between body and mind, what we consider purely psychological realities can have real and measurable influences on the physical self.

Ways to Relieve Stress

Only in recent years have we been able to scientifically measure some of the effects of stress on our bodies and discover antidotes to its insidious work. Fortunately, the methodical study of stress overload has led to numerous successful ways to relieve damaging levels of stress. Here are some of the techniques that experts in stress reduction suggest:

- Reduce the amount of pressure in your external world. Try to identify the elements of a given situation that cause you to feel stressed. Then brainstorm a list of actions that you might take to either decrease the pressure or increase your sense of control. In every circumstance or life event there is always at least some small change you can make that will ease the stress for you.

Are You Stressed Out?

One of the problems with stress is that its effects are usually invisible—you can't see it, and you can't see what it's doing to your body until you become sick. And many of us don't know when we've had too much. I've noticed that people who are overstressed tend to lose touch with their bodies because one common reaction to stress is to become desensitized. Some physical signs of overstress are:

Digestive upsets of all kinds

Hair loss

Unexplained fatigue

Chronic body aches in the morning

Sleeplessness

Heart palpitations

Dizziness

Continuous sighing

Loss of appetite

Difficulty swallowing

Frequent urination

Rashes and itching

Some emotional signs of stress are:

Hair-trigger temper

Loss of concentration

Memory loss

Crying

• Is it lack of time or a too-tight deadline that is stressing you out? Can you manage your time differently in some way? Try saying no to new commitments until you feel less pressured.

• Are you overwhelmed by work and responsibilities? Try breaking down a big task into small steps, and take them one by one.

• Is an awkward or uncomfortable working or living space creating pressure for you? Can you change your physical environment?

• Is money a constant worry? Should you attend a seminar or course in personal financial management?

• When faced with a high-stress problem, remember to ask yourself, "Whose problem is this?" If the answer is that it isn't yours, you may not have to solve it.

• In reading this chapter you have probably thought of hassles and stresses in your own life. Look back on some unwelcome event in your life, the memory of which still causes you anxiety and unhappiness—and find some way in which your life has been enriched because of it.

• Tackle harmful habits that undermine your health, especially smoking, drug use, alcohol abuse, and binge-starve patterns of eating. It's usually best to work on these one at a time, and to get professional help if you need it.

• Try to recognize when you are being negative and self-defeating.

• If stress and tension are chronic in your life, don't hesitate to seek professional counseling or therapy. It often takes someone else to help us identify the stress points and see a way out.

• All experts in stress relief advise that we should try for healthy balances in our lives. What they mean by this is balancing effort with rest, work with leisure, structured with unstructured time. Look for ways to restore the harmony between your body and mind.

• Take the time to pay attention to the quality of your life—with particular attention to nutrition and exercise. People who exercise regularly deal better with stress. They also sleep better and manage weight control better. Plan time for relaxation and pleasure, and stick to it. Some suggestions are a daily walk or an afternoon nap, daily relaxation exercises, regular workouts, and balanced, well-timed meals. All these activities can add harmony to life and keep moods on a more even keel.

Meditation and Relaxation Techniques

Relaxation can mean many things—yoga, meditation, deep breathing, or other relaxation methods. It can mean taking a long walk or counting backward from one hundred. Whatever form they come in, relaxation techniques can provide relief from stress by lowering blood pressure and heart rate. They also appear to reduce stimulation of gastric secretion and in general relax the gut.

In his landmark work. *The Relaxation Response,* Dr. Herbert Benson proved that meditation could help people who had high blood pressure because it produced a physiological response directly the opposite of "fight or flight." Meditating and other relaxation responses have been shown to decrease blood lactate, a substance strongly linked to anxiety. During the first ten minutes of meditation, blood lactate levels drop rapidly and remain extremely low throughout meditation. This effect may block the stress mechanism that some researchers believe to cause many different ailments.

Relaxation techniques have also been shown to help regulate glucose in some people with adult-onset diabetes, to open constricted air passages in those with chronic, nonseasonal asthma of the upper airways, and to lower elevated cholesterol levels.

Regular exercise workouts also provide great release from stress. The endorphins released into the bloodstream during strenuous exercise create an almost palpable sense of well-being.

The trick to stress relief is to find a relaxation technique that's right for you and fits into your lifestyle.

PART THREE

Quick Fixes with OTC Products

*E*veryone and anyone can have a sudden GI problem—from simple indigestion to diarrhea and vomiting. People who have chronic GI problems may have a sudden flare-up of their symptoms even when they follow the Self-Help Nutritional Program. So it's good to know how to help yourself get immediate relief from a sudden attack by using over-the-counter (OTC) drugs.

Unfortunately, many of the traditional remedies believed to aid digestive upsets may actually make things worse for GI patients. For example, swallowing a bubbling, aspirin-containing Alka-Seltzer for an upset stomach can irritate the stomach lining and make ulcer patients suffer.

Using OTC Products

OTC drugs, like prescriptions drugs, have benefits as well as potential problems. OTC drugs are easy to purchase and, when used appropriately, can often provide some relief of GI problems. Drugs often become OTC by lowering the dose of a prescription drug, which usually makes them safer, but also can make them weaker and less effective. There are many OTC drugs on the market that either have no efficacy in treating a particular disease or are labeled "possibly effective."

Unless an OTC drug has been recommended by your physician, it's up to you to diagnose your problem correctly and then choose the best OTC drug to treat it. There is a lot of room for error in this method, and OTC drugs can cause problems. Even though weaker than prescription drugs, OTC remedies can still have side effects, and may even lead to life-threatening complications in people with GI problems. For instance, aspirin and nonsteriodal and inflammatory drugs (NSAIDs) like ibuprofen can cause serious ulceration of the stomach lining and lead to gastrointestinal bleeding.

All in all, self-diagnosis and drugs of any kind make a bad combination. If you have GI symptoms you should always be evaluated by a physician. Based on the diagnosis, your physician can advise you about which OTC drugs will be most helpful for you if you need them.

That said, many people are still going to purchase OTC medications to relieve symptoms. Here is some information about common OTC medicines and their effect on GI disorders.

Commonly Used OTC Remedies

• Antacids

Antacids, commonly used to help relieve heartburn, are one of the most widely used OTC drugs on the market. Antacids work by neutralizing stomach acid, and antacids that contain simethicone can also relieve gas pains.

Antacids come in tablet or liquid form. We used to recommend liquid over tablets because liquids had a better neutralizing capacity, but newer tablet formulations are nearly equivalent in their capacity to neutralize acids, so the two preparations can be used almost interchangeably.

All antacids work the same way, but different products contain different ingredients. Both tablets and liquids contain either magnesium, aluminum, calcium, or a combination. There can be some side effects when these products are used on a regular basis.

Magnesium-containing antacids (e.g., Maalox or Mylanta) taken frequently may cause diarrhea. Those containing aluminum, such as ALternaGEL, may cause constipation. I usually recommend that my patients who take antacids regularly alternate one with another to offset the potential side effects of each.

Theoretically, calcium-containing antacids have the potential to stimulate more acid secretion over the long run. But women who would like extra calcium to help prevent osteoporosis might prefer calcium-containing antacids like Tums or Titralac. The best advice is to experiment with various products and discover which ones seem to work best for you without producing side effects.

Antacids come in regular strength and extra strength. Extra-strength preparations should be used only when the recommended dosage of a regular antacid does not fully control symptoms. The equivalent volume of an extra-strength preparation will produce a greater incidence of side effects such as diarrhea.

Some brands of antacids that carry the suffix "plus" or use the word "gas"—for example, Mylanta Gas—contain simethicone, which absorbs gas. People who suffer from gas pain are often helped by simethicone-containing antacids. Simethicone is also available without an antacid (Mylicon or Gas X) for people who suffer from gas but not acid-related problems. Gaviscon contains alginic acid, which foams up when exposed to acid. With a person in the erect position, the foam stays in the upper stomach and acts as a barrier to acid reflux.

People who suffer from intermittent heartburn take antacids on an as-needed basis. This is a good idea if your heartburn is usually well managed on the Self-Help Nutritional Program but you still experience occasional heartburn. In general, full doses of antacids should not be taken for more than two weeks without your physician's advice. People who have any kind of kidney disease should not take antacids except under a doctor's supervision.

If you are using antacids to ward off heartburn or dyspepsia, the best time to take the drug is one hour after meals and at bedtime. Antacids should not be taken at the same time as other medications because they may alter the body's ability to absorb certain drugs.

If you use antacids to supplement other forms of ulcer therapy, take them only when you need pain relief.

• Pepto-Bismol

One of the most versatile of all OTC products, Pepto-Bismol can soothe heartburn and indigestion as well as help settle an upset stomach and ease nausea. It is widely used to control routine diarrhea, as well as traveler's diarrhea, and is part of the standard triple therapy regimen to treat *Helicobacter pylori* (see chapter 6). The active ingredient in Pepto-Bismol is bismuth subsalicylate, which suppresses the growth of bacteria, particularly *H. plyori,* often found in the stomach in patients with ulcers. Pepto-Bismol contains aspirin and can cause ringing in the ears if you take the medication frequently.

• Pain Relievers

Even though many GI diseases cause pain, pain relief is often achieved without traditional painkillers. For example, antacids relieve the pain of heartburn and ulcers better than painkillers. An antispasmodic such as

Bentyl or Levsin, both prescription drugs, probably works better than aspirin or acetaminophen for the pain associated with attacks of IBS.

However, people with GI conditions occasionally suffer from other kinds of pain—headaches, joint pains, muscle aches—that are best helped by traditional painkillers. What kind of painkiller can you use that won't make your GI problem worse?

Two common painkillers are aspirin and nonsteriodal anti-inflammatory drugs (NSAIDs) such as ibuprofen, found in Advil, Nuprin, and several prescription drugs. Both aspirin and NSAIDs block the production of prostaglandin—the hormone that protects the stomach lining—and ulcers may form. As a result, people who already have upper GI problems, specifically ulcers, are at even higher risk of suffering complications. Other people at risk are those over sixty years of age, women, those taking steroids plus NSAIDs, smokers, and those with rheumatioid arthritis. Even buffered or enteric-coated products do not fully protect the stomach. So if you have upper GI problems, you should avoid aspirin and NSAIDs, if possible.

One alternative is acetaminophen (Tylenol), a painkiller that does not irritate the stomach lining. Even acetaminophen has drawbacks if overused, however. In massive doses it can cause serious liver damage. High but conventional doses taken over a long period of time can also damage the liver if you also consume excessive amounts of alcohol. The damaging effects of Tylenol and alcohol appear to be cumulative, so if you take Tylenol on a regular basis it's important not to drink alcohol. As long as you avoid alcohol and take no more than 4 grams of Tylenol a day, it's unlikely that you will suffer any kind of liver damage (two extra-strength Tylenol equal 1 gram).

One problem is that Tylenol is not anti-inflammatory, and while people do take if for arthritis, it is not as effective as aspirin or prescription-strength NSAIDs. If you have an upper GI problem and you need aspirin or NSAIDs for arthritis, ask your physician about a drug called misoprostol (Cytotec). Standard ulcer drugs like Zantac, Tagamet, Pepcid, Axid, and Carafate offer the stomach little or no protection from aspirin and NSAIDs but do protect the duodenum. The proton pump inhibitors (Prilosec, Prevacid, Aciphex, Protonix, and Nexium) protect the stomach and duodenum from NSAID-induced ulcers but except for Prevacid are not yet approved by the FDA for this indication. Arthritis patients with a history of NSAID-induced ulcer are now able to use the selective COX-2 inhibitors Celebrex, Bextra, and Mobic. However, recent concern about COX-2 inhibitors increasing the risk of heart attack and stroke have limited their use. In the case of Vioxx, the drug was withdrawn from the market. (See chapter 6 for more information on NSAID-induced ulcers.)

Quick Fixes with OTC Products

For more information on antacids, Pepto-Bismol, laxatives, antidiarrheals, hemorrhoid products, and other OTC drugs, see the table below.

Before using any OTC or prescription medication, read the instructions and package insert carefully. The dosage recommendations given here are typical for the average adult. Pregnant women should not use any medication without the advice of their physician. The following is only a partial list of the OTC drugs useful in treating gastrointestinal disorders. Complete information can be found in the *Physicians' Desk Reference for Nonprescription Drugs* (Montvale, N.J.: Medical Economics Company).

Symptom	OTC Remedy	Dosage
Gas pain (without heartburn)	Gas-X Extra-strength Gas-X	*Chewable tablets* Chew thoroughly and swallow 1–2 tablets as needed after meals or at bedtime not to exceed 6 Gas-X chewable tablets or 4 Extra-strength Gas-X chewable tablets in 24 hrs.
		Extra-strength Soft Gel Tablet Swallow with water, 1 or 2 soft gels as needed after meals or at bedtime
		Extra-strength Gas-X Liquid 2–4 tsp. as needed after meals or at bedtime, not to exceed 10 tsp. in 24 hrs.
	Extra-strength Phazyme-125	1–2 soft gels as needed after meals, not to exceed 4 per day
	Maximum-strength Gas Aid Soft Gels	1–2 soft gels as needed after meals and at bedtime Do not exceed more than 4 soft gels per day
Upper abdominal gas pain (with heartburn)	Maalox Antacid/ Antigas	2–4 tsp. or chewable tablets after meals and at bedtime
	Mylanta Gas	1–2 chewable tablets or soft gels as needed after meals and at bedtime, not to exceed 4 tablets per day

Symptom	OTC Remedy	Dosage	
Heartburn not relieved with regular antacids	Extra-strength Mylanta	*For frequent episodes* 2–4 tsp. liquid; 2–4 chewable ultra tablets or gelcaps between meals and at bedtime Do not take more than 10 tablets or 12 gelcaps in a 24 hr. period	
	Maalox Max Maximum-strength Antacid/Antigas	*As needed for occasional episodes* 2–4 tsp. 4 times a day, not to exceed 12 tsp. in 24 hrs. or 1–2 chewable quick-dissolving tablets, not to exceed 8 in a 24 hr. period	
Heartburn	H$_2$ blockers	*Heartburn Prevention*	*Heartburn Treatment*
	Tagamet HB 200	200 mg tablet, $\frac{1}{2}$ hr. before a meal	1 tablet up to twice daily
	Pepcid AC	10 mg tablet, 1 hr. before a meal	1 tablet up to twice daily
	Maximum-strength Pepcid AC	20 mg tablet 1 hr. before a meal or as needed	1 tablet up to twice daily
	Pepcid Complete		1 tablet up to twice daily
	Zantac 75	Not indicated	1 tablet up to twice daily
	Axid AR	75 mg $\frac{1}{2}$–1 hr. before a meal	1 tablet up to twice daily
Nausea	Emetrol	1–2 tbsp. Every 15 min. until distress subsides	
	Pepto-Bismol	2 tbsp. or tablets every $\frac{1}{2}$–1 hr., if needed, not to exceed 8 doses in 24 hrs. (4 doses if using maximum-strength formulation)	

Symptom	OTC Remedy	Dosage
	Dramamine or Bonine	1–2 tablets every 4–6 hrs., not to exceed 8 tablets in 24 hrs.
Traveler's diarrhea, *Treatment*	Pepto-Bismol	2 tablets or 2 tbsp. liquid, 6 times a day
Traveler's diarrhea, *Prevention*	Pepto-Bismol	2 tablets, 4 times a day, beginning 24 hrs. before trip, continuing until 2 days after return, not to exceed 21 days.
Constipation	Metamucil	1 tsp. or tbsp. depending on formulation in 8 oz. water 1 to 3 times a day as needed
	FiberCon	2 capsules up to 4 a day, take each dose with 8 oz. of water
	Phillips' Milk of Magnesia	2–4 tbsp. at bedtime or at rising, followed by 8 oz. of liquid
	Colace (stool softener)	1 100 mg capsule twice a day
	Perdiem	1–2 tsp. swallowed with 8 oz. water, 1–2 times a day
	Citrucil	1 tbsp. with 8 oz. cold water up to 3 times a day
IBS		
Diarrhea	Pepto-Bismol	2 tbsp. or tablets every $\frac{1}{2}$–1 hr, if needed, to a max. of 8 doses in 24 hrs. (4 doses using maximum-strength formulation)
	Imodium A.D.	4 tsp. or 2 caplets after first loose BM. If needed take 2 tsp. or 1 caplet after each subsequent BM. Do not exceed 8 tsp. or 4 caplets per day
	Kaopectate	2 tbsp. or caplets after each loose BM, not to exceed 12 tbsp. or 12 caplets in 24 hrs.

Symptom	OTC Remedy	Dosage
Cramps	Donnagel	2 tbsp. or 2 chewable tablets after each BM, not to exceed 7 doses in 24 hrs.
Lower abdominal gas pain/flatulence	Beano	5 drops per food serving containing beans or 3 tablets per meal
	Regular-strength Lactacid (mild intolerance)	3 caplets with first bite of dairy food (never take more than 6 caplets of original-strength at a time)
Hemorrhoids	Anusol HC-1	1 suppository, rectally, up to 3–4 times daily
	Preparation H	Apply ointment, cream, or rectal suppository up to 4 times a day
	Nupercainal	Apply ointment, cream, or rectal suppository 3–4 times a day
	Tucks	Use up to 6 times daily or after each BM

PART FOUR

Dietary Supplements, Herbs, and Integrative Health: Beyond the Basics

—Liz Zorzanello Emery, M.S., R.D., C.N.S.D., L.D.N.

*I*f you've been searching for an alternative remedy for your gastrointestinal symptoms, you're not alone. Many people who suffer from gastrointestinal problems have turned to dietary supplements, herbs, and other treatments to gain relief from their discomfort. Each year, Americans spend millions of dollars seeking help beyond the boundaries of traditional medical care. This chapter attempts to sort through the ever-growing sea of information on the use of alternative treatments for gastrointestinal health. Is it safe to self-medicate? Can I trust what the label says? Should I be concerned about herb-drug interactions? Issues inherent to the use of supplements and complementary treatments will be outlined here.

Tinctures, Teas, Potions, and Pills: Safety and Efficacy Issues

One of the driving forces behind the growing use of dietary supplements and herbs has been the basic law of supply and demand. The Dietary Supplement Health and Education Act, or DSHEA, passed in 1994, has had a major impact on our use of supplements by fueling product development in the supplement industry. Prior to its passage, only one-third of the public had used dietary supplements, and sales were estimated at $8.8 billion dollars per year. Today, with the increased availability of products and heightened interest in self-help, at least 80 percent of Americans have used or are using these supplements, with sales reaching $15.7 billion in the year 2000.

According to DSHEA, dietary supplements are defined as products intended to supplement the diet that contain one or more of the following: a vitamin, a mineral, an herb or botanical, or an amino acid. They are intended to be taken in pill, capsule, tablet, or liquid form. They are considered neither foods nor medicines, and are regulated differently from either. Supplements that you buy from the drugstore, grocery store, or Internet must adhere to certain labeling guidelines but do not have to be proven to be safe or effective prior to marketing. A supplement can carry a "structure-function claim," such as "supports gastrointestinal health," but does not have to undergo clinical trials to prove that it works. Thus, the buyer must beware. Educating yourself to be a savvy consumer is essential.

Pre-, Pro-, and Synbiotics: The World of Friendly Bacteria

One of the fastest growing categories for supplements related to gastrointestinal health is that of prebiotics, probiotics, and synbiotics. Probiotics are otherwise known as the "friendly bacteria" that live in our gastrointestinal tract and help to maintain the proper internal environment. Prebiotics are the fuels that help the probiotic organisms to flourish. Synbiotics is a relatively new term that refers to a combination of pre- and pro- biotics intended to maximize microfloral balance.

The use of microorganisms in foods and medicine has a long history, dating back to biblical times. Use of fermented foods such as kefir and yogurt for medicinal purposes, and the use of fermentation for food preservation spans thousands of years and many world cultures. We now know that our bodies carry whole colonies of "friendly bacteria" and maintain a delicate equilibrium between host and microorganisms. From birth, a baby's gastrointestinal tract becomes colonized with bacteria that help its immune and digestive systems to develop normally. As adults, we carry such a large number of live microorganisms within our bodies that the number of microscopic bacterial cells actually exceeds the number of human cells present! It is no wonder that any upset to this balance can affect us adversely. Increased use of antibiotics, improved sanitation and hygiene, and advances in vaccinations have all changed the character of bacterial challenges that we face on a daily basis. These factors have the potential to alter the microbial balance in our intestines. Furthermore, gastrointestinal illnesses can render our bodies more susceptible to alterations in the normal intestinal microflora. Under some circumstances, supplemental use of probiotic organisms has been shown to be beneficial in restoring health.

Several types of probiotic bacteria have been studied, most notably various strains of *Lactobacillus* and *Bifidobacterium*. Research-grade preparations that are not yet available to consumers have been used in some of these studies. Overall, emerging data supports the use of probiotics in maintaining remission in both pouchitis and Crohn's disease; data for ulcerative colits is suggestive but not as clear. Probiotics may also be useful in preventing antibiotic-related diarrhea and diarrhea caused by rotavirus.

Pouchitis may occur after a surgical procedure known as an ileal-anal anastomosis has been performed for ulcerative colitis. Inflammation of the pouch is treated with antibiotics, but often recurs. Several studies have demonstrated prolonged remission in those patients given a mixture including several strains of *Lactobacillus* and *Bifidobacterium I* (use of VSL#3), or a combination of the probiotic *Lactobacillus GG* with the prebiotic fructooligosaccharide. In Crohn's disease, preliminary data suggests that particular probiotics, including the yeast *S. boulardii* and a probiotic mixture including several strains of *Lactobacillus* and *Bifidobacterium*, may be beneficial in reducing disease activity. In one study from the Mayo Clinic, VSL#3 was shown to help abdominal bloating in patients with diarrhea-predominant irritable bowel syndrome.

The ideal probiotic is one that gives sufficient quantities of viable organisms that can survive the acidic environment of the stomach and go on to colonize the large intestine. Products should contain at least 1 billion live organisms per daily dose. The probiotic VSL#3 contains 450 billion bacteria per dose, which may explain why it seems to work so well. In a January 2003 study by ConsumerLab.com, one-third of probiotic products tested contained less than 1 percent of the expected dose of live bacteria. If you want to purchase probiotics, ask for proof that the product contains live bacteria.

Most commercially available yogurts and acidophilus milk contain relatively small but potentially helpful amounts of live cultures. Fermented soy products such as miso and tempeh can provide minor amounts as well.

Although the data is promising that probiotics can reduce intestinal inflammation, we still do not know with certainty which organisms should be used, what the optimal dose is, or how long they need to be taken. Probiotics are generally thought to be safe, but should be used with caution in persons who are immuno-suppressed. No data exists on use during pregnancy or lactation.

A Sea of Hope

Fish oil supplements have been investigated over the last decade, and although not all researchers agree, many support the use of fish oils for inflammatory bowel diseases like Crohn's disease and ulcerative colitis. Fish oils contain potent Omega-3 fatty acids that act as anti-inflammatory agents

Sample Probiotic Formulations

Product Name	Bacteria Strains*	Live Organisms per Serving*	Comments
Actimel®	S. thermophilus L. bulgaricus L. casei	10 billion	A cultured dairy drink available in selected markets in the U.S.
Culturelle®	L rhamnosus GG (Lactobacillus GG)	10 billion	Also contains inulin, a prebiotic ingredient
Nature Made® Acidophilus	L. acidophilus	1 billion	Contains 500 million cells per tablet
Puritan's Pride® Acidophilus	L. acidophilus, L. bifidus, L. rhamnosus	2.4–3 billion	Also available with pectin, a soluble fiber
Stonyfield Farms yogurt	L. bulgaricus S. thermophilus L. acidophilus L. bifidus L. casei L. reuteri	Proprietary information, not available from manufacturer	This yogurt contains added probiotics
VSL#3™	L. acidophilus L. plantarum L. casei L. bulgaricus B. breve B. longum B. infantis S. salivaris	450 billion	High potency

* According to manufacturer

in the body. They have been shown to reduce disease activity and the need for anti-inflammatory medications in ulcerative colitis and to help prevent relapse in Crohn's disease.

If you want to use fish oil, look for an enteric-coated brand. The coating prevents the fish oil from dissolving in the stomach, and minimizes one of the more unpleasant side effects of this supplement, "fish burps." Fish oil can thin the blood, so if you are taking any blood thinners such as Warfarin, make sure that you discuss the fish oil with your doctor beforehand. Because of their tendency to thin the blood, fish oils should be discontinued one week to ten days prior to surgery, endoscopy, or colonoscopy. Diabetics who take fish oil should watch for any change in their blood glucose levels and notify their doctors. Children, pregnant women, and nursing mothers should take fish oils only if monitored by a physician.

Walking Through the Garden of Herbs

A variety of herbs have been used to promote gastrointestinal health. Herbs have been used for centuries as medicines, and, indeed, many of our modern-day medicines, such as the heart medication Digitalis and the chemotherapy drug Taxol®, were originally derived from plants. Plants contain many bioactive substances that have the potential to alter bodily processes. In most cases, the active constituents of plants are not single components, but combinations of natural elements that work synergistically as Mother Nature packaged them together. Therefore, many herbalists recommend using products derived from whole leaves, in the form of tinctures, freeze-dried extracts, and teas. Tinctures are made from alcohol extraction, and teas are made from hot-water extraction. To prepare an herbal tea, combine two tablespoons of fresh herb with eight ounces of freshly boiled water in a glass or china cup. Cover to prevent evaporation of essential oils, and steep for five to ten minutes. Pills made from standardized extracts may be useful but may not contain all of the active components of a whole plant.

Scientific evidence supporting the use of herbs is limited, in large part because there is little financial incentive to study natural substances. In the past few years we have seen a proliferation of professional literature addressing the medical use of herbs. We have confirmation that some herbs do indeed act like medicines in the body, and we have also learned that some herbs can interact with prescription medications. St. John's Wort, considered useful for mild to moderate depression, speeds up the body's metabolism of many drugs, thus lowering their effectiveness. St. John's Wort can reduce blood levels of birth control pills, drugs used after organ transplant, and drugs used to treat HIV infection. Garlic, ginkgo, and ginger can interfere with blood clotting. They can increase the effect of blood thinners, and should be discontinued at least one week before surgery, endoscopy, or colonoscopy. Valerian can potentiate the effects of anesthesia and should also be discontinued several days prior to procedures.

Herbs that may help relieve gastrointestinal distress are listed in the chart that follows. Herbs generally recommended for gastrointestinal conditions include carminatives such as peppermint, chamomile, and lemon balm. Carminatives help to calm the muscles of the digestive tract and aid in expelling gas. Many carminatives are also purported to ease localized inflammation and act as anti-microbials. For gastrointestinal conditions, the local effects of the herbs on the actual tissue of the GI tract are thought to be as beneficial as possible systemic effects of the herbs. Nervine herbs such as chamomile and valerian can help to alleviate stress and reduce muscle spasms. In addition to their value when taken orally, decoctions of these herbs can be added to a relaxing warm bath, which can soothe your symptoms as well.

Mind over Matter?

We could all use a little escape from the pressures of everyday life now and then. In today's fast-paced world, stress often correlates with physical symptoms. The good news on this topic is that there is real scientific evidence that methods such as relaxation, hypnotherapy, counseling, and behavior therapy can help people gain the respite they deserve from their GI symptoms.

The brain talks to the body through nerve impulses, hormones, and chemicals called neuropeptides. Muscle activity of the gut can be altered by stress signals coming from the brain. Alleviating stress can normalize the portion of our gastrointestinal function that relies on the brain.

Basic techniques such as counseling, guided imagery, and progressive relaxation can be helpful in coping with stress. Progressive relaxation can be done with a professional, with the help of a guided audiotape, or, with training, on your own. Progressive relaxation involves relaxing the muscles in your body, one by one. Start by tightening the muscles of your toes, then concentrate on releasing all of your tension. Next, tighten your feet, release, and move up your body until you are fully relaxed. Before you stand up, take a few deep breaths and visualize yourself feeling healthy and energized. Regular use of these techniques can help you to feel better all over. Several scientific studies have documented significant improvement in symptoms, including abdominal pain, bowel dysfunction, anxiety, and depression with counseling, psychotherapy, stress management, and relaxation therapy. Quality of life has also been shown to improve with these therapies.

Recently, hypnosis has come into the limelight for persons suffering from irritable bowel syndrome (IBS). Hypnotherapy is performed by a trained professional, who helps you to enter a relaxed state and then guides you to imagine your intestinal muscles becoming smooth and calm. In a six-year study recently completed in the U.K. IBS patients who had undergone a 12-week gut-targeted hypnotherapy program reported improvement in symptoms, a decrease in anxiety and depression, and an improved quality of life. Most important, this study found that improvements were sustained over several years.

Although acupuncture has been shown to give relief from some forms of chronic pain, results evaluating acupuncture for use in gastrointestinal conditions have been less convincing. Still, some people do use acupuncture to help relax muscle spasms and normalize bowel function. If you decide to try acupuncture, look for a practitioner who is licensed and experienced.

Alternative or Complementary?

The most important thing to remember if you try any non-traditional treatments is that you should not venture out alone. Don't delay medical evaluation for severe pain or a change in your condition. Do tell your physician about herbs and supplements that you are taking. It is important to know about any substances that could interfere with your prescription medications or procedures. "Natural" does not always mean "safe," and herbal products and dietary supplements can have side effects. Nontraditional treatments, when they are used, should be integrated into your medical care rather than viewed as an alternative.

Selected Herbs for Gastrointestinal Health

Herb	Action	Suggested Use	Contraindications and Side Effects
Peppermint (*Mentha piperita*)	Calms smooth muscles of the digestive tract; relieves gas, stimulates bile flow; antibacterial	As hot tea used in moderation, or 0.6 ml essential oil in enteric-coated form, taken in divided doses	Avoid use with obstruction of gall bladder or gallstones; non-enteric-coated form can cause heartburn
Chamomile (*Matricaria recututa*)	Antispasmodic, antibacterial, anti-inflammatory; relieves gas	As hot tea used in moderation, or 10–15 grams daily, or per package directions	Possible allergic reactions
Lemon Balm (*Melissa officinalis*)	Relieves gas; mild sedative	As hot tea used in moderation, or 1.5–4.5 grams daily	None known
Valerian (*Valeriana officinalis*)	Sedative, relieves smooth-muscle spasms and relaxes muscles	As hot tea, one cup to several cups daily, or per package directions	Avoid taking with sedative and anti-seizure medications; avoid taking with alcohol. Do not mix with the herb skull-cap. May interact with anesthesia, so discontinue at least 1 week before surgery
Ginger (*Zingiber officinale*)	Anti-emetic	For nausea, 2–4 grams of fresh root daily in tea, or 1.5–3.0 mls tincture daily	Avoid use with obstruction of gallbladder or gallstones; can prolong blood clotting time; use with care in combination with blood thinners and discontinue at least one week before surgery

PART FIVE

The Self-Help Nutritional Program: The Two-Week Master Program

*T*he Self-Help Nutritional Program for GI disorders uses state-of-the-art information to create a nutritional plan that can be used by almost everyone with GI problems.* It brings together in one program all the knowledge gained in the past two decades about how food behaves and reacts within the gastrointestinal tract.

The Two-Week Master Program

In a standard American diet, 35 to 45 percent of the daily calories come from fat; 12 to 20 percent from protein; and 40 to 50 percent from carbohydrates. In the Two-Week Master Program the goal is to shift the emphasis of your diet so that less than 30 percent of daily calories come from fat; 12 to 20 percent come from protein; and 55 to 60 percent or more come from carbohydrates.

The Two-Week Master Program will help you choose foods that offer good nutritional value for the calories, while steering clear of the foods that create problems for you.

Food has seven constituents: proteins, fats, carbohydrates, fiber, water, vitamins, and minerals. The program contains all seven constituents in the amounts necessary for good health. At the same time it provides them in a balance that the digestive tract can handle without stress.

In my years of working with patients suffering from GI problems of all kinds, and also with overweight patients, I've learned a great deal about what *doesn't* work as far as diets are concerned. My patients have told me

*The program is not recommended for people with acute diverticulitis or moderate to severe inflammatory bowel disease (Crohn's disease, ulcerative colitis) unless directed by a physician.

time and again that they are discouraged by complicated diets. They don't want to look up calories or memorize food exchanges. And they don't want to face the same boring food day after day.

With that in mind, and with the help of Cheryl Clifford Marco, R.D., I've tried to make the Master Program as simple as possible and as delicious as possible. By offering varied menus, the program avoids the spartan and monotonous fare that has characterized nutritional treatment of GI disorders in the past. These menus will quickly disprove the idea that foods easy on your digestive system must necessarily be bland and boring. If you cannot imagine life without Mexican food or other colorful, entertaining menus, all is not lost. The best part of this program is that it's made up of foods that everyone else eats. In the surprised words of one of my patients, "I'm finally eating real food again!"

The Two-Week Master Program uses many of the recipes in this book, as well as everyday foods that you are probably accustomed to eating. It may seem that you will have to learn a lot of new recipes, but most of them are simple and quick, easy to learn and easy to remember. A little organized shopping will put you in a position to prepare all of them.

• About the Recipes

The recipes in the last section of this book have been designed for quick and easy meal preparation. With a little practice you will be able to prepare them automatically without even looking at the book. To ensure good results, every recipe has been carefully kitchen-tested and retested several times during development.

On many days, you will eat animal protein only once, and the portions are smaller than what you are probably accustomed to. Be assured that your diet is nutritionally balanced and that you are getting more than enough protein on any given day.

To help you calculate, every recipe contains the following nutritional information.

Calories Per Serving.   Most recipes are for four servings, but all indicate their yield.

Percent of Carbohydrate.   This is the percentage of calories derived from carbohydrate. Overall, the meal plans are designed to be high in carbohydrate: 55 to 60 percent of your total daily calorie intake should be derived from carbohydrate. Some recipes are almost all carbohydrate, although others are fairly low.

Percent of Protein.   This is the percentage of calories derived from protein. About 12 to 15 percent of your total daily calories should be derived from protein. Although this is probably less animal protein than you are accustomed to eating, it is more than enough for the average man or woman.

Percent of Fat.   This is the percentage of calories derived from fat. Less than 30 percent of calories in the diet are derived from fat. Although the fat content of the diet is low overall, some individual recipes are higher than others. A good rule of thumb when purchasing prepared foods is to buy products with no more than 3 grams of fat per 100 calories.

Grams of Fat.   This is the total grams of fat per serving. There are 9 calories in 1 gram of fat. Some recipes appear to have a high percentage of fat calories, but because total calories are so low, the grams of fat are also quite low. This is particularly true of the salad recipes, which are predominantly low-cal vegetables, but have some oil or mayonnaise in their dressings.

Grams of Fiber.   This is the total grams of dietary fiber per serving. It is recommended that 20 to 30 grams of fiber be consumed daily.

• How Many Meals a Day?

Three standard meals a day is the way to go for most people with GI disorders. However, certain conditions may benefit from several smaller meals each day.

People who have had stomach surgery for peptic ulcer disease may find that since they no longer have a pyloric sphincter, which controls the amount of food from the stomach that enters the small intestine, a large volume of food is deposited into the small intestines at once. This "dumping syndrome" can cause several problems, including diarrhea, too rapid absorption of glucose, excessive insulin release, and low blood sugar a few hours after the meal. Some people with long-standing diabetes fill up easily and are unable to eat large meals. And some people with IBS, especially those who have an exaggerated, almost uncontrollable urge to move their bowels after a meal, do much better if they eat smaller meals. For these people, breaking the three basic meals into smaller units and eating several times a day may be helpful.

A word of caution: At no time should you eat *fewer* than three meals a day.

• Snacks Between Meals

Snacks are not included in the meal plans, and for most people they will be unnecessary. If you are interested in adding snacks to the basic meal plan, make sure you stay within the recommended guidelines of the diet. Also, if you have difficulty eating the recommended portions at one sitting, you can stretch the same amount of food into five or six smaller meals. Remember, though, that snacks should not be eaten in the evening or just before bedtime because food late at night can increase GI distress.

• Beverages

Noncaloric soft drinks are not included in the meal plans, but you may have them if you wish. If your GI complaint permits it, coffee and tea may be used (see chapter 26). Water is probably the best beverage you can drink with your meals, or at any other time.

Whenever milk is specified in a meal plan, it is 1 percent low-fat milk. You may substitute lactose-free low-fat milk products in any of these menu plans (see chapter 33).

After Two Weeks

The Two-Week Master Program gives you calorie, fat, and fiber content for each recipe and meal plan. This means that after you have followed the program for two weeks you can begin to pick and choose recipes that personally appeal to you, and also suit your particular requirements. You can also begin to invent or adapt your own recipes, using the guidelines set out in the chapters that follow.

Overall, the Self-Help Nutritional Program for GI disorders is so normal that you will be able to incorporate its nutritional guidelines easily into your family's lifestyle.

Once you have completed the Two-Week Master Program, the recipes are intended to become a part of your everyday cooking for yourself, for family, and for friends. It's important that everyone in your family can enjoy the same food. The tenets of the program are good for all ages—reduced fat and cholesterol, increased complex carbohydrates. Just as important to you and your family, these recipes taste good, provide variety, and are nutritionally sound. Eating habits are formed early in life. When you choose a healthy diet for yourself to help your GI problems, you can be assured you are also having a positive impact on the health and lifestyle of others you live with, including children.

It may seem hard to shift from old eating habits to a new style of eating. Change is never easy. But in this case changing your diet will bring you immediate rewards. You will begin to feel better and find relief from discomfort that may have been going on for years.

Even George, the attorney who needed his mother to help him through the Two-Week Master Program and who didn't know a pot from a potato, was able to stay with the diet because it helped him make a gradual shift in his eating habits. After following the Two-Week Master Program fairly rigidly, he returned to his old eating habits—with some important changes. He cut down on spices, fats, and regular milk products. Then he tried preparing a couple of the recipes himself. He paid more attention to what he was doing and increased his repertoire. Within a few weeks, the benefits of the new program had begun to settle in and he found he had made the transition.

The key to good nutrition is flexibility. Any nutritional plan should become an integral part of your overall lifestyle. Whether you grab lunch in a diner or dine in a four-star restaurant, you should still be able to stick to the fundamental principles of this program. The idea is to choose foods that offer good nutritional value for the calories, while steering clear of the foods that create problems for you. If you follow the six principles of the Self-Help Nutritional Program, you should succeed in mastering your GI complaint.

High fiber, low fat, low lactose, low spice, low gas-forming foods, and low calories: it's important to understand the principles behind each of these concepts before incorporating them into recipes and menu plans. These are the six elements that you will use every day for the rest of your life.

The program that follows contains an average of 1,850 calories a day. Some people will need more calories and some less, depending on their height and body build. See chapter 28 for information about adjusting the calorie content of the program to your needs.

Menus

Day 1
1735 calories
54 grams of fat (28% of calories)
29 grams of fiber

BREAKFAST   *Frosted Melon Cooler
2 slices whole wheat toast
2 teaspoons margarine or butter
1 tablespoon jelly or jam

LUNCH   2 whole wheat pita pockets stuffed with
1 cup or more fresh vegetables, such as grated carrots,
bean sprouts, cucumber, pepper, and tomato
2 ounces grated cheese
*2 tablespoons Basic Vinaigrette Dressing
1 cup 1% low-fat milk

DINNER   *Sweet and Sour Shrimp
1 cup noodles, preferably whole wheat
*Snow Pea Salad
1 kiwi, ½ cup raspberries

Day 2

1934 calories
47 grams of fat (22% of calories)
22 grams of fiber

BREAKFAST   *Orangy French Toast
1 cup 1% low-fat milk

LUNCH   *Eggless Salad
2 slices whole grain bread
1 pear

DINNER   *Marinated and Grilled Chicken Breast
*Potato Salad
Tossed green salad
*2 tablespoons Basic Vinaigrette Dressing
*Blueberry Apple Crumble

Day 3

1846 calories
50 grams of fat (25% of calories)
29 grams of fiber

BREAKFAST   *Blueberry Apple Crumble (leftover from Day 2)
½ cup plain low-fat yogurt
1 cup 1% low-fat milk

LUNCH   *Rice Salad
2 whole wheat rolls
2 teaspoons margarine or butter
1 popsicle
1 orange

*Asterisk indicates a recipe you will find in Part Nine.

DINNER
*Marinated and Grilled Flank Steak
*Eggplant in Rich Tomato Sauce
*Cold Barley Salad
1 whole wheat roll
1 teaspoon margarine or butter
*Banana Dream Pie

Day 4

1814 calories
42 grams of fat (21% of calories)
31 grams of fiber

BREAKFAST
2 cups whole grain cold cereal
1 cup 1% low-fat milk
½ cup blueberries
1 slice whole wheat toast
1 teaspoon butter or margarine

LUNCH
*Marinated and Grilled Flank Steak (leftover from
Day 3) on
2 slices French bread
1 tablespoon catsup
½ cup applesauce

DINNER
*Acorn Squash Soup
*Chicken and Herbs Baked in Foil
*Kasha and Corn
Tossed green salad
*2 tablespoons Basic Vinaigrette Dressing
1 banana

Day 5

1748 calories
50 grams of fat (26% of calories)
26 grams of fiber

BREAKFAST
½ melon
1 cup oatmeal
1 cup 1% low-fat milk
2 slices whole wheat toast
2 teaspoons of margarine or butter
1 tablespoon jelly or jam

LUNCH
*Acorn Squash Soup (leftover from Day 4)
1 bagel
1 tablespoon cream cheese
½ cup pineapple (packed in its own juice)

DINNER   *Veal with Sun-Dried Tomatoes
              *Lemony Potatoes
              Tossed green salad
              *2 tablespoons Basic Vinaigrette Dressing
              *Patriotic Pizzazz

Day 6   1834 calories
              42 grams of fat (21% of calories)
              22 grams of fiber

BREAKFAST   *Strawberry Pancakes
              2 teaspoons margarine or butter
              3 tablespoons maple syrup
              1 cup 1% low-fat milk

LUNCH   *Beautiful Bow Tie Pasta
              1 whole grapefruit

DINNER   *Flounder in a Flash
              *Cinnamon Rice
              *Broiled Tomato Halves
              Tossed green salad
              *2 tablespoons Basic Vinaigrette Dressing
              *Apricot Apples

Day 7   1778 calories
              53 grams of fat (27% of calories)
              24 grams of fiber

BREAKFAST   *Granola Cereal
              ½ cup strawberries
              1 cup 1% low-fat milk
              1 slice whole wheat toast
              1 teaspoon margarine or butter

LUNCH   *Tuna Patties on hamburger roll
              1 peach
              2 plums

DINNER   *Oriental Barbecued Chicken
              *Veggie Stir-fry
              *2 slices Easy Cornbread
              *1 Peanut Butter Bar

Day 8   2011 calories
              52 grams of fat (23% of calories)
              24 grams of fiber

BREAKFAST   ½ melon
             *2 Oatmeal Raisin Muffins
             2 teaspoons margarine or butter
             1 cup 1% low-fat milk

LUNCH   *Turkey Meatball Soup
             *1 slice Easy Cornbread (leftover from Day 7)
             *1 Peanut Butter Bar (leftover from Day 7)
             1 cup 1% low-fat milk

DINNER   *Fettuccini with Clam Sauce
             1 whole grain roll
             1 teaspoon margarine or butter
             *Spinach Salad
             1 peach

Day 9

1978 calories
46 grams of fat (21% of calories)
29 grams of fiber

BREAKFAST   *Hot Buckwheat Cereal
             1 slice of whole wheat toast
             1 teaspoon margarine or butter
             1 tablespoon jelly or jam
             1 cup 1% low-fat milk

LUNCH   *Fettuccini with Clam Sauce (leftover from Day 8)
             1 whole grain roll
             1 teaspoon margarine or butter
             1 banana

DINNER   2 baked pork chops
             *Boiled Potatoes with Apples
             *Cucumber-Radish Salad
             *2 Oat Biscuits
             1 orange

Day 10

1857 calories
46 grams of fat (22% of calories)
26 grams of fiber

BREAKFAST   *Fruit Cup
             1 bagel
             1 tablespoon cream cheese
             1 tablespoon jelly or jam

LUNCH　　　*Fruited Chicken Salad
　　　　　　2 whole wheat pita pockets
　　　　　　1 cup 1% low-fat milk

DINNER　　　*Teriyaki Salmon Kabobs
　　　　　　1 cup brown rice
　　　　　　*Apple Salad
　　　　　　*4 Oatmeal Drop Cookies

Day 11

1847 calories
59 grams of fat (29% of calories)
24 grams of fiber

BREAKFAST　*Tomato, Mushroom, and Basil Omelet
　　　　　　2 slices whole wheat toast
　　　　　　2 teaspoons margarine or butter
　　　　　　1 tablespoon jelly or jam
　　　　　　1 cup orange juice

LUNCH　　　2 cups whole wheat spaghetti with
　　　　　　1 cup chopped fresh vegetables, such as carrots,
　　　　　　　　peppers, tomatoes, zucchini, mushrooms
　　　　　　*2 tablespoons Basic Vinaigrette Dressing (over pasta
　　　　　　　　and vegetables)
　　　　　　*2 Oatmeal Drop Cookies (leftover from Day 10)

DINNER　　　*Lemonade Chicken
　　　　　　*Vegetable Kabob
　　　　　　*Cold Bulgur Wheat Salad
　　　　　　*Fruit Cup (leftover from Day 10)

Day 12

1915 calories
50 grams of fat (23% of calories)
30 grams of fiber

BREAKFAST　½ grapefruit
　　　　　　*3 slices Banana Bran Bread
　　　　　　1 cup 1% low-fat milk

LUNCH　　　*Wheat Berry Salad
　　　　　　1 whole wheat pita pocket
　　　　　　1 banana

DINNER　　　*Salmon Mousse on 4 slices cocktail rye bread
　　　　　　*Creole Topped Potato
　　　　　　Tossed green salad

*2 tablespoons Basic Vinaigrette Dressing
1 whole grain roll
1 teaspoon margarine or butter
½ cup sherbet

Day 13

1820 calories
49 grams of fat (24% of calories)
25 grams of fiber

BREAKFAST   *Lemon Pancakes
2 teaspoons margarine or butter
1 cup 1% low-fat milk

LUNCH   *Snappy Seafood Salad
1 whole wheat pita pocket
1 pear

DINNER   *Stuffed Bell Peppers
*Green Salad
1 whole grain roll
1 teaspoon margarine or butter
*Apple Cake
1 cup 1% low-fat milk

Day 14

1865 calories
50 grams of fat (24% of calories)
28 grams of fiber

BREAKFAST   *1 slice Blueberry Orange Bread
*Berry Banana Smoothie

LUNCH   *Tomato Basil Soup
2 ounces boiled ham
1 ounce cheese (preferably a lower-fat cheese)
2 slices whole grain bread
mustard

DINNER   *Chicken Breasts in Creamy Mustard Sauce
*Dilly Carrots
1 cup noodles, preferably whole wheat
2 plums
*Apple Cake (leftover from Day 13)
1 cup 1% low-fat milk

PART SIX

The Principles Behind the Self-Help Nutritional Program

19 Increasing Fiber

In the 1950s, D. P. Burkett, the British surgeon and epidemiologist, observed that low-fiber diets seemed to be associated with an increased incidence of appendicitis, colon cancer, diverticulosis, and hiatal hernia. He went to Africa to study populations where these ailments were almost unknown, and compared their diet with the British diet. At the same time, he methodically collected, measured, and compared stool specimens from both populations. He found that the typical Englishman produced 200 grams of stool a day, while the African tribesman produced over 600 grams a day. The reason, Burkett concluded, was that the Africans consumed large quantities of natural fiber in the form of whole grains, seeds, and nuts, while the English consumed very little.

A low-fiber diet is also low in residue, causing food wastes to pass slowly through the bowel, with serious consequences. Irritable bowel syndrome, diverticulitis, diverticular bleeding, and perforation are all associated with low-residue diets. Cancer of the colon may be linked to low-fiber diets because there is more time for carcinogens present in the stool to come in contact with the gut wall.

Positive Effects of Fiber

Conversely, high-fiber diets increase the bulk in stool and cause it to pass through the bowel more quickly. High-fiber foods also absorb toxins and prevent pollutants from being absorbed into the body. In one animal study, rats were fed either a low-fiber diet or a high-fiber diet along with a variety of possibly harmful food additives and/or toxic chemicals. The rats that ate a high-fiber diet lived longer and in better health, despite the addition of toxins, than those fed a low-fiber diet.

In another unusual animal study, researchers fed rats small amounts of three potentially harmful food additives. None were harmed when given individual food additives. With two additives in the diet, however, the animals experienced various symptoms, including balding, scruffy fur, diarrhea, and poor weight gain. When another group of animals were fed all three additives at once, they all died within two weeks. Yet when a control group of animals were fed all three additives *plus* a high-fiber diet, all survived unharmed.

The benefits of high-fiber diets was illustrated in a long-term study at Memorial Sloan-Kettering Center and Cornell University—New York Hospital. Over a period of four years, researchers found that high-fiber diets inhibited the growth of rectal polyps, which can lead to cancer, in people with an inherited tendency toward such polyps. A more recent study from Harvard showed no protective effect of dietary fiber against colon cancer or polyps.

Nevertheless, a diet high in fiber is now recommended by the National Cancer Institute, the Food and Nutrition Board, and the National Academy of Sciences.

Fiber is a near miraculous protector of the intestinal tract and improves GI problems across the board.

- Fiber relieves constipation by making the stool bulkier and softer.
- Fiber stops diarrhea by absorbing excess water in the stool. For the same reason, it helps mild cases of colitis.
- Fiber helps relieve hemorrhoids, diverticulosis discomfort, and IBS.
- Fiber provides some protection against the formation of gallstones.
- Fiber can help heal and prevent ulcers.
- A high-fiber diet helps control weight, reduce blood cholesterol, and control blood sugar levels.

What Kind of Fiber

Fiber is material from plant cell walls that resists digestion and is largely excreted in the stool. Some fiber ferments in the digestive tract, producing small-chain fatty acids, the major nutrient for the colon.

There are two main categories of fiber: water insoluble and water soluble. Both kinds are found in the same foods, but the ratio varies. We've only recently realized that different fibers have different effects.

• Insoluble Fiber

Insoluble fiber primarily increases stool bulk and water content, speeding transit of stool through the bowel. Because it is a natural laxative, insoluble fiber is effective in preventing diverticulitis and treating irritable bowel syndrome and hemorrhoids. Insoluble fiber is also believed to lessen the risk of colon cancer, possibly by reducing the amount of time carcinogens remain in the GI system. Some insoluble fibers also decrease the amount of bile acids in the stomach, which may prevent the development of ulcers. Wheat bran is the most concentrated form of insoluble fiber, but all whole grains and many fruits and vegetables also contain large quantities.

• Soluble Fiber

Soluble fiber absorbs water and slows down food transit from the stomach. The greatest benefit of soluble fiber is that it helps decrease cholesterol levels in your blood by washing bile acids from the intestinal tract. Because it gives a feeling of fullness for a longer period of time, soluble fiber controls appetite and enhances weight-loss diets, even in obese people. Soluble fiber also helps protect against both hypoglycemia and hyperglycemia because it helps your system maintain an even level of blood sugar. Dried beans, whole oats, and oat bran are the most concentrated forms of soluble fiber. (Dried beans and legumes may cause gas, however. See chapter 24 for tips on how to reduce gas.)

Insoluble Fibers	Soluble Fibers
Wheat bran	Oat bran
Corn bran	Whole oats
Whole grains	Rice bran
Dried beans and peas	Dried beans
Popcorn	Chick peas, black-eyed peas
Seeds and nuts	Lentils
Most fruit and vegetables, especially carrots, white potatoes, sweet potatoes, artichokes, broccoli, leeks, parsnips	Sesame seeds
	All fruits and vegetables, especially citrus fruits, apples, pears, sweet potatoes, carrots, okra, cauliflower, corn, bananas

Using Fiber to Help GI Disorders

The goal of the Self-Help Nutritional Program is to change your diet to include more foods naturally high in fiber. Fiber is found in carbohydrates—

grains and cereals, fruits and vegetables. Carbohydrates may be either simple or complex. Complex carbohydrates require quite a bit of processing by the digestive tract to break them down into absorbable nutrients. Grains and cereals fall into this category, and this is the kind of complex carbohydrates your muscular GI system likes best. Fruits and vegetables, which have more sugars, also contain complex carbohydrates and are also good sources of fiber.

Because different fibers have different beneficial effects, the Self-Help Nutritional Program recommends using a wide variety of complex carbohydrates daily—whole grains, cereals, fresh fruits and vegetables. Such a wide range of ingredients also adds color and interest to recipes, and helps keep you feeling satisfied. Deriving fiber from several different sources also prevents the gassiness and abdominal discomfort sometimes associated with wheat bran alone.

• About Bran

Bran, the outer shell of wheat, oats, rice, and other whole grains, is the most concentrated form of both soluble and insoluble fiber. The natural fibers found inside fruits, vegetables, and grains have exactly the same benefits attributed to bran, although in a less concentrated form. Obviously, bran is present in all whole grains. Various brans can also be purchased separately.

When you consume a diet that emphasizes fiber-rich foods across the board there is no need to consume additional quantities of bran. A bowl of cooked oat bran cereal is fine if you like it, but a bowl of oatmeal is every bit as good. You may also add bran to your own recipe creations if you wish, but the recipes in this program are designed to provide substantial amounts of fiber, and it's unnecessary to add wheat bran or oat bran to recipes and foods that are already naturally fiber-filled.

If you do choose to add bran to your recipes, however, it's important to remember that soluble bran such as oat bran seems to work best when it's cooked. Insoluble bran, such as wheat bran, tends to be more effective when it is uncooked. Coarsely ground wheat bran also appears to work better than finely ground bran, even though the two are chemically identical.

• Vegetables Against Free Radicals

Vegetables are an excellent source of fiber. Eating vegetables of all kinds on a regular basis helps a wide range of GI problems, and also plays a vital role in preventing other diseases. For instance, beta-carotene and other carotenoids—pigments found in many yellow, orange, and red vegetables and dark green leafy vegetables (beet greens, broccoli, carrots, spinach)— help combat cancers of the mouth, throat, lung, stomach, and bladder, and possibly cancer of the colon and cervix. These disease-fighting carotenoids are thought to protect healthy cells of the body against damage by molecules known as free radicals, which are found in air pollution and food additives.

In the body, free radicals cause a chemical reaction (oxidation) that can produce disease by changing the structure of cells. Carotenoids are *antioxidants*—they destroy free radicals before they can do harm. Because we are exposed to free radicals every day, we need to eat plenty of carotenoid-rich vegetables like broccoli and carrots. Vegetables rich in vitamins C and E, such as asparagus, cabbage, and sweet potatoes, are also potent antioxidants and may fight many types of cancer.

A few of these cancer-fighting vegetables, particularly cabbage, are known to aggravate some GI disorders. You will notice that the Two-Week Master Program uses asparagus and sweet potatoes to supply antioxidants, but avoids cabbage. Check your Flag Foods carefully and experiment with vegetables. Fortunately, there are many carotenoid-rich vegetables that the GI tract likes.

Drinking More Water

Most people don't think of water as food, but all of us need a certain amount of water to maintain life. About half of the human body is made of water. Every single cell needs water to maintain itself. Much of our water is in foods; we also consume large amounts of water in the form of coffee, tea, soft drinks, milk, and other liquids.

Since fiber absorbs considerable amounts of water, it is important that you drink plenty of water with the Self-Help Nutritional Program. You need about 30 cubic centimeters of water per kilogram of body weight every day, or 1 cc for every calorie that you consume. Therefore, if you consume an average of 2,000 calories a day, you need 2,000 cc of fluid each day—or eight 8-ounce glasses of water. (By the way, drinking water will not increase your body's fluid retention. And it won't make you feel heavy and bloated.)

20 *Lowering Fat*

*F*ats have many jobs to perform in the body: small quantities are used for body repair and growth of tissues; fat also provides fatty tissues for insulation and is essential to the body's use of certain vitamins. Fats also provide energy.

Too much fat, however, causes problems for the digestive tract. Fat makes the gallbladder work hard, which is a problem if you have gallstones or gallbladder disease. It relaxes the LES valve, which lets stomach acids back up into the esophagus. Fat also stimulates the pancreas, which can cause pain if you have pancreatitis. High-fat diets are associated with increased risk of many chronic diseases, including cancer and heart disease.

Fat is also by far the most concentrated source of calories, with more than twice as many calories per gram as protein or carbohydrate. Studies on overweight people show that the degree of obesity has more to do with the percentage of fat intake than with surplus calories from all sources. Furthermore, fat calories are stored more efficiently than carbohydrate or protein calories, which makes it easy for the body to convert dietary fat into body fat, and very hard for the body to convert carbohydrates into fat.

Help for GI Problems

Reducing fat in the diet relieves heartburn, prevents gallbladder attacks, and aids pancreatitis. A low-fat diet also helps prevent colon cancer and the development of kidney stones in people with Crohn's disease. A low-fat diet will usually prevent the cramps and diarrhea some people with IBS experience after eating. Reducing *total* fat helps control weight and also helps prevent other diseases associated with high-fat diets such as heart disease and certain cancers, including breast cancer.

How Many Grams of Fat?

The goal is to derive less than 30 percent of your daily calories from fat. To discover how much fat you can eat each day and stay within the guideline, do this simple calculation:

1. Multiply your daily calories by .3
2. Divide the result by 9, the number of calories in each gram of fat

The result is the total number of grams of fat you can eat per day. Only one-third of this total should come from saturated fat (described further below). Following are some examples.

Calories per Day	Grams of Fat per Day	Grams of Saturated Fat per Day
1200	40 or less	13 or less
1500	50 or less	17 or less
1800	60 or less	20 or less
2100	70 or less	23 or less
2400	80 or less	27 or less

How Much Is a Gram?*

Many packaged food products offer nutritional information, including number of grams of fat. For quick reference, there are 5 grams of fat in each of the following:

1 teaspoon of oil, margarine, mayonnaise, or butter

1 tablespoon of regular salad dressings, diet margarine, or diet mayonnaise

1 tablespoon of cashews

5 large olives

10 large peanuts

⅛ avocado

2 whole walnuts or pecans

6 whole almonds

*Adapted from the American Dietetic Association and the American Diabetic Association Exchange List for Meal Planning.

The primary goal of the Self-Help Nutritional Program is to decrease the *total fat* in your diet. In the Two-Week Master Program, all kinds of fats are minimized. The program supplies only 21 to 28 percent of calories from fat each day, even less than the amount recommended by the National Cancer Institute. Your lifelong objective is to maintain this low consumption.

It is much easier to monitor your fat intake by counting grams than by calculating percentages. The box on the previous page gives you a quick way to keep track of your daily fat intake.

Fats can be reduced by decreasing the amount, eliminating the fat, or employing cooking methods that do not require fat. The fats used in the Master Program are usually from vegetable oils; if a recipe calls for a saturated fat such as butter, a very small amount is used.

Good Fats vs. Bad Fats

All fats are high in calories and used slowly by the body; however, some fats are more deleterious than others.

Fats are either saturated or unsaturated. Saturated fats can elevate blood cholesterol; unsaturated fats do not increase blood cholesterol. For the most part, saturated fats are derived from animal foods—meat, milk and butter; unsaturated fats are found in vegetable oils. There are a few critical exceptions.

• Polyunsaturated Vegetable Oils

For more than two decades polyunsaturated vegetable oils have been recognized as heart-healthy alternatives to butter and other fats derived from animal products. But new research indicates that what might be good for the heart is bad for the immune system. Polyunsaturated oils are high in omega-6 fatty acids. New findings from animal studies show that diets high in omega-6 stimulated the growth of tumors of the breast, pancreas, and colon.

• Tropical Vegetable Oils

Vegetable oils derived from coconut, palm, and palm kernel are highly saturated. Nondairy creamers, cookies, and other baked products and snack foods are typical products that contain tropical oils. Food companies have recently been under pressure to remove highly saturated tropical oils from

processed foods. Tropical oils are often replaced with partially hydrogenated oils that contain trans fatty acids. New studies suggest that these
trans fats are just as harmful as saturated fat and tropical oils.

• Margarine and Solid Shortenings

Trans fatty acids are produced when liquid vegetable oil is hardened, or
hydrogenated, to produce margarine or solid vegetable shortening. When
vegetable oil is hydrogenated, some fatty acids become more saturated,
while others are changed into trans fatty acids. Researchers believe that
these trans fatty acids act like saturated fats to lower the good form of cholesterol—high-density lipoprotein, or HDL—that protects against heart disease, while increasing the level of harmful cholesterol—low-density
lipoprotein, or LDL.

Any processed food that contains partially hydrogenated oil contains
trans fats: crackers, cookies, pastries, cakes, doughnuts, french fries, potato
chips, puddings, and graham crackers.

If you use margarine, choose tub margarine, which is lower in both saturated and trans fatty acids. (Stick margarine generally has twice as much
fatty acids as softer tub margarines.) Margarines or spreads that list liquid
oil as the first ingredient are a better choice than those that list partially hydrogenated oil first. Liquid squeeze margarines are the lowest in saturated
and trans fats. Liquid oils and foods like corn oil or mayonnaise that list liquid oils as the first ingredient are also low in saturated and trans fats.

• Olive and Canola Oil: Monounsaturates

Monounsaturated fat has become the "fat of choice." Like the polyunsaturates, monounsaturates lower *total* cholesterol. They may do even more
to protect your heart, however, because they are more selective when they
go to work on cholesterol. Cholesterol is broken into several different factors. Generally, HDLs are good factors, working to keep arteries clean;
LDLs cause the artery-clogging damage. Monounsaturated fats lower total
cholesterol without lowering the good HDLs. Not all monounsaturates have
this effect, however.

Olive oil is a good choice for cooking because it is one of the richest
sources of monounsaturated fat in the diet. More than three-quarters of its
fat is monounsaturated, virtually none of it in the trans form. Canola oil
(rapeseed oil) is almost as high in monounsaturated fat but is lower in saturated fat than olive oil.

Peanut oil and avocado oil, although monounsaturates, are saturated to the extent that they provide a neutral effect. They are not harmful, but don't provide the same benefit as olive oil or canola oil.

• Omega-3 Fatty Acids

Omega-3 fatty acids, found in fish oils, benefit the body in several ways. They have the reverse effect of omega-6, slowing tumor growth. Omega-3 fatty acids are also heart-healthy. Early observations in Greenland showed that Eskimos, despite a diet high in fat and cholesterol, had a low incidence of heart disease. Closer examination showed that while their total cholesterol was high, their triglycerides, another blood fat linked to heart disease, were low. The Eskimos also had high HDLs, the good cholesterol. This good ratio of cholesterol factors was traced to the high proportion of omega-3 fatty acids in the traditional Eskimo diet of fish and other marine animals.

Omega-3 fatty acids also reduce clotting of the blood, which helps prevent the progression of coronary artery disease. Certain fishes are high in omega-3 fatty acids, especially salmon, tuna, mackerel, herring, sardines, halibut, and trout.

Omega-3 fatty acids are converted to a class of prostaglandins in the body that helps to decrease inflammation. They may be helpful in diseases such as rheumatoid arthritis and immune disorders. Excessive intake of omega-3 fatty acids can potentially increase your risk of bleeding, however, so supplements should not be used without consulting your physician.

• Fat and Heart Disease

The major risk factors for heart disease are high blood pressure, cigarette smoking, obesity, and high blood cholesterol. Dietary fat, especially animal fat, increases the level of cholesterol in your blood. Certain lower-fat foods can also boost cholesterol in the blood, even though they tend to have less impact than dietary fat: egg yolks, organ meats such as liver and kidney, caviar, fish roe, and shellfish all contain large quantities of cholesterol.

Cholesterol is a natural fatty substance manufactured in the liver and also present in many foods that we eat. When the body doesn't burn all its fats, cholesterol is laid down like silt along the inside of the arteries where it forms a hard pastelike deposit, which narrows the arteries and as a result increases your risk of heart disease and premature death.

About 25 percent of Americans between the ages of twenty and seventy-four have high blood cholesterol, which translates into at least 40 million people. Anyone at any age can have high blood cholesterol. For unknown reasons, not everyone who eats a high-fat diet has elevated cholesterol, and some people who eat an exceedingly low-fat diet do have elevated blood cholesterol. The answer to this mysterious paradox may lie in genetics: some people use cholesterol more efficiently than others. It's also an interesting fact that cholesterol levels tend to jump when you are under stress.

One thing we know for sure: many people can lower their blood cholesterol levels by making alterations in their diet. These include reducing fat and increasing fiber, particularly soluble fiber (in the form of oat bran, whole oats, and dried beans), which acts like a sponge to mop up excess cholesterol and transport it out of the bloodstream.

A federal advisory panel has labeled total blood cholesterol above 240 milligrams per deciliter of blood as high blood cholesterol, 200 to 239 as borderline, and below 200 as desirable. The panel advises everyone over age twenty to have total cholesterol measured at least once very five years, and those classified borderline to have the test repeated. There is new evidence that even children can have elevated cholesterol, which can lead to problems later in life. At this time, children probably do not need to have their cholesterol checked routinely unless there is a strong history of high cholesterol and early heart attack in the family.

Cholesterol-lowering drugs are now available, but are usually recommended only for those with the highest risk of heart disease or when changes in diet fail to do the job.

• Fat and Cancer

The role of fat in cancer is not yet well documented, but it appears that high-fat diets may stimulate the production of substances that increase the risk of various cancers. For example, dietary fat stimulates the release of bile acids from the gallbladder. These acids are then more readily converted to a carcinogen, or cancer-causing substance. Bile acids may also injure healthy tissue in the colon. Both mechanisms may play a role in increasing the risk of colon cancer. Dietary fat may also stimulate hormones that promote tumor growth. Thus, high-fat diets have been associated with an increased risk of cancer of the breast and endometrium in women, the prostate in men, and the colon in both men and women.

To reduce the risk of heart disease and cancer, the National Cancer Institute has advised Americans to reduce their intake of fat from all sources

Which Fats Are Which?

Monounsaturated	Polyunsaturated	Saturated
Olive oil	Safflower oil	Butter
Canola oil	Sunflower oil	Meat fat
Peanut oil	Corn oil	Lard (pork fat)
Avocados	Soybean oil	Hydrogenated fats§
Olives	Cottonseed oil	Cream
Peanuts	Margarines†	Cheese
Peanut butter*	Sesame oil	Whole milk
Cashews	Mayonnaise	Coconut oil
Almonds	Walnuts	Palm kernel oil
Pecans	Fish oils‡	Palm oil

*Peanut butter that is natural, ground from pure peanuts, contains monounsaturated fat. Peanut butter that has been hydrogenated has been processed in a way that makes its fats more saturated. Most commercially made peanut butters available at your supermarket are hydrogenated. In natural peanut butters the oil rises to the top; to decrease total fat content, pour off oil before using.

†Margarines differ in their ratio of saturated to unsaturated fat. Generally, the softer the margarine, the higher the polyunsaturates. If the first ingredient listed on the label is a hydrogenated vegetable oil, then the product is higher in saturated fat. Look for a liquid oil as the first ingredient on the margarine label. Ingredients on all labels are listed in order of decreasing predominance.

‡Fish oils are high in the omega-3 fatty acids that fight cholesterol.

§Hydrogenated fats are polyunsaturated fats that have been processed to make them solid. The processing also makes them saturated.

to less than 30 percent of total daily calories. According to the National Cancer Institute, not everything you eat needs to be less than 30 percent fat. The 30 percent figure is for the entire day. Therefore, if you eat an ice cream cone that is 80 percent fat, you can balance it against a dish with much less fat. For people with GI disorders, however, it is much better to avoid high-fat foods across the board, because a single serving of high-fat food can act as a trigger on the GI tract.

Avoid Cholesterol-Packed Foods

Many foods that raise blood cholesterol also have a negative effect on the GI tract. You can do double duty—protect your arteries and soothe your digestive disorder—if you avoid or use sparingly foods that promote cholesterol in the blood:

Beef—ground chuck, short ribs, processed meats such as corned beef, salami, sausage, bologna, frankfurters

Veal—breast (other cuts have less fat and cholesterol)

Lamb—chops and ribs

Pork—shoulder, loin, sausage, chitterlings, spareribs, salami

All fried foods

Whole-milk dairy products, cheeses with more than 5 grams of fat per ounce, ice cream, cream, butter

Nondairy creamers

Processed foods—especially those that contain coconut oil, palm kernel or palm oil, animal fat, or hydrogenated oils

Sauces such as hollandaise and béarnaise, quiche lorraine

Egg yolks—limit yourself to three or four a week, or substitute egg whites for whole eggs in recipes

21 *Reducing Lactose*

A low-lactose diet helps those who suffer from intestinal gas and lactose intolerance, one of the world's most common GI complaints (see chapter 10). The gas and diarrhea resulting from "milk" intolerance is caused by the milk sugar lactose, and not the milk itself or its fat content. Skim milk will cause as much trouble in lactose-intolerant people as whole milk with regard to GI symptoms.

Lactose is found in all dairy products, which are also a major source of calcium and other beneficial nutrients. Fortunately, it isn't necessary to abandon dairy products on the Self-Help Nutritional Program, even if you are lactose intolerant. There are several alternatives to regular dairy products that can be used by those who are lactose intolerant.

Acidophilus Milk

Acidophilus milk is regular milk with active lactobacillus added to it. This bacterial culture has the ability to make lactase, the enzyme that allows us to digest lactose. Warmed in your digestive system, acidophilus starts to work to break down lactose.

This milk cannot be used in cooking or added to a hot drink, because heat kills the lactobacillus. If you choose acidophilus milk, use it for drinking. Acidophilus milk is available at your supermarket or health food store. It tastes the same as regular milk.

Lactaid Milk

Ready-made milk called Lactaid comes with lactase, the enzyme that digests lactose, already in it. You can buy 1 percent low-fat, skim, or chocolate

210

Lactaid milk in your supermarket. Reduced-lactose milk is marketed under several other brands as well (Dairy-Ease).

Lactaid milk tends to stay fresher and taste sweeter than regular milk because the enzyme has pre-split the milk sugar lactose into sweeter-tasting glucose and galactose. Because this milk is predigested, it is heat stable—you can heat it and it will still help symptoms of lactose intolerance. However, Lactaid milk usually breaks down only about 70 percent of the lactose in milk. Most people can handle the remaining 30 percent. Some people, however, are so lactose intolerant that they require milk products that are 100 percent lactose-free. A new 100 percent lactose-free milk is now sold by Lactaid.

Lactase Enzyme: Drops and Tablets

The lactase enzyme is available as a liquid that can be added to milk (if you can't find Lactaid milk) or in a tablet form that can be taken when you ingest milk products. Both are sold under various brand names at your health food store or pharmacy.

Instructions for the liquid lactase enzyme are given on the package label, but you will probably need to use more than the recommended amount to make the milk as close to 100 percent lactose-free as possible. After adding the drops to milk, allow the mixture to sit in the refrigerator for twenty-four hours before using it. You may then use the lactose-free milk for drinking or in any recipe that calls for milk.

Instead of treating the milk with drops, you can treat your digestive tract with lactase enzyme tablets. Take one or two tablets whenever you drink untreated milk or eat cheese, ice cream, or any products or dishes made with dairy products.

Fermented Milk Products

Even people who are lactose intolerant can usually tolerate small amounts of lactose. Fermented or processed milk products such as yogurt, butter, hard and soft ripened cheeses, buttermilk, and sour cream usually do not cause digestive problems. In these products the lactobacilli have predigested some of the lactose. Yogurt that contains live cultures is even easier to digest. (Yogurt that isn't made with live cultures will probably have the same effect as milk.)

Adjusting Lactose in Your Diet

For those who suffer from gas, we recommend that when first starting the Two-Week Master Program you purchase lactase enzyme liquid or tablets. (All of the recipes in the recipe section indicate how many lactase enzyme tablets to take with the meal.)

You can begin to discover your personal tolerance level by gradually adding small amounts of regular milk products to your diet, while observing for symptoms of flatulence, diarrhea, or abdominal cramps. Try using regular milk in your coffee, or experimenting with fermented milk products such as yogurt and cheese. If no symptoms occur, begin to use regular milk products in your recipes.

22 *Lowering Spice Content*

Spicy foods may stimulate acid secretion and cause sudden spasms of the esophagus in certain people predisposed to spasms. Spices may also aggravate preexisting digestive disorders, such as esophagitis and IBS, and exacerbate their symptoms.

Documentation of the negative effects of specific spices on the GI tract are scarce, however. One study that tracked the effect of spices in the diets of ulcer patients showed that the spices most strongly linked to gastric distress are black pepper, chili pepper, mustard seed, cloves, and nutmeg. Symptoms are generally worse if spicy foods are eaten on an empty stomach. Garlic, chili, and curry powder are also irritating spices for many people with GI complaints.

Not all spices are irritating to the stomach. Those least likely to exert a harmful effect are cinnamon, allspice, mace, thyme, sage, paprika, and caraway seed.

Overall, a low-spice regimen can be expected to benefit heartburn, ulcers, and IBS. Most of the recipes in the Self-Help Nutritional Program have been developed without spices. If you are able to tolerate spices, use your imagination and add them whenever you wish. Herbs such as thyme, rosemary, basil, sage, and others may be added to, or substituted in, recipes to suit your own taste.

Effect of Spices on the GI Tract

Most Aggravating	Least Aggravating
Black pepper	Allspice
Chili pepper	Caraway seed
Chili powder	Cinnamon
Cloves	Mace
Curry powder	Paprika
Garlic	Sage
Mustard seed	Thyme
Nutmeg	

23 *Reducing Fructose*

An often overlooked culprit in the cause of abdominal pain, bloating, and diarrhea is the simple sugar fructose. Fructose is present in fruits and vegetables, but it is also added in large quantities to soft drinks, beverages, and many foods in the form of high-fructose corn syrup. The absorption capacity for fructose is limited, and many people experience incomplete absorption of this sugar. When unabsorbed, fructose can draw fluid into the intestine and cause bloating, abdominal pain, and discomfort. When the unabsorbed sugar reaches the colon, it is fermented by bacteria there, and can produce excessive amounts of gas and diarrhea.

Fructose consumption is on the rise in the United States. In 2002, Americans consumed over 9 million tons of high-fructose corn syrup, much of that in sweetened beverages. Fructose also comes in honey, fruits and fruit juices, and selected other foods. Recent studies have shown that persons who are fructose intolerant can get relief by eliminating fructose from their diet. Fructose intolerance can be diagnosed by a breath test.

A strict low-fructose diet requires counseling from a registered dietitian and careful planning to ensure nutritional adequacy. This type of diet should not be followed unless true fructose intolerance is diagnosed by a physician. If you simply want to try reducing fructose in your diet, this can be done rather easily by eliminating sodas, fruit drinks, wine coolers, dried and canned fruits, honey, and processed foods sweetened with high-fructose corn syrup.

24 *Reducing Gas-Forming Legumes*

*T*he process of digestion always produces gas, but some people—especially people with GI disorders—may react adversely to even small amounts of gas in the GI tract. For example, even a little excessive gas for someone who suffers from IBS can produce spasm and pain.

We know that certain foods create more gas than others, and that reducing these gas-forming foods in the diet can help improve certain GI conditions. Unfortunately, many of the worst offenders are also good for you. Beans, for example, are nourishing, inexpensive, and so versatile that they are used in every kind of cuisine. They are also major producers of flatus because their carbohydrates are so difficult to digest that gas-producing bacteria in the colon have a field day. The disease-fighting cruciferous vegetables, which include the cabbage family, also tend to be gas producers. If you suffer from excessive gas you'll need to experiment with foods. Each person is different, and there is no need to eliminate foods that don't bother you.

Some people can reduce excessive gas simply by making the above changes. I had one patient who began suffering from excessive gas seemingly without cause. Lisa had never complained of gas before, but on a routine visit told me that she had noticed that she was always "gassy" and it was starting to bother her. I showed Lisa the list below, and she checked seven out of nine items. She was surprised, and so was I. The only two risk factors she *didn't* have were constipation and air swallowing. Lisa had recently been under a lot of stress and had fallen into poor eating habits, a combination of factors that produced excessive gas. She gulped her meals, overate once or twice a day, drank quantities of club soda, and used food to calm her anxiety. She got almost no exercise. Lisa didn't have to change the types of food she ate, but she did have to change the way she ate them. This proved to be a simple adjustment for her to make.

Steps to Reduce Excessive Gas

Many people find that if they eat legumes and cruciferous vegetables several times a week in small quantities, gas production subsides. You can also reduce the gas production of beans by changing the way you prepare them. Cook dried beans using the quick-soak method: Bring dried beans to a boil for 2 minutes, then turn off heat and let stand for 1 hour. Drain water. Add fresh water, then cook beans as usual. This cooking method reduces gas production by about 20 percent.

Here are some further steps you can take to prevent the occurrence of excessive gas.

1. Eat slowly.
2. Chew your food well.
3. Avoid eating when you feel tense or upset.
4. Don't overload your stomach. Keep meal sizes moderate.
5. Limit fluids with meals.
6. Avoid constipation.
7. Limit carbonated beverages.
8. Exercise.
9. Eliminate gum chewing, smoking, sucking on hard candies, drinking through straws or from bottles, and gulping large quantities of fluid. All these activities encourage air swallowing.

The strategy we used to create recipes for the Self-Help Nutritional Program was to avoid beans altogether, and use very few legumes. This was accomplished for the most part by substituting whole grains, such as bulgur wheat and kasha, and other vegetables for beans and legumes. Some foods such as broccoli, known to be gas-forming, are used in the recipes for the Two-Week Master Program. However, these foods are marked as Flag Foods, and a substitute such as carrots is offered for people who have trouble with gas.

Beano, a new product from the makers of Lactaid, contains the enzyme α-galactosidase, which aids in the digestion of beans and legumes. It can be purchased OTC at your pharmacy.

25   *Low Calories/High Nutrition*

*O*ne of the most important goals of the Self-Help Nutritional Program is to control your calorie intake so that you maintain a desirable body weight. Overeating and excess weight can have a devastating effect on GI disorders, including heartburn and gallstones.

Problems Associated with Being Overweight

Extra weight in the abdomen increases pressure under the LES valve, the one-way valve located between the esophagus and the stomach, and causes acid to back up. Clothes that fit tightly around the waist also increase pressure on the abdomen, which in turn builds up the pressure under the LES. People who are overweight often wear clothes that are too tight because of recent weight gain, or the wishful notion that if they buy the same size as they always have they haven't really gained weight. But even if your clothes are a perfect fit, you are still more likely to have heartburn if you are overweight. Fat isn't deposited only under the skin where you can feel it and see it, it is also deposited deep within the body. Fat accumulates around internal organs, especially around the intestines and the abdominal lining. As fat fills up the interior of the abdomen, pressure builds up under the LES, causing reflux. Losing weight may not be as easy as chewing antacid tablets, but it's a much more effective and long-lasting way to treat heartburn.

Intestinal gas and flatulence are also common GI responses to excess weight. People who overeat, especially if they eat large quantities of food in one sitting, produce excessive gas. Overeating can also cause distress if you have IBS.

Belching is another by-product of excess weight. The more you weigh, the more difficult it is to exercise; the less exercise you do, the more weight you gain. When you do exert yourself, there is a lot of huffing and puffing, and you tend to swallow more air than usual. Just as extra weight in the abdomen causes stomach acid to back up into the esophagus, it also causes excess air to back up. Losing weight encourages you to be more active, makes breathing easier, and belching usually subsides.

When you are overweight, fat may also infiltrate vital organs, although fatty infiltration doesn't cause specific GI problems for most people. Severely obese people may lose some function of the pancreas. Since the pancreas normally produces far more enzymes than are necessary to digest food, however, some loss of function usually doesn't pose any problem. Even people who have had most of the pancreas surgically removed because of chronic pancreatitis or cancer still have normal digestive function.

Fatty infiltration of the liver, however, is another story. Like the pancreas, the liver usually continues to function normally up to a point because there is a tremendous reserve of function. Occasionally, however, a fatty liver becomes inflamed, a process called steatohepatitis, which sets up a potentially dangerous condition. Inflammation can lead to scarring and, in some cases, cirrhosis. The worst part is that liver inflammation may not produce any noticeable symptoms. The surest cure is prevention by losing weight before the condition develops. (Once scarring has occurred, the damage is irreversible.)

Obesity is strongly associated with gallstones. The liver manufactures bile, which is then stored in the gallbladder and released as needed to digest fats. Bile is mainly composed of bile salts, phospholipids, and cholesterol. When you are overweight, bile becomes supersaturated with cholesterol. Stored in the gallbladder, the cholesterol-rich bile begins to crystallize and the particles join together to form a stone. Stones can cause serious problems if they migrate out of the gallbladder and get stuck in the bile ducts.

Maintaining ideal weight definitely prevents the formation of gallstones. In a study published in the *New England Journal of Medicine,* investigators at Harvard University reported a one-to-one correlation between weight and risk for gallstones. The more you weigh, the higher the risk. But surprisingly, *losing* weight may increase the risk of getting stones. Prolonged fasting or modified fasting as part of a rapid weight-loss program causes the gallbladder to become inactive because very little fat (1–2 grams per day) is being processed. Bile that would normally be ejected to help digest fats stagnates in the gallbladder, becomes more saturated with cholesterol, and makes stone formation more likely.

Excess weight is also associated with other medical conditions—heart disease; adult onset diabetes mellitus; high blood pressure; cancer of the breast, endometrium, and prostate; cancer of the colon and rectum; arthritis of the knees and hips; varicose veins; gout; and respiratory problems.

Self-Help

The Self-Help Nutritional Program is a naturally low-calorie program because it reduces fat calories. It also increases carbohydrates and controls the amount of protein you consume. Many people believe that a low-calorie diet should emphasize protein to guarantee nutritional health. They believe that a high-fiber, low-calorie combination will leave out essential nutrients. The secret lies in getting maximum nutrition from minimal calories.

• Proteins and Carbohydrates

Proteins are the compounds that form the basic structure of all living matter. A regular daily intake of protein helps all body cells and tissues repair and replace themselves and grow. Protein is important for making hormones and enzymes, and for proper immune function.

There are two kinds of protein: animal-derived proteins (meat, fish, eggs, and dairy products) and vegetable proteins (peas, beans and other legumes, and grains). Animal protein is often called high-quality protein because it is made in precisely the form the body requires. However, animal protein is inevitably accompanied by high quantities of fats. Vegetable proteins, on the other hand, when combined, can add up to valuable protein without the excess fat.

Some people think that protein is less fattening than starchy carbohydrates. This isn't true: gram for gram, protein and carbohydrate contain the same amount of calories. But because animal protein is dense, it doesn't take much volume to add up to a lot of calories and it's easy to eat more protein than you actually need at any one time. If you eat more protein than you require for replacement of body tissues, the excess is used to provide extra energy or is stored in the body as fat.

• How Much Protein?

The average American consumes about 100 grams of protein daily, almost twice as much as most adults need. Depending on your size, you need only 50 to 80 grams of protein a day to maintain good health. Protein needs are calculated at .8 grams per kilogram (2.2 pounds) of body weight per day. So if you weigh 130 pounds you need less than 50 grams of protein a day.

You will obtain 7 grams of protein from each ounce of meat, fish, poultry, or cheese that you eat. An 8-ounce glass of milk contains 8 grams of protein. You also obtain protein from the cereals, grains, and vegetables that you eat. As you can see, your protein intake can add up very quickly to meet your needs. In fact, it is difficult *not* to meet your daily protein needs (see box).

The American Heart Association recommends no more than 6 cooked ounces of animal protein such as fish, poultry, meat, or cheese daily. This is because animal protein contains fat and because excess protein is likely to be converted into fat by the body. This is similar to the amount of protein recommended by the Self-Help Nutritional Program.

People who suffer from certain serious GI diseases—inflammatory bowel disease, Crohn's disease, pancreatic disease—may need twice as much protein, however, because absorption of nutrients from the bowel is impaired or the inflammatory stressful state eats up a lot of the body's protein (nitrogen) stores. Unless protein intake is increased, a state of "negative nitrogen balance" will result and weight loss will come from muscle as well as fat.

The Two-Week Master Program supplies more than enough protein to meet your needs, regardless of your weight or physical condition: 55 to 75 grams of protein each day, on average, depending on portion size.

Low-Carbohydrate, High-Protein Diets

Low-carbohydrate diets are gaining popularity, but they are not always a good choice for people with gastrointestinal problems. In fact, side effects of low-carbohydrate diets often include gastrointestinal symptoms. Due to their low fiber and high fat content, low-carbohydrate diets can cause constipation, worsening of irritable bowel symptoms, gastroesophageal reflux, gallbladder attacks if gallstones are present, and increased abdominal pain in patients suffering from chronic pancreatitis.

People lose weight quickly on low-carbohydrate diets because the initial weight loss is water, not fat. Normally our bodies store some carbohydrate as an energy reserve in the form of glycogen. With glycogen, we also store water. Low-carbohydrate diets cause rapid depletion of body glycogen, energy, and water. The first week of a low-carbohydrate diet is accompanied by a large water diuresis, which appears on the scale as several pounds of weight loss. When we diet to lose weight, however, what we really want is to lose body fat. That can be accomplished only by taking in fewer calories than we burn in a day, through permanent changes in eating and exercise habits. The slow but steady approach of the Two-Week Master Program is the best choice for people with gastrointestinal disorders.

Vitamin and Mineral Supplements

We need some forty vitamins and minerals to maintain health. In their proper dosages, these vitamins and minerals are necessary to promote growth, reproduction, and maintenance of cell life. The amounts needed to do this job are well supplied in a good basic diet, and most of us can obtain all the vitamins and minerals we need from food.

It's true that some nutrients in food may be lost during storage or preparation, may be improperly absorbed by the body, or may be excreted too hastily as a result of many complex factors. For this reason millions of healthy people take vitamin and mineral supplements, often in massive doses. For the most part, I believe that vitamin and mineral supplements are unnecessary. Even worse, when dosages are abused, supplements can be dangerous. Although too little of any essential nutrient can produce deficiency, too much can result in toxicity.

Fat-soluble vitamins—A, D, E, and K—are stored by the body, which means they can accumulate and become toxic if you ingest too much. High doses of vitamin A, for example, can cause bone pain and headache due to increased intracranial pressure.

Grams of Protein in Common Foods

Food	Serving Size	Grams of Protein
Barley	¼ cup raw	4.1
Bean curd (tofu)	1 piece (4 ounces)	9.4
Beans, kidney	½ cup cooked	7.2
Beans, lima	½ cup cooked	6.5
Beans, navy	½ cup cooked	7.4
Bean sprouts, mung	½ cup, raw or cooked	2.0
Beef, lean ground	¼ pound raw	23.4
Bran flakes (40%)	1 cup	3.6
Bread, white	1 slice	2.4
Bread, whole wheat	1 slice	2.6
Broccoli	1 cup cooked	8.4
Bulgur	1 cup cooked	2.7
Cheese, American	1 ounce	6.6
Cheese, cheddar	1 ounce	7.1

Food	Serving Size	Grams of Protein
Cheese, cottage	½ cup	15.0
Chicken	1 drumstick	12.2
Corn	½ cup kernels	3.2
Eggs	2 medium	11.4
Farina	½ cup cooked in water	3.2
Flounder	3 ounces	25.5
Frankfurter	1 (2 ounces)	7.1
Ham, boiled	3 slices (3 ounces)	16.2
Lamb, rib chop	3 ounces	17.9
Lentils	½ cup cooked	7.8
Liver, chicken	1 liver	6.6
Macaroni	1 cup cooked	6.5
Mackerel	3 ounces	17.9
Milk, skim	1 cup	8.8
Noodles, egg	1 cup cooked	6.6
Oatmeal	1 cup cooked in water	4.8
Pancakes	3 4-inch cakes	5.7
Peanut butter	2 tablespoons	8.0
Peas, green	½ cup cooked	4.3
Pork, loin	3 ounces	20.8
Pork sausage	2 links (2 ounces)	5.4
Potato	7 ounces baked	4.0
Rice, brown	1 cup cooked	4.9
Rice, white	1 cup cooked	4.1
Scallops	3 ounces	16.0
Sesame seeds	1 tablespoon	1.5
Shrimp	3 ounces	11.6
Soup, bean with pork	1 cup, made with water	8.0
Soup, tomato	1 cup, made with milk	6.5
Soybeans	½ cup cooked	9.9
Spaghetti	1 cup cooked al dente	6.5
Squash, acorn	1 cup baked	3.9
Sweet potato	5 ounces baked	2.4

Food	Serving Size	Grams of Protein
Tuna, canned	3 ounces, drained	24.4
Turkey	3 ounces	26.8
Veal, stew meat	3 ounces	23.7
Walnuts	10 large	7.3
Wheat flakes	1 cup	3.1
Wheat, shredded	1 cup	5.0
Yogurt	1 cup	8.3

Adapted from *Nutritive Value of American Foods,* Agriculture Handbook No. 456 (Washington, D.C.: U.S. Government Printing Office, 1975).

Water-soluble vitamins—C and B vitamins—are rapidly absorbed and rapidly excreted. Rapid excretion in the urine means that it's hard to overdose on these vitamins, although it is possible. Megadoses of vitamin B6, for example, can cause nerve damage. When taken in large amounts, almost any nutrient becomes toxic.

Minerals are derived from metals and salts such as iron and calcium, sodium chloride and phosphorus. We need most minerals only in minute quantities and, like vitamins, excesses can do more harm than good.

• When to Take Supplements

For the majority of people with GI problems, the Two-Week Master Program supplies all the nutrients necessary and they will not require supplemental vitamins and minerals. However, there are certain exceptions. Supplemental vitamins and minerals may be good for people who have diseases such as ileitis or Crohn's disease, which are often accompanied by deficiencies. A person who has GI bleeding from ulcers may need iron supplements.

Another exception would be if you are severely cutting calories to lose weight. If your caloric intake is less than 1200 calories a day, you should take a multivitamin supplement that includes iron, as well as a calcium supplement. Certainly if you are pregnant, you will probably want to take a high-potency vitamin as prescribed by your obstetrician.

Calcium supplements may be of value for women at risk for osteoporosis. Calcium has also proved beneficial for preventing colonic polyps. So if you have a family history of colonic polyps or colon cancer, you may want to take calcium supplements.

• Vitamin C and GI Disorders

Vitamin C usually does not make heartburn or ulcers worse, even though it is an acid. It doesn't seem to matter much which form of vitamin C you take. Some people think that vitamin C from rose hips is easier on the digestive system than regular ascorbic acid, but rose hips contain ascorbic acid too. If you took pure rose hips to give you a megadose of vitamin C, the pill would be the size of a golf ball. So it doesn't seem to matter to the GI tract which kind of vitamin C you ingest. Chewable ascorbic acid tablets may erode tooth enamel, so I would choose the regular tablets that you swallow whole.

Whether megadoses of vitamins, especially vitamin C, can actually promote health by preventing viral illness and cancer remains controversial. Proponents of orthomolecular medicine (which theorizes that people have inherited a biochemistry that requires very high vitamin intake, and that without supplements sickness of mind or body sets in) extol the value of 1 to 2 grams or more of vitamin C a day, but in my view convincing proof is lacking.

One word of caution: if you decide to take large doses of vitamin C (more than 1 gram a day) you may have more frequent bowel movements or notice that your stools become looser because of its laxative effect.

*Y*our GI tract needs both macronutrients (carbohydrate, protein, and fat) and micronutrients (vitamins and minerals) to manufacture new cells. If the GI tract is deprived of certain essential nutrients, the small intestine can shrink, which results in poor absorption, diarrhea, and increased risk of infection. Deficiencies ultimately affect every organ in the body, including the immune system. True deficiency diseases are rare because of the wide variety of foods that are available to us in the United States. (We are much more likely to suffer from overconsumption of nutrients, particularly fat.) For your body to function at peak performance over your lifetime, you need to avoid either overconsumption or underconsumption of essential nutrients.

26
Flag Foods for Fine-Tuning

*T*he perfect GI diet would reduce the formation of stomach acid and intestinal gas, promote GI motility and proper elimination while avoiding spasms or cramps, prevent reflux of stomach acid, and reduce stimulation of the gallbladder and pancreas. Even though many people have two or more GI complaints, I've never known anyone to need all of the above features at the same time. Furthermore, people with the same symptoms may react in different ways to the same food. If the Two-Week Master Program eliminated every known gastrointestinal irritant, you might wind up with nothing to eat.

An obvious example is milk. Milk doesn't pose a problem for a person with IBS (unless that person is lactose intolerant). But milk can cause a problem for ulcer patients because it increases the production of stomach acid.

Decades of clinical research have isolated foods that tend to irritate the lining of the GI tract, cause spasm, stimulate acid secretion, or produce gas. By the time these studies circulate piecemeal through the professional medical community and trickle down to the consumer, it is impossible for the average person, or even the average doctor, to systematically apply them to a therapeutic nutritional plan.

The key to making any GI nutritional program work is to discover the specific foods that aggravate *your* particular symptoms. Flag Foods solve that problem, providing a way to personalize the Self-Help Nutritional Program.

Flag Foods are the specific foods that trigger particular GI disorders. The Flag Foods for your particular GI problem will soon become so familiar to you that they will be like bells going off any time you encounter them.

Flag Foods help you adjust the program in another important way. Different people suffering with the same GI complaint may require more severe dietary restraints than others. Flag Foods let you "tune" the Two-Week Master Program to make it more or less restrictive. If you find one of your Flag Foods listed in a recipe, you can eliminate or substitute for that ingredient when you prepare your meal. For example, those who are lactose intolerant may find that they can tolerate some milk products; others will have to eliminate milk products completely. (In the recipe section, every Flag Food carries an asterisk.)

The following lists present the Flag Foods that are specific irritants for each GI problem. To design your personal list, look under headings for your particular disorder(s).

You may find with experience that some Flag Foods on your list really don't bother you. If so, it's perfectly all right to include them in your diet. If they don't bother you, they probably aren't hurting your GI system.

Conversely, you may have a problem with certain foods that *don't* appear on your Flag Food list. Peppers, for example, may help stimulate the defense mechanism of the stomach lining, so they are not included on the Flag Food list for ulcers. If you think peppers are a problem for you, try eating them. If they bother you, add them to your Flag Foods list and avoid them in the future.

Heartburn

The Flag Foods for heartburn, sometimes called reflux esophagitis or gastroesophageal reflux disease (GERD), are listed in three categories. It is a good idea to (1) eliminate foods that relax the LES, (2) reduce foods that irritate the esophagus, and (3) reduce foods that form stomach acid and gas.

Flag Foods That Relax the LES

Fatty or greasy foods, including:
    Fried foods
    High-fat meats
    Untrimmed meats, poultry skin
    Butter, margarine, mayonnaise
    Cream, cream sauces
    Salad dressings
    Pastries, most desserts
    Whole-milk dairy products

Chocolate

Nuts

Peppermint

Caffeine-containing beverages, including:
    Soft drinks
    Coffee
    Cocoa
    Tea

Flag Foods That Irritate the Esophagus

Alcohol

Chili powder

Black pepper

Fruit juices, including:
    Tomato juice
    Orange juice
    Grapefruit juice

Flag Foods That Produce Stomach Acid and Gas

Caffeine beverages

Decaffeinated coffee

Milk, cream

Carbonated beverages

Note: Remember, if you have heartburn, avoid late-night snacks before bedtime, and try to keep the head of your bed elevated to prevent acid reflux.

Peptic Ulcer Disease

Flag Foods for peptic ulcer disease are similar to those for heartburn except that there is no need to eliminate foods that relax the LES, unless reflux is also a problem for you. Once you have started medication for peptic ulcer disease you may find you can eat all the Flag Foods that may aggravate patients with peptic ulcer disease.

Flag Foods for Peptic Ulcer Disease

Alcohol

Chili powder

Black pepper

Citrus juices

Decaffeinated coffee

Milk, cream

Carbonated beverages

Caffeine-containing beverages

Intestinal Gas

Intestinal gas may produce flatulence, belching, or simply pain in the abdomen. All categories of food can produce gas. It's largely a matter of discovering which specific foods bother you.

Flag Foods "Hot List" for Intestinal Gas

Milk and milk products, except lactose-reduced or lactose-free

Dried beans, peas, and lentils, including soybeans

Apricots

Broccoli

Brussels sprouts

Cabbage

Cauliflower

Corn

Grapes

Prune juice

Raisins

Turnips

Nuts

Wheat germ

Wine

Food sweetened with sorbitol

Flag Foods That Cause Gas in Some People

Fruits

Bananas	Melons
Citrus fruits	Peaches
Berries	Pears
Dried fruits	Prunes
Apples, applesauce, apple juice	

Vegetables

Asparagus

Avocado

Carrots

Celery

Cucumbers

Eggplants

Green peppers

Lettuce

Onions

Potatoes

Radishes

Sauerkraut

Scallions

Shallots

Tomatoes

Zucchini

Other

Graham crackers

Popcorn

Corn and potato chips

Soft drinks

Pastries

Wheat products

Milk Intolerance

If you suffer from milk intolerance, also called lactase deficiency, you will have to restrict your consumption of foods containing lactose. The degree of restriction varies with each person. When you begin the Two-Week Master Program, you should avoid lactose completely. Gradually, you should add small amounts of lactose to the diet while observing for symptoms of flatulence, diarrhea, and abdominal cramps.

Fermented dairy products are often well tolerated by lactase-deficient individuals and are a good source of dietary calcium, so by all means experiment with low-fat yogurt, low-fat cheese, and low-fat cultured buttermilk.

Lactaid or Lactrace, supplemental lactase enzymes, when added to milk in the recommended dose, will reduce the lactose by 70 to 100 percent.

Flag Foods "Hot List" for Milk Intolerance

Milk, skim, low-fat, or regular (except lactose-reduced or lactose-free)

Cream

Cottage cheese, ricotta cheese

Ice cream, ice milk

Frozen yogurt

Flag Foods That Most People Can Use in Moderation

Yogurt

Aged cheese

Cultured buttermilk

Chronic Pancreatitis

Flag Foods for Chronic Pancreatitis

Fatty or greasy foods, including:
  Fried foods
  High-fat meats and untrimmed meats
  Butter, margarine, mayonnaise
  Cream, cream sauces
  Chocolate, pastries, most desserts
  Salad dressings
  Whole milk dairy products

High-protein foods, including:

Nuts	Seafood
Tofu	Peanut butter
Meat	Poultry
Fish	Eggs

Constipation, Diverticulosis, IBS

The following foods (except bananas) tend to cause constipation because they are usually eaten in place of unrefined carbohydrates.

Flag Foods for Constipation, Diverticulosis, IBS

Refined sugar

Pastries

Candy

Bananas

Baked goods made with white flour

Too much meat

People who have IBS and also have gas should also avoid Flag Foods listed for intestinal gas.

Hemorrhoids

At the first sign of a hemorrhoid attack, it might be helpful to switch to a low-fiber, low-residue diet until the acute symptoms of pain and itching subside, but you should return to the Self-Help Nutritional Program as soon as possible. The following foods are known to irritate hemorrhoids.

Flag Foods for Hemorrhoids

Any hot, spicy food
Peppers

27 *Smoking, Alcohol, and Caffeine and Digestive Disorders*

Smoking and GI Disorders

The premature death rate from all diseases is much higher among smokers than nonsmokers. The mechanism by which smoking affects disease and premature death is complex and in some cases not well understood, but the statistics speak loudly and the facts are inescapable. According to statistics first released by the American Cancer Society more than twenty-five years ago, a person who smokes two packs of cigarettes a day has a premature death rate ninety times higher than that of nonsmokers.

A survey by the National Institute of Health determined that even living with people who smoke doubles a person's risk of developing cancer. The risk goes up according to how many smokers a person lives with. In fact, *smokers* living with other smokers increase their own risk of cancer, because secondhand smoke may be more toxic and laden with more carcinogens than directly inhaled smoke.

Although most people know that smoking tobacco increases the risk of cancer and heart attacks, its effects on nutrition are not as well known. We know that tobacco use hinders calcium metabolism and may accelerate osteoporosis. Many smokers use cigarettes to keep from eating, and as a result may suffer nutritional deficiencies. Other substance abuse is also known to interfere with nutrition. Cocaine alters appetite, and heavy users often develop nutritional deficiencies. The same is true of heroin addicts and people who abuse other drugs.

When it comes to GI disorders, cigarette smoking is equally hazardous. Smoking makes heartburn worse by reducing the pressure of the LES and letting acid reflux more easily. Because smoking increases the urgency to defecate, it can aggravate the symptoms of IBS. Cigarette smoking also increases the likelihood of getting ulcers, especially those caused by aspirin or ibuprofen, makes ulcers harder to heal even with strong medication, and increases the likelihood that ulcers will return after healing. Finally, smoking increases the risk of cancer of the tongue, esophagus, pancreas, and bladder.

Recent information indicates that smoking can aggravate Crohn's disease causing more frequent flares and making individuals less responsive to treatment. The exact opposite is true in ulcerative colitis. Several studies have now confirmed that ulcerative colitis will often flare when someone stops smoking. Those individuals may benefit from a nicotine patch in order to control their symptoms of ulcerative colitis; however, no doctor ever recommends a patient to commence smoking again.

Alcohol and GI Disorders

In moderation, alcohol seems to have little harmful effect on most healthy nonpregnant adults, although some recent studies dispute this. Some studies suggest that alcohol may even have several beneficial effects: it raises HDL, the good high-density lipoproteins in cholesterol, and relieves stress by relaxing tense muscles. But if a little alcohol may be helpful, a lot can be devastating.

Alcohol contributes to 10 percent of all deaths in the United States each year, including those associated with diseases affecting the liver, heart, and other vital organs, as well as accidental death and homicide.

Women are particularly vulnerable to the ill effects of alcohol because they have lower amounts of the enzyme that breaks down alcohol in their stomachs, and therefore their bodies absorb more alcohol. This may be the reason that in women the liver, the clearing-house for alcohol, is more readily damaged by alcohol. Pregnant women must be especially wary because alcohol easily crosses the placenta and damages the fetus. Babies born to alcoholic women are at high risk for fetal alcohol syndrome, a cluster of severe physical and mental defects that accounts for half of all birth defects. Even women who drink a modest, or perhaps any, amount of alcohol during pregnancy may increase their baby's risk of birth defects and of being born underweight.

Alcohol is one of the dietary factors most frequently associated with GI illness. Alcohol can damage the entire length of the GI tract and makes existing GI ailments worse across the board. Alcohol abuse creates a cancer risk, especially in the body parts that are exposed to the alcohol, such as the esophagus. In a study of more than 8,000 Japanese men living in Hawaii, those who consumed more than 16 ounces of beer daily had an increased risk of rectal cancer. Alcohol is an irritant to the stomach by damaging the stomach lining. While alcohol probably doesn't cause ulcers, it certainly can cause gastritis and can make existing ulcers worse. Because alcohol can also damage the lining of the small intestine, the absorption of nutrients may be impaired, leading to malnutrition and diarrhea. Even if alcoholics eat good diets they may still have nutritional deficiencies because the nutrients aren't absorbed.

Alcohol also causes various other nutritional problems. Excessive alcohol consumption interferes with metabolism and reduces appetite, leading to weight loss. People who drink also tend to consume quantities of caffeine and nicotine.

All the alcohol you ingest must be detoxified by the liver. So if you drink, drink in quantities that the liver can handle. The liver can normally process about 1 ounce of alcohol per hour, which translates into about 4 ounces of wine, 12 ounces of beer, or 1 ounce of distilled liquor. If you drink more than that in one hour, the liver has to work harder to clear your blood of toxic alcohol. Prolonged heavy drinking can lead to chronic inflammation and eventually scarring of the liver (cirrhosis) and death. Complications from liver disease are the ninth leading cause of death in the United States.

There is really no role for alcohol in the Self-Help Nutritional Program. While many people can tolerate small amounts of alcohol on a daily basis without having significant GI symptoms, for the most part alcohol aggravates GI conditions, particularly reflux esophagitis, gastritis, peptic ulcer disease, and sometimes gallbladder disease and IBS.

Caffeine and GI Disorders

In terms of the body as a whole, caffeine appears to produce beneficial effects when used in moderation and negative effects when used in excess. When you drink a cup of coffee, the caffeine in it is absorbed immediately. The brain is stimulated and blood flow is increased to the heart. This direct effect picks you up when you feel tired, but makes you jittery when you consume too much caffeine. Caffeine raises the basal metabolic rate so your body burns calories faster. But it also triggers the release of insulin, which makes you feel hungry. Caffeine stimulates the heart muscle and can make the heart a more efficient pump. But at high doses it can cause a too-rapid heartbeat and irregular heart rhythms.

Very little good can be said about caffeine when it comes to GI problems. Caffeine relaxes the muscles of the digestive tract and blood vessels, making the kidneys increase urinary output. Thus, caffeine can dehydrate body cells. Large amounts of coffee can cause intestinal secretion and diarrhea, while the tannins in tea can cause constipation. Caffeine also promotes the secretion of acid in the stomach. One well-designed study showed that both *regular and decaffeinated* coffee can stimulate acid secretion, so ulcer patients are advised to avoid coffee in any form.

Coffee is also notorious for its ability to induce heartburn, especially if consumed on an empty stomach. Ohio State University researchers showed that this can happen even after drinking decaffeinated coffee. All coffees cause a drop in pressure in the valve at the end of the esophagus (lower esophageal sphincter, or LES). As the LES relaxes, it allows some of the acidic stomach contents to back up, producing the typical burning effects of heartburn and indigestion. The researchers related this effect not to caffeine but to the large variety of acids, including tannic, acetic, nicotinic, formic, and citric acids, found in coffee. Tea also contains acid, in particular tannic acid, that can irritate the digestive tract. The effect of tannic acid can be countered by adding milk to tea.

Heavy coffee drinking may also cause symptoms that mimic an anxiety attack, including headache, jitteriness, upset stomach, and difficulty sleeping. Since anxiety is a trigger factor for many GI disorders, drinking coffee may set up a chain reaction: coffee leads to anxiety, anxiety leads to a reaction in the digestive system.

• Foods with Caffeine

Most obviously, caffeine is found in coffee. A 5-ounce cup of percolated coffee contains about 110 milligrams of caffeine. The same cup of coffee prepared by the drip method contains 146 milligrams of caffeine. Instant coffee, on the other hand, has about half the caffeine of regular coffee—60 milligrams in a 5-ounce cup.

On the whole, tea contains less caffeine than coffee, although some "power" teas may contain as much or even more than regular coffee. Tea brewed in bags has slightly more caffeine than loose tea, and in general, domestic brands of tea have less caffeine than the imported black teas. The longer you brew the tea, the more caffeine it contains. A cup of tea brewed with a tea bag for five minutes contains 46 milligrams of caffeine. Brewed for only one minute it contains 28 milligrams of caffeine.

Cola drinks are another source of caffeine. Although the amount of caffeine in cola drinks is much less than in coffee—ranging from 17 to 26 milligrams in 6 ounces—the serving size of soda is typically 12 ounces, which gives a caffeine dose of 34 to 53 milligrams. Cocoa and chocolate contain lesser amounts of caffeine (13 milligrams to 5 ounces).

• Alternatives to Caffeine

Decaffeinated coffee is not a useful alternative to regular coffee with regard to prevention of GI symptoms, but grain-based substitutes, such as Postum and Pero, should be all right. Some coffee substitutes are made from bran, wheat, and molasses; others are made from barley, rye, chicory, and beets. As with coffee, however, excessive consumption of grain-based products may have a laxative effect or cause flatulence.

Herbal teas may be safe substitutes for coffee, but you will need to experiment with these to see if they produce any negative effects for you. Some herbal teas can be toxic in large quantities, and all herbal teas should be used with caution.

• Breaking the Caffeine Addiction

Are you addicted to caffeine? Some people who drink only one or two cups of coffee in the morning ("Just enough to get my heart started") are addicted. One quick way to tell: Skip your morning coffee, and avoid caffeine the rest of the day. If you feel well all day, you are not addicted. If you start to develop severe headache and nausea by early afternoon, you are addicted.

The way to break a caffeine habit without turning your system upside down is to trail off slowly. Reduce your coffee consumption by one or two cups a day until you're totally off caffeine. You may have a day or two when you feel a little groggy, but it will pass quickly, and things soon return to normal. People who give up caffeine are just as alert, and function just as well, as those who consume caffeine.

PART SEVEN

Weight Considerations

28

How to Adjust Calories for Your Needs

Some of us are taller or shorter than others; some too heavy and others too thin. The Two-Week Master Program averages about 1850 calories a day—which may not be enough for some people, and may be a little too much for others. For this reason, it's important to be able to adjust the program upward or downward to suit your own needs.

Calculating Your Caloric Needs

Before making any adjustment in the diet, you should take a few minutes to discover exactly how much you should weigh and how many calories you need each day to maintain your ideal body weight.

Most people don't even come close to making an accurate assessment of how much they eat. In a study of diet histories, men underestimated their calorie intake by an average of 500 calories daily, while women missed the mark by an average of 900 calories daily. When you consider that you might need only about 1800 calories to maintain your ideal body weight, these wild guesses can become significant.

• Adding Calories

If you need more calories than are provided by these meal plans, you can increase your portions and add a little more of the high-calorie foods such as olive or canola oil and 100 percent fruit juices. If you find you are losing more weight than you wish, or if you want to gain weight, increase your portions and snack between meals on low-fat foods such as fruit, low-fat yogurt, bagels, whole-grain bread with jelly or jam, fig bars, or other

Your Most Desirable Body Weight

Most of us know when we are at our ideal body weight. But given the changing fashion dictates of our time, as well as the social demand for thinness, it's easy to get a distorted view of just how thin we should be. People who suffer from anorexia typically have a distorted view of their bodies, seeing themselves as fat even when they are bone thin.

An easy way to find out how much you should weigh is to check a height-and-weight chart such as that provided by the Metropolitan Life Insurance Company. The problem with this table and others like it is that it's based on averages and doesn't allow for individual adjustments. You can make your own quick calculation by using the following rules of thumb.

Find Your Body Frame

Wrap your thumb and index finger around the smallest part of your wrist. If your thumb and index finger touch, you are medium build. If you cannot close your fingers around your wrist, you have a large body build. And if your fingers overlap, you have a small body build.

Find Your Body Weight

WOMEN: 100 pounds for the first 5 feet
                    5 pounds for each additional inch
                    Example: 5 foot 3 inch woman
                    100 pounds + (5 × 3) = 115 pounds

MEN: 106 pounds for the first 5 feet
                    6 pounds for each additional inch
                    Example: 5 foot 11 inch man
                    106 pounds + (6 × 11) = 172 pounds

Adjust for Body Build

For small body frame—deduct 10 percent from estimated weight.
For large body frame—add 10 percent to estimated weight.

Adjust for Age

If you are more than 50 years old, add 10 percent to estimated weight.

Thus, a 5 foot 3 inch woman of medium build, age 55 years old, should weigh about 115 + 11.5 (10%) = 126.5 pounds.

How Many Calories?

It's difficult to calculate how many calories you need to reach and maintain your ideal body weight, because many variables are in play. You can have your caloric needs charted by a qualified professional in a hospital, weight loss center, or exercise physiology center. The technique involves measuring oxygen consumption and carbon dioxide production. Sometimes centers use standardized formulas to calculate caloric needs. This kind of detailed calculation is usually reserved for severely malnourished or severely obese people. Most people do not need to know their caloric needs so precisely. The following formula can give you a fairly accurate ballpark figure, without investing in an expensive testing procedure. To calculate how many calories you need, you first need to assess your activity level.

• What Is Your Activity Level?

Sedentary—mostly sitting throughout the day: office work, studying, lab work, teaching, and no regular exercise program

Moderately active—mostly standing and walking, very little sitting in your job; or if your job is sedentary, you exercise about three times a week

Very active—daily vigorous exercise or sports

• Calculate Your Calorie Needs

Sedentary—13 calories per pound

Moderately active—14 calories per pound

Very active—15 calories per pound

Thus, a sedentary woman weighing 115 pounds needs 1495 (115×13) calories a day to maintain her weight.

low-fat cookies (see recipes). In other words, eat all of the same foods as on the Two-Week Master Program, but eat more of them.

Note: If you are underweight as a result of your GI disorder and need to gain weight, be sure to read chapter 31.

Subtracting Calories

A low-fat diet such as the Two-Week Master Program is automatically good for weight control. Most people who follow the program will lose weight or control weight easily without counting calories. Most of the calories come from carbohydrates, which are more readily turned into energy than fat calories.

However, if the 1850-calorie level is too high for you, there are three easy ways to cut calories without losing the digestive benefits of the diet.

1   You can reduce calories most efficiently by eliminating or decreasing the added fats—margarines, mayonnaise, oil—and by using a lower-fat salad dressing. (Recipes are given in chapter 45 for both a moderate-fat and a low-fat dressing.)

2   You can reduce the portion size of the recipes. If you do reduce portion sizes, you should make up for any possible loss of nutrients by taking a multivitamin and mineral supplement.

3   You can choose those recipes with the least fat content. Even though all GI recipes are fairly low in fat, some have almost no fat at all. Stick with those extremely low-fat recipes to give you the most nutrition for your calories. We have included the fat content in every recipe for your convenience.

All recipes in the last section of this book have their calorie content listed, and their macronutrients itemized. Every recipe and meal plan provides information about fat, protein, carbohydrate, fiber, and calorie values. This means that you can pick and choose recipes that appeal to you, meet the requirements of your GI problem, and provide the number of calories you wish to consume each day.

29 *Losing Weight*

*I*f you have GI complaints and are overweight, one of the best things you can do for yourself is shed excess pounds. Extra weight aggravates many GI problems, especially heartburn, excessive intestinal gas, belching, and gallstones. Obesity may also have a damaging effect on the liver (see chapter 25).

Obesity is associated with many other significant health problems. If you are more than 20 percent above your ideal body weight you have a higher than normal risk of developing high blood pressure, heart disease, diabetes, high cholesterol, and several types of cancer, including colon, breast, and uterine cancer in women, and prostate cancer in men. Your risk is higher if you carry the extra weight around your middle rather than around your hips or thighs. (So you may need to exercise to get rid of a spare tire, even if you aren't obese.)

By contrast, weight control has been proved to be an important factor in lowering the risk of coronary heart disease, high blood pressure, and diabetes, and it plays an important role in any cholesterol-lowering plan. Obese individuals tend to have low HDL-cholesterol levels, the good cholesterol that helps fight heart disease. Weight loss can raise HDL cholesterol, lower the bad LDL cholesterol, and improve the cholesterol ratio. Studies have documented many cases in which patients have shown significant improvement in serum cholesterol, triglycerides, and blood sugar, as well as blood pressure, after losing only one-quarter of the weight they needed to lose to reach their ideal weight goal. So even modest weight loss is important for improving health.

Causes of Weight Problems

Our ability to eat almost everything and turn it into usable fuel has its down side. We have developed a taste for a bewildering variety of foods, and as a result some of us are attracted to the low end of the nutritional scale, and many of us overeat. In America one person in four is overweight.

Lifestyle influences weight problems. In a large study of families where regular activity and proper eating habits were encouraged, children had better nutritional habits and were slimmer and more active. Economics also plays a part. Large surveys show that low-income women are more likely to have a weight problem than more affluent women. Why? One might speculate that with less money to spend on quality foods and several mouths to feed, poor women purchase the least expensive and subsequently least nutritious foods. Self-image and social habits probably play a part, also. We know that people who watch a lot of television are fatter than those who don't. TV viewing burns almost no calories and encourages continual trips to the refrigerator.

All of that being said, there's more to excess weight than eating habits and lifestyle. Several new scientific studies have shown the strong genetic basis of obesity, proving that obesity is a real disease, not a personality disorder. One large study of more than 6,000 adults found that overweight people did not eat more than their normal-weight peers, even when exercise levels were taken into consideration. Different people burn calories at different rates. And some people are born with more fat cells than others, which makes it easier for them to gain weight.

Fat cells are the cells that make up adipose tissue (fat). You are born with a certain number of fat cells. Overfeeding in infancy can increase weight by increasing the number of fat cells. But as an adult, the number of your fat cells is generally fixed, and weight gain occurs as the size of each fat cell increases. That's why if the fat cells are removed surgically (suction lipectomy), they tend not to come back.

Yet even with this strong new evidence pointing straight at genetics, most of us still believe that if fat people would just stop eating so much they would be thin. We assume that heavy people have less willpower than thin people. Even overweight people themselves and, more surprisingly, doctors, believe that being fat is the individual's fault and that somehow they are weak people.

People who are overweight in modern American society have a tough social scenario to live with. Thin is in, fat is out, and this social dictate appears to be securely entrenched. Overweight people, even those within ten to twenty pounds of their ideal weight, are subject to close social scrutiny. Go to any party or social gathering and listen to the immediate comments on weight gain or weight loss: "Lois, you look wonderful. Have you lost weight?" "Max, good to see you. You've put on a few pounds, haven't you?" "Jane, I feel I have to say this to you, you need to lose some weight."

We even do it to ourselves. "Sarah, how are you?" "Okay, I guess, but I've got to lose ten pounds." Growing up with this burden of guilt can obviously be a source of great anxiety and stress.

The causes of obesity are many and complex: genetics, faulty appetite control, poor eating habits and food choices, emotional and cultural factors. A better knowledge of nutrition and how it works, along with exercise, are the keys to healthy weight control. But many of us still turn to drastic dieting as a solution. About 34 million Americans are overweight, but at least 70 million think they should be on a diet!

Bad News Diets

At any given time, some 20 million of us actually are on some sort of weight-loss diet, and this obsession has led us into some dangerous eating habits—eating binges alternating with fasting.

People who are overweight tend to bounce from one weight-loss plan to another, doing much damage to their bodies in the process. Many very-low-calorie diets are unsafe and ultimately ineffective. Constipation and intolerance to cold can result from very-low-calorie diets. Gout, abdominal cramps, and fainting spells may result from fasting. Many of the early liquid diets provided such low-quality protein that vital body organs became starved, and in a few instances death resulted. Such diets caused depletion of important vitamins and minerals such as calcium, magnesium, sodium, and potassium, leading to disastrous shifts in electrolyte balance. The worst problem, from the dieter's point of view, is that after such struggling and deprivation they eventually regain all of the lost weight, and often more. Many studies have shown that 95 percent of those who lose weight will regain it over the next two years.

The Good News

While the Self-Help Nutritional Program is primarily a therapeutic diet designed to prevent and treat digestive disorders, it is also an excellent weight-loss vehicle. It is high in nutrition, but lower in fat—and calories—than standard American fare. At the same time it rates high on the satisfaction scale.

Hunger is the number-one diet breaker. The high fiber content of the Self-Help Nutritional Program means that you probably won't feel hunger pangs even though you are eating less. Most people who follow the program to lose weight never feel deprived, even though they are consuming fewer calories than usual.

When you eat high-fiber foods, fluid causes the fiber to expand and occupy a greater volume in the stomach. When the stomach is distended, signals pass through nerve endings in the stomach walls, up the central nervous system to the brain, and the brain senses that you are full. Soluble fiber slows down the rate at which the stomach empties, which means that you feel fuller for a longer time. Thus, a high-fiber program provides greater satisfaction with fewer calories, a big help in reducing the stress associated with dieting. Many people on a high-fiber diet even forget they are dieting.

Because high-fiber foods are also complex carbohydrates, most people seem to lose their desire for desserts and candy. High-fiber intake lowers the level of blood insulin, which reduces your desire for food, especially sweets.

Beyond all of these weight-loss benefits, and even more important from a health standpoint, including high-fiber foods in your diet can help make weight control a permanent part of your life. Finding a way to control weight with the foods that also enhance and extend our lives is an important goal.

Fats vs. Carbohydrates

Overweight people who begin the Two-Week Master Program almost always lose weight automatically because, gram for gram, vegetables, fruits, grains, and other complex carbohydrates contain fewer calories than fats. Every gram of carbohydrate has 4 calories, while every gram of fat has more than twice that number. There are 454 grams in a pound, so a pound of carbohydrate contains 1816 calories. But a pound of fat contains 4086 calories!

By replacing fat with complex carbohydrates, you reduce calories, even though you may actually be eating *more* food. We speak of the number of calories per unit of weight as *caloric density*. Fatty food has greater caloric density than any other food. Since our program is low in fat, it has low caloric density—which means it is ideal for weight loss.

In addition, the body doesn't have to work very hard to store fat as opposed to carbohydrate. The body stores fat so efficiently that it uses only 3 calories to convert 100 calories of dietary fat into body fat. In contrast, the body must spend 23 calories to convert 100 calories of dietary carbohydrate into body fat. This means that you burn less energy after a fatty meal than after a carbohydrate-enriched meal, another factor leading to weight gain.

Overall, by concentrating on complex carbohydrates, the Two-Week Master Program is set up to give you minimum caloric density, at the same time that it forces the body to burn maximum calories to process the food it takes in.

Cutting Calories

The Two-Week Master Program provides about 1850 calories per day. If you now eat more than 3000 calories per day—and many people do—you can expect to lose a significant amount of weight on the program simply by following the recommended meal plans. If you now eat 2500 calories per day, you can expect to lose about 5½ pounds a month on the program.

If you want to lose weight but don't know how many calories you now consume every day, try this method: begin the Two-Week Master Program, follow portion allocations carefully, and keep track of your weight twice a week. If your weight remains the same, repeat the program for two more weeks, adjusting the calorie count downward (see chapter 6).

If you haven't lost weight after one month, consult your physician or a registered dietitian to help you design a personal weight-loss program that incorporates the principles of the program.

Diet Isn't Always Enough

Following the Two-Week Master Program is only part of a good weight-control program. Every person has a unique biochemical makeup, a preprogrammed rate at which their body burns calories. And this programming can make even the lowest-calorie diet virtually useless. A combination of your genetic makeup, the number of fat cells accumulated in your body as a child, and your current eating habits determines the weight your body would like to be. This is called "set point."

Everyone has a personal set point and it is enough to drive any dedicated dieter crazy. The more strenuously you diet, the less weight you lose as the body strives to maintain its hold on the status quo. You cut back a little more. And a little more. After several weeks of arduous calorie-cutting, you have lost a total of five or six pounds, and you can't bear the deprivation any more. You say to yourself, "If this is what it takes to lose weight, I'd rather be fat."

This set point business is part of our marvelous evolutionary advantage. When you reduce your calorie intake, your body compensates by slowing down your metabolism. The lungs use less oxygen. Cell replacement and building slow down. Vital organs reduce their demand for calories. The whole body goes into a state of semihibernation.

The set point has allowed the human species to survive periods of starvation and poor nutrition. Even now it works in our favor. For example, if you overeat on a weekend cruise, your body will start to burn calories faster because the set point speeds up your metabolism to process the unexpected excess. But if your ship goes down and you are cast adrift in a lifeboat, the set point will protect you by lowering your metabolism to burn energy slowly. Unhappily, if you cut calories on purpose to lose weight, your set point will also try to protect you against loss.

People who go off and on diets frequently are in even worse shape. Resupplied with food after a period of deprivation, the body immediately sets to work to convert as much food as possible to fat, to store up in case of yet another bout of deprivation. Yo-yo dieters may have a permanently slower metabolism because their set point is trying to keep things under control. They may have to restrict calories to 1000 calories a day or even less to lose weight.

Everyone wants a magic food that will effortlessly lower the set point and increase metabolism. Is it grapefruit? Is it protein? It might as well be a bird or a plane.

While the set point makes things more difficult, it is not invincible. The good news is that you can affect your body's set point and you can shake your metabolism free from its doldrums, but the magic isn't food. It's exercise (see following chapter).

Some individuals take diet drugs to lose weight. Phenylpropanolamine, an OTC drug, and phentermine (Ionamin, Adipex-P), a prescription drug, stimulate the sympathetic nervous system and may cause certain gastrointestinal side effects including dry mouth, diarrhea, constipation, and nausea. Similar side effects can be seen with sibutramine (Meridia), a relatively new prescription drug. The newest anti-obesity drug, orlistat (Xenical), interferes with the digestion of dietary fat. About one-third of the fat ingested doesn't get absorbed, resulting in greasy stools.

30 *Exercise to Control Weight and Improve Digestive Function*

*E*xercise is the most efficient way to lower your body's set point and raise your metabolism. Exercise gives you energy, elevates your metabolism to burn fat more quickly, and lets you eat more without gaining weight. Furthermore, exercise can help people with irritable bowel syndrome and constipation because it promotes laxation and generally makes you feel better. Exercise also helps reduce stress, the great aggravator of most GI problems (see chapter 18).

Exercise, the Mood Lifter

One great appeal of exercise, in terms of improved quality of life, is the remarkable sense of well-being it produces. Theoretically, this response is caused by the body's reaction to strong muscular activity: extra brain chemicals, called endorphins, are released to make the exertion less painful. The longer muscular effort continues, the more chemicals are released and the more euphoric you feel. These same chemicals tend to improve gastrointestinal motility.

Exercise is also a good antidote to boredom, one common reason that many of us overeat. Another interesting side benefit is that smokers who actively engage in such activities as swimming and jogging tend to quit smoking cigarettes, thereby eliminating a devastating risk factor for many life-threatening diseases, and a major culprit when it comes to digestive problems.

The Many Ways Exercise Helps Weight Loss

We used to believe that exercise helped weight loss simply by burning more calories. Now we know that regular exercise enhances weight loss in a host of different ways.

- Exercise burns calories. To lose a pound of fat, you must burn 3500 calories. Anything that helps burn calories is a good adjunct to dieting.
- Exercise speeds up your metabolic rate. The good effect lasts hours after you've finished exercising so that you continue to burn calories at a higher rate. If you exercise before you eat you'll benefit not only from the calories burned during exercise but from additional calories burned after the meal.
- Exercise helps control your appetite by stabilizing insulin and blood sugar.
- Exercise increases muscle mass. Muscle is the major calorie-using tissue in the body. The more muscle you have, the more food you can eat without adding body fat.
- Exercise maintains lean muscle tissue, tones up the body, and makes you look better and feel stronger.
- Exercise elevates your mood. Because you feel better when you exercise, it's easier to stick with your weight-loss diet.
- Exercise helps relieve stress.

Besides helping you lose weight, exercise protects your heart by helping to lower blood pressure and cholesterol.

A special note: Exercise is clearly beneficial, but it cannot overcome the damage done by a fatty diet. You cannot get away with a steady diet of burgers, french fries, and shakes and hope to exercise off the fat and cholesterol.

What Kind of Exercise?

The best exercises for helping both the heart and the digestive system are swimming, walking, and bicycling. Swimming is the least stressful of this aerobic group of exercises. Walking is better than jogging because it places minimal strain on the heels, ankles, shins, and knee joints, so the walker seldom suffers the pain of ligament damage.

A word of caution about running: recent research has confirmed what many joggers have suspected all along, that vigorous exercise, especially running, can cause heartburn even if you have not eaten recently.

Running appears to induce more reflux than exercises that involve less agitation. Dr. Donald Castell, current president of the American Gastroenterological Association, and his previous group at Bowman Gray

Medical School of Wake Forest University in Winston-Salem, N.C., observed the acid levels of seven men and five women as they performed a one-hour exercise routine after a day of fasting and one hour after eating a small meal. Running consistently caused the most reflux. Weight lifting caused less reflux, and bicycling caused the least. The findings suggest that people who suffer indigestion might benefit from less jostling activities, such as bicycling.

The chest pain some people experience during exercise, which is a primary indicator of angina, may be caused by heartburn. If the chest pain is accompanied by belching or regurgitation, the problem is probably in the stomach, not the heart. However, anyone who experiences chest pain during exercise should see a doctor for evaluation and diagnosis.

How Much Exercise?

How much exercise you need to maintain health and control weight remains controversial. It appears that a less rigorous workout may be just as beneficial as strenuous activities. A continuing study of 17,000 Harvard College alumni also suggests that moderate physical exercise can increase life expectancy. In a nutshell, even moderate exercise carried out on a fairly regular basis is good for you. In terms of heart benefits, the regularity of the exercise is more important than the type of physical activity you choose. You're better off taking a brisk walk every day than playing tennis once a week. Most experts recommend a steady aerobic workout for about thirty minutes, three to five times a week.

How hard should you work out? You don't have to exercise at maximum exertion. When you must gasp for breath, the body turns up the burners on carbohydrate. That's not so good. Carbohydrates burn fast enough as it is. When you get enough air, the body uses mostly fat for fuel. That's better. So, if you must gasp to speak, you're working too hard and need to slow things down. Keep your exercise at a level that lets you speak if necessary, but not chatter on indefinitely.

Getting Started

Regular exercise should be a part of everyone's lifestyle, yet statistics from the Centers for Disease Control show that 59 percent of Americans get less than twenty minutes of physical activity three times a week.

Many people find it hard to get started. Once they do get started, they

Take a Walk

Walking is almost the perfect exercise, chiefly because it fits in with most people's lifestyle and can easily be carried out in a consistent manner. Walking makes the whole body function more efficiently, and there is no doubt that walking can reduce stress and improve general well-being.

CALORIES USED UP IN ONE HOUR'S WALK

Walking Speed (miles per hour)	*Your Weight in Pounds*						
	100	120	140	160	180	200	220
2	130	160	185	210	240	265	290
2½	155	185	220	250	280	310	345
3	180	215	250	285	325	360	395
3½	205	248	290	330	375	415	455
4	235	280	325	375	420	470	515
4½	310	370	435	495	550	620	680
5	385	460	540	615	690	770	845

Although walking won't help you lose weight fast, over time it can make a difference. The trick is to be consistent, and keep your feet moving at a brisk pace. Taking a stroll and window shopping doesn't count. Neither does meandering up and down the aisles of the supermarket, unless you're going at a dead run. A brisk one-hour walk can burn more than 300 calories an hour—the faster you walk, the more calories you burn. One-half hour of brisk walking every day can result in a 15-pound weight loss in the period of one year.

find it difficult to continue. Part of the problem may be our perception that exercise must be performed at a specific time and in a specific place. It's true that a regular workout is ideal, but a lot of us are in the midst of playing catch-up with our daily lives. Our obligations are many, time still comes in the same twenty-four-hour allotments, and doing *anything* at precisely the same time three times a week may seem impossible. So we don't exercise at all.

If you are having trouble getting a regular program going, remember that even erratic physical activity is better than being completely sedentary. And any kind of activity is better than nothing at all. Some of us have access to gym equipment or swimming pools. Some of us enjoy sports and

Everyday Ways to Lower Your Body's Set Point

One way to begin to lower your body's set point is to sneak up on it. Think about physical activities that you enjoy and that are readily accessible to you. Dancing is good exercise, and so is table tennis. So is mopping the floor and washing the car, if you like to do it. Here are some recommendations from physical trainers of simple ways to incorporate more physical activity into daily life.

• If you work at a sedentary job, make a point of getting up every hour for a couple of minutes and walking somewhere in the office building. Climb up and down a flight of stairs, for example.

• Leave home earlier in the morning and walk to a farther bus stop than usual. On your way home, get off the bus a couple of stops before your regular stop. Instead of parking your car in the most convenient place, park it in the least convenient, the spot that makes you walk a little to reach your destination.

• Engage in at least one specific exercise session one day a week. Choose an aerobic exercise that uses your whole body. Swim or work out on a regular day, or try an exercise class at lunch hour or after work. If you get bored with the exercise you have chosen, change it. Change it every week if you like, but do some form of real exercise on your Exercise Day.

• On your Exercise Day, don't attempt too much too soon. If you choose swimming, for example, settle for doing a couple of laps the first time you go. Work up gradually until you reach the time and distance where you feel most comfortable. If you get one regular Exercise Day started and it feels good, increase it to two and then three days when you're ready.

• Run through a series of easy stretching exercises or calisthenics when you get out of bed in the morning.

• Take a brisk walk every day, no matter how brief.

• Buy a stationary exercise bike or a treadmill for your use at home. (Make sure you remember to get on it.) If you use an exercise bike, you may have to take short frequent breaks when you first begin. But if you stick with it you can extend your riding time until eventually you will be cycling more than you are resting.

• Try to find a sport you like to play. If you are competitive by nature (Type A's take heed), make sure you take it easy on your opponents until you get into good condition. Then go for it.

• After every exercise session, no matter what it is, take a little time to completely relax physically.

have the opportunity to play frequently. And some of us have none of these things. But with a little imagination it should be possible for everyone to engage in some kind of physical activity. Try to make it as regular as you can. The one thing to avoid is extreme physical exercise on an occasional basis.

Exercise will not only help you lose or control your weight, it offers very specific benefits to the GI tract. Exercise is excellent for constipation because it improves bowel function. (But marathon runners may get diarrhea because vigorous exercise can improve bowel function *too* much.) Because it helps relieve stress, exercise may decrease the incidence of ulcers and the symptoms of IBS.

There is a triad of good health prescriptives that goes like this: weight control, exercise, and stress reduction. They are interrelated. Exercise and weight maintenance are closely tied together. Exercise and stress relief are also closely linked. And all three components can have considerable impact on your health, particularly your risk for heart disease and GI problems. Of the three, stress is the most mysterious, and the most critically involved with digestive problems.

A Word of Caution

If you are over the age of thirty-five or if you have a family history of heart disease, you should consult your physician before starting an exercise program. Also, if you are in very poor condition, if you are a heavy smoker, seriously overweight, or under treatment for a medical condition, check with your doctor before embarking on an exercise regimen. You may first need to undertake supervised exercise with a trainer to work yourself into better condition. If you haven't done any physical exercise in a while, be certain to start off slowly and gradually increase your tolerance.

Don't ever go from a resting state to hard exercise. Warm-up exercises are essential to get muscles working. Similarly, after exercise, cool-down exercises will keep muscles relaxed and warm until they are fully rested.

If you feel sick or dizzy, feel a tightness in your chest, get a severe headache, or see spots, stop exercising at once and check with your doctor as soon as possible. You may have an underlying problem that needs treatment. Never push yourself beyond what feels reasonable. Exercise is never better if it hurts. After an exercise session you should feel invigorated, not devastated.

31 *If You Need to Gain Weight*

*B*elieve it or not, some people have a problem maintaining adequate weight. Many people are thin for genetic reasons—that's just the way they are and it is normal for them. Thinness can also be caused by poor eating habits. Many underweight people eat virtually nothing throughout the day and only a small meal at night. Erratic eating habits are another common cause. Sometimes people become underweight because, under temporary stress or illness, they just stop eating.

These kinds of weight-loss problems are usually fairly easy to correct. But sometimes weight loss can be a symptom that requires special attention because it can signify a serious underlying disease state.

Unexplained Weight Loss

Many digestive problems can prevent nutrients from being absorbed and properly used. Any serious disease—cancer, severe lung, heart, or kidney disorder—can cause loss of appetite and weight loss. In fact, weight loss can be caused by virtually any disease of any body system. Severe depression, for example, may lead to weight loss. (A little stress may make us eat more, but a lot of stress often makes us lose our appetite.) Anorexia nervosa, a kind of self-induced starvation undertaken by some women who perceive themselves as fat no matter how thin they become, also leads to dangerously low weight levels.

Just as obesity can create digestive problems, too little weight is also a feature of some GI problems. Because the digestive tract is responsible for the intake, digestion, and processing of food, it is not surprising that when things go wrong with the tract itself, weight loss is sometimes a by-product.

• Painful Swallowing

In many cases, weight loss is caused by poor intake of food. For example, heartburn may be so severe that swallowing becomes painful, or certain foods burn on the way down, so people stop eating. The Self-Help Nutritional Program can help relieve acid reflux, the cause of an inflamed esophagus.

If scar tissue builds up inside the esophagus and causes narrowing, it may be difficult to swallow solid foods. Liquids may go down fairly well, but any food particle larger than the esophageal opening will stick. Weight loss may be the result.

Difficult swallowing can also occur if the esophagus doesn't contract properly. The esophagus may look perfectly normal, but instead of squeezing ingested foods along in an orderly fashion, it may contract erratically, causing food to stick along the route. With this kind of problem, known as a motility disorder, even liquids may cause difficulties. Drug therapy is often needed to control the spasm. The Self-Help Nutritional Program can also help by preventing the acid reflux that triggers the spasm.

Difficulty swallowing can also be caused by tumors of the esophagus, and painful swallowing can be caused by fungal and viral infections of the esophagus, so it is important to see your doctor for any swallowing problems.

• Early Satiety

Weight loss can also be caused by stomach disorders. In this case a hungry person feels full after eating only a small amount. The stomach, which acts as a reservoir, is designed to expand to accommodate food. Stomach tumors make it difficult for the stomach to expand; therefore an early feeling of fullness is a common symptom. Some people always eat small meals, but if you notice a change in your eating pattern, it's important to pay attention. People who have long-standing diabetes may also develop early satiety and weight loss due to defective emptying of the stomach. Otherwise normal individuals may also have early satiety from defective emptying of the stomach, called gastroparesis (see chapter 6).

Early satiety and difficult swallowing are two important symptoms that require prompt evaluation by a physician because they may be caused by serious underlying disease.

• A Damaged Small Intestine

Any damage to the small intestine can affect food absorption and lead to weight loss. Crohn's disease (ileitis) and gluten-sensitive enteropathy (sprue), a wheat allergy, are two examples. Diseases of the small intestine can be quite serious. In mild disease, the Self-Help Nutritional Program may be helpful. But for most patients, treatment involves a highly individualized dietary and medical regimen designed by a physician working closely with a nutritionist. (In severe Crohn's disease, for example, the patient may have to be fed intravenously at first, then, with improvement, eventually progress to a low-residue, low-lactose, low-fat diet.)

Diseases of the large intestine generally do not cause weight loss because by the time food reaches the colon most of the nutrients have been absorbed. Only if the condition is severe enough to cause general sickness throughout the body, as in colon cancer or severe colitis, is weight loss likely to result.

How to Gain Weight

When otherwise healthy people are underweight, the problem can usually be corrected by stabilizing eating patterns, so that they eat three meals a day, and increasing calorie intake. This does not mean adding empty calories found in desserts and junk foods. It means concentrating on foods that are high in vitamins, minerals, and calories. Examples are whole grains, nuts, seeds, and dried fruits. Those following the Self-Help Nutritional Program can increase their portions and concentrate on the recipes that are somewhat higher in calories.

Dietary Supplements

Some people with digestive disorders associated with weight loss may need more than the Self-Help Nutritional Program. A wide variety of dietary supplements, with varying amounts of protein, fat, and lactose, are on the market, each designed to help overcome a specific nutritional and digestive problem. A supplement may be high in fiber or low in fiber. It may be high in fat or low in fat. Supplements are selected to match the individual's medical and nutritional needs. For example, certain conditions require extra protein. Some require a low-fiber, low-residue supplement. Some need extra fat.

If you are underweight because of any medical problem and require supplements to maintain body weight, it is essential that you contact your physician or a registered dietitian—or both—to make sure you choose a supplement designed to treat your condition.

As long as you have a normal or near normal small intestine and a stomach that empties reasonably well you will be able to use a standard polymeric formulation if you need extra calories in your diet. Polymeric formulations contain whole protein, fat, and carbohydrates just like in a regular diet except in liquid form. Therefore, you need a normal or near normal gastrointestinal tract in order to digest and absorb a polymeric nutritional supplement. Examples of polymeric formulations are Ensure and Sustacal. Ensure and Sustacal are designed to be palatable (taste good) so they can be taken by mouth. If you are being fed with a polymeric formulation through a gastrostomy tube or jejunostomy tube, there is no need to use the more expensive palatable formulations. Unpalatable products such as Isocal or Jevity should be used.

If your intestines are significantly damaged either by Crohn's disease or radiation, or if you have had surgical removal of a large portion of your small intestine, you may need what is called a chemically defined formulation. This preparation contains partially digested food in the form of amino acids and peptides instead of protein, and glucose instead of carbohydrates. These formulations tend to be unpalatable. If you want to take them by mouth rather than via a nasogastric tube or gastrostomy tube, ask a dietitian about adding flavor packets to improve taste. Subdue is a new chemically defined formulation that actually tastes good. These preparations may also be useful for those patients who have diarrhea and those who have a low serum albumin level who may not tolerate polymeric formulations. Examples of chemical defined formulations are Vital, Peptamen, and Riabolin.

Those individuals who have a severely compromised gut may require an elemental diet that contains just fatty acids, amino acids, and sugar. This preparation is predigested and easy to absorb. These preparations, such as Vivonex-TEN, are not palatable and usually require administration through a nasogastric, gastrostomy, or jejunostomy tube. Elemental diets have a high osmolality and are more likely to cause diarrhea than other preparations.

If you are being fed through a tube, remember that jejunostomy feedings need to be given by continuous infusion, whereas feedings through a nasogastric tube and gastrostomy tube can be given either by continuous infusion or by bolus (a large number of calories over a short period of time) infusion. Patients fed by a jejunostomy tube are usually those individuals who have impaired stomach emptying and those individuals who tend to choke on regurgitated feedings when infused into the stomach.

Occasionally, your diet may be deficient in one particular macronutrient (fat, protein, or carbohydrate) and in this case your doctor may prescribe a modular nutritional supplement. If you need supplemental protein, a modular feeding such as Promod, which just contains protein, may be prescribed. If you just need supplemental calories, a modular feeding of Polycose containing glucose polymers may be recommended. If you have a short or diseased small intestine, you may have difficulty absorbing long-chain fatty acids, the usual digestion product of dietary fat. In this case your doctor may prescribe MCT oil (medium-chain triglycerides), which is more easily absorbed by the small intestines.

Total Parenteral Nutrition

Occasionally, the small intestine is so diseased that a person is not able to derive enough calories from food taken orally or infused through a feeding tube and the nutrition must be given intravenously (through a vein). The vein usually chosen is the subclavian vein located just below the collarbone. If total parenteral nutrition is contemplated on a long-term basis a special catheter called a Hickman catheter or a Port-a-Cath is placed. Since total parenteral nutrition is extremely expensive and fraught with complication—such as blood clots in the veins, infection, metabolic abnormalities (abnormal blood chemistry), and liver disease—it should be used only when absolutely necessary. Those individuals who require total parenteral nutrition at home should contact the Oley Foundation.

PART EIGHT

Your Gastrointestinal Maintenance Plan

32   *Keeping Track of Your Progress*

*T*he goal of the Self-Help Nutritional Program is to reduce the frequency and severity of GI symptoms. The more frequent and severe the symptoms before starting the diet, the easier it will be to measure the results. Relief from milder symptoms usually cannot be measured in such a dramatic manner. However, measuring your success with the program is a good way to motivate yourself and maintain your success.

The best way to assess your progress is to keep a diary of your symptoms before and after starting the Two-Week Master Program. This doesn't mean that you will have to make diary entries forever. Keep the diary for several days before starting the program to get an average "baseline." After starting the program, continue to maintain the diary for two full weeks. This way you can easily determine how much progress you are making.

When you have completed the first two weeks, continue to incorporate the principles of the Master Program into your normal eating routine, and continue to keep track of your progress in your diary. At first you may feel compulsive about making entries, tracking even minor symptoms. Eventually, you will probably slow down and record only those symptoms that seem significant to you.

The diary will help you maintain your motivation after your symptoms have decreased. When you are feeling well and are free of pain and discomfort, it's easy to believe that it was always thus. Looking at your diary occasionally will help you remember what it was like before you started the Self-Help Nutritional Program.

Charting Your Progress

To begin, note the times of day you eat. Then record the symptoms as they occur.

Use any code that's easy for you. We use simple initials to denote:

B   Belching

C   Constipation

Cr   Cramps

D   Diarrhea

F   Flatulence

H   Heartburn

P   Pain

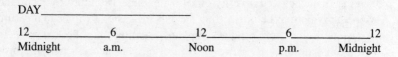

Here's an example of how to use the daily chart. Bill suffered from gastroesophageal reflux disease (GERD). He would wake up in the middle of the night coughing and have a sour taste in his mouth. His voice was hoarse. He would get heartburn when he lay down and when bending over. He also suffered from frequent belching.

Before starting the Two-Week Master Program, Bill's daily chart looked like this:

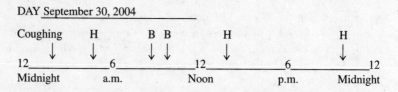

After one week on the program, antacids, and elevation of his bed, his chart looked like this:

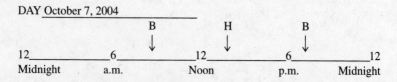

After completing two weeks, it looked like this:

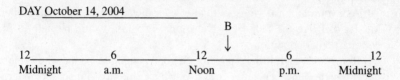

DAY October 14, 2004

Working with Your Doctor

The proper diagnosis and treatment of your digestive problem, as well as preventive maintenance, depends on a close, open, and effective working relationship between you and your doctor. This is true whether your doctor is a general practitioner, family physician, or internist, or a specialist in digestive diseases. You and your doctor are partners in the care of your GI disorder.

• Your Responsibilities as Patient

See Your Doctor When Symptoms Develop. It always amazes me how some people will take their pet to the veterinarian at the drop of a hat, or their child to a pediatrician at the first sniffle, but ignore potentially serious symptoms of disease in themselves. Part of this is a normal denial that we are sick, or an irrational feeling of being immortal. Some people don't like to spend money on themselves, and put their needs low on the priority list. In the case of some men, it's a case of "macho men don't get sick." This is particularly unfortunate when it comes to GI disorders because men tend to have more serious organic causes of GI disease than women do. So when symptoms occur, see your doctor sooner rather than later.

Be as Open as Possible with Your Doctor. Your description of your symptoms is 80 percent of the diagnosis. When it comes to GI disorders, your doctor usually cannot find out what's wrong with you just by tapping on your chest or pushing on your stomach. You need to describe your problem in detail. Don't withhold information because you think it's insignificant. Or embarrassing. No matter how embarrassing the symptoms, you must tell your doctor in order to get a diagnosis based on all the facts.

Question Your Doctor. It's important for you to understand the nature of your problem, why you need certain tests, and what they are like, including potential risks. Ask your doctor about the safety and effectiveness of any medication prescribed and what side effects to look out for.

Ask your doctor if you should alter your diet, and whether a high-fiber, low-fat diet like the Self-Help Nutritional Program would be helpful for your particular condition.

Remember, an informed patient is a good patient, someone who is more likely to experience a positive result. When it comes to GI disorders that require lifetime maintenance to avoid symptoms, your full cooperation and understanding are crucial.

Follow Your Doctor's Recommendations.   It's important for you to be as compliant as possible with your doctor's recommendations. It's fairly common for patients to come to our hospital after not improving on treatment instituted elsewhere. Often the diagnosis was correct, the treatment plan was correct, but somewhere along the way a breakdown in communications occurred, and the patients weren't doing what they were supposed to do. When it comes to GI disorders, a patient has to take most of the responsibility for the treatment program. Some people may subconsciously want to maintain their sick role because of the secondary gains that are associated with being sick (more attention, relief from household chores, etc.). While these secondary gains may seem attractive in the short term, ultimately maintaining a healthy mind and body will make you a more happy and successful person.

• Responsibilities of Your Doctor

See You as Soon as Possible When You Have Symptoms.   If you have serious symptoms like profuse rectal bleeding, vomiting of blood, severe abdominal pain, jaundice, or fever and chills, you should call your doctor immediately. If the doctor's secretary gives you an appointment two weeks down the road, that is inappropriate. Ask to speak to the doctor; if you cannot be seen right away, you may be directed to an emergency room.

On the other hand, if your complaint is belching, flatulence, or lifelong constipation that hasn't recently changed, waiting a few weeks for an appointment is probably medically safe.

Be Nonjudgmental.   You should feel comfortable telling your doctor all of your problems. Doctors need to know about intravenous drug abuse, homosexuality, and other behavior associated with high risk for diseases such as hepatitis, chronic diarrhea, and AIDS.

Allow Enough Time.   If the doctor doesn't allow enough time for an open exchange, much important information may be lost. Furthermore, if your doctor tries to direct the conversation, you may never get to some points you want to make. Doctors tend to do this at times to avoid listening to the details of every morsel of food a patient has eaten in the last week or to an entire treatise devoted to bowel function. However, important details are often embedded in these long exhortations. If you tend to be long-winded, unfocused, or just have difficulty talking to your doctor—or if your doctor tends to rush you—make a list of the things you think are important prior to your visit. That way you won't forget anything important, and your doctor won't be able to ignore the points you have written down.

The goal is to develop a smooth working relationship with your doctor, rather than an adversarial one.

Inform You About Tests.   Your doctor should inform you in detail about the diagnostic tests recommended, their necessity, discomfort, risk, cost, and likelihood of making a difference in the outcome of the problem.

Design a Therapeutic Plan.   An important part of your doctor's job is to formulate a therapeutic plan that is realistic for you. Asking a patient with hemorrhoids to take eight sitz baths a day is impractical if that person has a full-time job.

The treatment plan should include nutritional management in addition to drug therapy.

Keep Track of Your Progress.   Your doctor should follow up on your treatment to make sure you are improving and that the working diagnosis was correct.

As you can see, if you have a GI disorder, working with your doctor is more than just making an appointment, taking some pills, and going back to your normal life. Successful diagnosis and management of a GI problem so that impairment is minimized and healthy function maximized depends on an open and trusting doctor-patient relationship.

33   *Your Everyday Cooking*

*T*he following tips about shopping and food preparation will help you incorporate the principles of the Two-Week Master Program into your everyday cooking. With a little experience you will be able to adapt your favorite recipes, and even invent new ones.

Increase Fiber

Take a trip to your local health food or bulk food store and stock up on whole grains. Brown rice, whole wheat pasta, bulgur wheat, buckwheat, whole wheat couscous, wheat berries, whole wheat flour, whole grain cereals, and whole oat products are some choices you might make. As the demand has increased, many supermarkets have also begun to carry more whole grain products.

Gradually begin to use more of these products in your cooking. Many of the recipes in the Two-Week Master Program include more whole grains than you may be accustomed to, and it's wise to make a gradual transition. If you are unaccustomed to cooking with whole grains, you may need to experiment a little with recipes to see how various grains react to the cooking process.

Also begin to increase your intake of fruits and vegetables. Begin to center meals around grains and vegetables, deemphasizing the animal protein portion of the meal. Get in the habit of using fruit as a dessert. And use the leftovers of the grain and vegetable portion of your dinner to make lunch the next day. The meal plans are designed to make use of leftovers as brown-bag meals.

Reduce Fats

Fats are typically added to diets in the form of butter, margarine, oil, mayonnaise, cream, nondairy cream, and salad dressing. Whole-milk dairy products, animal protein foods, nuts, seeds, and bakery goods are also sources of excess fat. It's easy to replace most of these items with healthier, low-fat alternatives.

Fats in Baking and Cooking.   It's difficult to bake without using any fat, but much of the fat used in baked goods can be replaced with fruit, pureed fruit, or fruit juice. Many of the recipe in this book demonstrate this concept.

Fats also can be reduced by increasing the use of cooking liquids. For example, you can "sauté" using vermouth, wine, defatted broth, tomato juice, low-sodium soy sauce, fruit juice, vegetable oil sprays, or any other nonfat liquid. Jellies, jams, and fruit butters can be used in place of margarine or butter on bread. Try low-fat yogurt instead of mayonnaise, or use half yogurt and half low-fat mayonnaise. Try the lower fat salad dressing recipes included here, or purchase a bottled low-fat dressing. Try mock sour cream (see chapter 45) instead of sour cream on your baked potato.

Foods containing "fake fats" (Olestra, Olean) can be used to lower fat consumption but can cause greasy stools and abdominal discomfort. Patients with diarrheal disorders including irritable bowel syndrome, inflammatory bowel disease, or malabsorption should avoid products containing Olestra. Similar side effects can be seen with the anti-obesity drug xenical (Orlistat), which should be available sometime in 1999. This drug should also be used cautiously by patients with gastrointestinal disorders.

Butter and Oil.   Since you will be using fat in smaller amounts, you might freeze your butter or margarine to make them last longer. Likewise, refrigerate your vegetable oils to prevent them from becoming rancid. Olive oil will thicken and may turn cloudy when refrigerated, but will return to its normal state of room temperature with no harm done.

Dairy Products.   All the dairy products you use in your daily cooking—including cottage cheese, yogurt, and milk—should be low-fat. Skim or 1 percent low-fat is recommended; 2 percent low-fat and whole milk are less acceptable. Cheeses should be used only in moderation. Even cheeses partially made with skim milk are not actually low in fat.

Frozen desserts vary in their fat content and can be very misleading. Ice cream is usually high in fat; ice milk is lower, but is not low in fat. Sherbet, sorbet, and fruit ices are lower in fat. Sherbet, which is made with milk, is not lactose-free, but sorbets and fruit ices are. Frozen yogurt may be low in fat, but check the label. Likewise, tofu frozen desserts may be low in fat, but many have vegetable oils added. Read the label to be sure. Tofu-based products are lactose-free.

Animal Fats.   Meat, poultry, fish, seafood, pork, and eggs are all animal proteins. Limit your consumption of animal protein to 6 to 8 ounces a day, in keeping with the overall concept of reducing animal protein and increasing complex carbohydrates.

You can further reduce the fat content of animal protein by following a few simple rules: skin poultry before cooking, cut off visible fat from meat, and use cooking methods that help remove fat—broiling, roasting, poaching, baking, steaming, or braising.

Nuts and Seeds.   Nuts and seeds are high-fat foods that should be used only as a garnish. Nuts and seeds are also gas producing, so many people will want to avoid them completely.

Reduce Lactose

All milk and milk products contain lactose. If you are lactose intolerant, or don't know if you are, use the dairy products recommended in chapter 21.

Even people who are lactose intolerant can usually tolerate small amounts of lactose in prepared foods. Aged cheese usually does not cause symptoms because fermented dairy products are often better tolerated. Yogurt is usually well tolerated by lactose-intolerant people as long as it has an active culture. Look for nonfat or low-fat yogurt with active cultures. If you do use dairy products, small portions along with a meal may be better tolerated than large portions consumed without other foods.

Substitute Herbs for Spices

Herbs can be used in place of spices in your everyday cooking. Add a small amount, taste, and add more to please your own taste. Herbs are fragile, so are usually added near the end of the cooking time.

Store herbs in a cool, dark cabinet. (Forget about the shelf above the stove where heat and light quickly destroy their flavor.) If possible, purchase herbs in a shop with a high product turnover so packages haven't been sitting for months on the shelf. Herbs available in bulk almost always taste better than prepackaged varieties. They will usually be fresher and less expensive. Bulk herbs are usually sold in ½- to 1-ounce portions, and you can easily store them in your own containers. Herbs can make a tremendous difference in flavor when you use few spices and less fat, so it's important to buy top quality. Seasonal fresh herbs are especially good. Better yet, start your own herb garden.

Reduce Legumes

Legumes such as dried beans and lentils are very healthy and good for you, but they are gas-forming. However, if your GI problem is not aggravated by gas, eat legumes as often as you want. Many people find that if they add small quantities of legumes to their diet several times a week their digestive systems adjust and produce less gas.

Lentils and split peas are the most easily tolerated. It also helps prevent gas if you discard the soaking liquid or the liquid legumes are canned in before using.

To Cook or Eat Raw

In general, the more you cook something the more vitamins and minerals are lost, especially the B vitamins and vitamin C. So for the most part, the less you cook vegetables the better. That being said, there are some exceptions.

Some plant foods must be cooked in order to burst the cell wall and derive nutrients from the food. Potatoes are an example. Raw potatoes provide little more than fluid and fiber. Cooked potatoes provide fluid, fiber, complex carbohydrates, vitamins, minerals, and some protein.

Carrots and beans are another example of high-fiber foods that do better if they are cooked longer. When they are cooked adequately these vegetables are more easily digested, and therefore their nutrients are better absorbed. This more efficient use of the food offsets some loss of nutrients in the cooking process.

The recipes in Part Nine will give you the experience you need to begin to modify all of your cooking and eating habits.

34   *Dining Out*

When it comes to dining, no man or woman is an island. Eating is our most social activity, usually performed in the company of anywhere from one to hundreds. Every occasion, great or small, is marked by a ritual sharing of food and drink. It could be a raise or a new job, birth, engagement, wedding, shower, confirmation, bat- or bar-mitzvah, graduation, new apartment or house, anniversary, retirement, or even death; it could be a picnic, potluck dinner, power breakfast, business lunch, romantic supper at an out-of-the way restaurant, or a catered affair. You get the idea. No event passes without celebration by breaking bread together. It has always been so. Our prehistoric ancestors gathered together around fires in front of caves to share the rewards of the hunt and celebrate the fact that yet another day had passed safely.

Celebrating life by sharing food is impossible to avoid for everyone but the most determined hermit. And this essential part of being human is one of our healthiest, most positive traits. But for people with GI problems, these events have often been uncomfortable or downright torture.

Let's assume you have carefully worked out your own diet, including the specific Flag Foods that you know will aggravate your GI problem. Deviating from that diet may not be dangerous, but taking a night off or splurging at lunch will often cause a reaction. It isn't so difficult to maintain your diet even at a party or a restaurant. It just takes some forethought.

Dinner Parties

We are all more nutrition and weight conscious these days than ever before in history. As a result, any get-together of two or more people is bound to include someone who has restrictions on his or her diet. It may be on a physician's advice or self-imposed, but there are many millions of people who avoid certain foods that they believe are harmful.

Today's party givers want their guests to enjoy themselves, and one thing that means is being flexible about menus. With so many health-conscious people, even cocktail parties that used to have only potato chips, dip, and peanuts for sustenance, now are likely to feature baskets of fresh vegetables, whole grain breads, and flavored seltzer as well as martinis.

One thing for you to bear in mind if you suffer from a GI disorder: managing diet at a dinner party or a restaurant is not just a whim or self-indulgence or a way to draw attention to yourself. It's as important for you to control your diet as it is for someone who is trying to manage diabetes or heart disease. You are entitled to be served foods that you can eat without becoming ill. At the same time, you don't want your host to have to do handstands to accommodate you.

So when the invitation to a dinner party arrives, it's a good idea to call your hosts and ask them for a general idea of what will be served. You can do this whether you know your hosts well or not at all. This is not so you can dictate the menu, but so you can prepare yourself in advance. By all means, explain why you're asking: you have to follow a somewhat restricted diet for medical reasons.

Obviously, if you're invited for a fish fry or a barbecue you aren't going to ask them to change the menu for your sake. But if your hosts are still preparing the menu, they are likely to ask you what restrictions you have and you can tell them in advance what your Flag Foods are.

What you don't want to do is arrive at a dinner party and spring your special dietary needs on an unsuspecting host at the last minute. I'll never forget one guest arriving at a dinner party that featured a main course of lamb navarin and announcing that he was a vegetarian. His host rushed frantically into the kitchen and prepared a vegetable and pasta dish while trying to serve dinner to eight other people.

So, if you are going to make your needs known, make them known with plenty of time to spare. Most people will be pleased to know in advance what foods their guests have to avoid.

If the menu is already set, you will know beforehand what you can eat plenty of and what you will have to stay away from. Even at the barbecue there are likely to be baked potatoes and vegetables. If it looks as if your selection is going to be severely restricted, you might want to have a snack before the party so you won't be tempted to wolf down food that will bring on an adverse reaction.

This may seem odd to you. But after all, if Scarlett O'Hara ate before the barbecue, why shouldn't you? In fact we go to dinner parties for a lot of reasons other than the food. Parties are enjoyable social occasions whether you eat much or not. Unless you're willing to eat something that's likely to trigger a GI reaction, fill yourself up before-hand on foods that you know are in line with your diet.

Fortunately, today's parties are often semibusiness engagements that are designed to satisfy a wide variety of special needs. Having a wide choice of such things as vegetables and interesting breads as well as a main course is one way for a host to make sure even the most finicky guests have something to eat.

One Los Angeles caterer always makes sure that there is plenty of extra-virgin olive oil, vegetables, fish, and plain fruit, which can satisfy most palates and stomachs. A New York caterer says the best hosts try not to serve pork, lamb, duck, or fried foods. They serve starches such as pasta, potatoes, and bread along with salad and vegetables and fruit for dessert.

Platter service, which allows guests to discreetly select what they're going to eat, and buffets, which offer variety, are popular today across the country. So chances are if you are invited to a party you will be able to manage pretty well. Restaurant dining, however, may require some skill on your part.

Restaurants

Dining in a restaurant used to be a special occasion, often to mark an important event in one's life. Today eating out is more likely to be an everyday event in many people's lives. What with lunches at restaurants near your workplace and more elaborate business lunches, Americans eat about one meal in three in restaurants.

Although many meals are eaten in fast-food restaurants where the selection is generally pretty limited and the accent is more on "fast" than "food," there is still a good chance that in most restaurants, even with GI problems, you can get a healthful, tasty meal without suffering afterward.

The same kind of forethought is necessary with restaurant meals as with partygoing. First of all, what sort of restaurant are you going to? Fast-food restaurants will not have a variety of foods for people on restrictive diets. Many items on the fast-food menu are high in saturated fats, from hamburgers with mayonnaise to french fries cooked in beef fat and shakes thickened with coconut oil. Even the fish and chicken dishes are often fried.

Most ethnic restaurants, on the other hand, have a much fresher and healthier selection of dishes for people with GI problems. This comes as a big surprise for many people who thought they would never be able to eat flavorful, tasty food again. But contrary to what you might believe, ethnic restaurants are definitely on your "go" list.

Chinese, Japanese, Mexican, Middle Eastern, and Italian restaurants all have many freshly prepared dishes that are high in fiber and low in saturated fat. Some people, depending on their Flag Foods, will have to avoid the spicier items, but even Mexican restaurants serve fish and rice dishes that are low in spice. All so-called peasant cuisines are based on combinations of inexpensive grains and vegetables that make complete dishes, high in complex carbohydrates and low in saturated fat.

It is best for anyone who has dietary restrictions to plan ahead. Restaurants are in business to give service along with good food. Call the restaurant you are planning to dine in and check out the menu over the phone. In a good restaurant you can talk to the manager or headwaiter about your dietary restrictions. They will be happy to help you plan a meal that will be both satisfying to your palate and easy on your GI system.

Many people these days dine out on the spur of the moment, in a casual neighborhood restaurant or other restaurant where you really can't call ahead and do any special ordering. In this case make it a habit to ask for low-fat dairy products and foods prepared without fats or salt. Ask for the sauces and salad dressings to be served on the side so you can control the amounts you use.

More important than these special requests is making a good selection to begin with. It helps to know as much as possible about the preparation of food and the language commonly used to describe dishes on restaurant menus. If you cook, you're ahead of the game, because you understand what goes into the preparation of most dishes. If you don't cook and are unfamiliar with cooking terms and food preparation, here's a quick course in menu terminology.

Menu Terminology to Watch Out For

French

aioli: garlic mayonnaise

beurre: butter

béarnaise: sauce of egg yolks and butter with herbs and shallots

béchamel: cream sauce (flour, milk, butter)

hollandaise: sauce of egg yolks and butter with lemon

Italian

pancetta: Italian bacon

burro: butter

olio: oil

parmigiano: Parmesan cheese

formaggio: cheese

frittata: omelet

Indian

samosa: small pastry

paratha: fried bread

poori: fried bread

ghee: clarified butter

Japanese

tempura: batter-coated deep-fried fish, shrimp, or vegetables

Good Menu Choices

Salads, dressings on the side

Melon, berries, other fresh fruits

Seafood cocktails (sauce on side)

Oysters or clams on half-shell

Broth- or tomato-based soups with noodles or vegetables

Gazpacho (will usually have onions and/or garlic)

Minestrone (usually has beans)

Clam chowder (Manhattan style)

Tomato juice (except for people with heartburn)

Fish, all varieties, broiled, poached, or steamed

Poultry (skin it before you eat it)

Red meat, lean cuts, broiled

Vegetables, all kinds (avoid broccoli, corn, cauliflower, cabbage, fried potatoes)

Pastas, brown rice, and whole grains, all kinds, plain or with tomato sauces, wine sauces, fish and seafood sauces, vegetables

Breadsticks, hard rolls, French and Italian bread, pita bread, whole wheat toasts, and whole grain breads

Angel food cake

Gelatin

Sorbet

Low-fat dairy products (lactose-intolerant individuals should bring lactase enzyme tablets with them when dining out)

PART NINE

Gastrointestinal-Healthy Recipes

35 *Appetizers and Soups*

===

Acorn Squash Soup

Basic Chicken Stock

Crab and Potato Chowder

Winter Vegetable Soup

Salmon Mousse

Tomato Basil Soup

Turkey Meatball Soup

Acorn Squash Soup
SERVES 4

This is a very elegant yet healthy "cream" soup. It's a great way to serve squash to those of us who are not squash lovers.

½ tablespoon butter or margarine
1 small onion, chopped
*2 garlic cloves, chopped
½ teaspoon ground coriander
¼ teaspoon ground cumin
*⅛ teaspoon ground black pepper
2 medium-sized acorn squash (about 1½ pounds total), peeled and coarsely chopped

1½ cups chicken stock, preferably homemade (see page 280)
1½ cups water
1 teaspoon sugar
1 teaspoon salt (omit if you used canned chicken broth)
**½ cup evaporated skimmed milk
*grated nutmeg

*Garlic, black pepper, and nutmeg must be avoided by many of you. The soup is quite acceptable even when they are omitted.
**If you are lactose intolerant, you may make low-lactose evaporated skimmed milk. Use two times your usual amount of lactase enzyme drops. The soup is also quite good without the milk, but the milk does add an extra dimension.

1 Melt butter in medium saucepan over medium high heat. Add onion, garlic, and spices and sauté for about 2 minutes. Add squash and stir to coat, about 1 minute. Add stock, water, sugar, and salt. Bring to a boil, turn heat to low, cover, and let simmer until squash is tender, about 10 to 15 minutes.

2 Allow squash to cool slightly and then puree in a blender or food processor.

3 Stir in evaporated skimmed milk and reheat, but do not allow to boil. Garnish with grated nutmeg and serve.

Nutritional information per serving*

171 calories	9% of calories from fat
77% of calories from carbohydrate	2 grams of fat
14% of calories from protein	5 grams of fiber

Basic Chicken Stock
YIELD: 5 TO 6 QUARTS

Defatted stock is a wonderful basis for low-fat cooking. It is rich and fla-vorful but virtually fat-free. Canned broth can be used as a substitute as long as it is first defatted (refrigerate the can overnight), but the results will not be as good. Homemade stock takes a long time to make, but it is not labor-intensive time, so you can make it while you are at home do-ing other things. Bones and chicken scraps can be obtained inexpensively from your butcher, or if you bone your own chicken, simply save the bones, skins, and scraps in a plastic bag in your freezer. You do not need to follow this recipe exactly; use vegetables and spices that are available to you, put them in a large stock pot with the chicken, and simply cover with cold water.

about 2½ pounds chicken bones, skins, scraps	3 celery stalks and leaves, washed
	3 bay leaves
2 medium carrots, washed, unpeeled, cut into quarters	several parsley sprigs
	several dill sprigs
2 medium onions, washed, unpeeled, cut in quarters	1 teaspoon dried thyme
	1 teaspoon dried tarragon
1 leek, green and white parts, well scrubbed	20 peppercorns (if desired)
	3 garlic cloves, peeled (if desired)

*Throughout this section, assume that one serving is based on the number served.

1 Put all of the above into a large stock pot. Cover with cold water (probably about 6 to 7 quarts). Cover pot.

2 Turn heat to medium high. Bring to a bare simmer, turn heat to medium low.

3 Simmer at this temperature for 3 to 6 hours. Skim if necessary.

4 Strain. Cool in refrigerator for several hours and remove hardened fat.

5 Freeze in various size containers, including ice cube trays. Remove from the ice cube trays when frozen and store in a plastic bag in your freezer. Use these cubes for fat-free "sautéing."

Nutritional information per serving (1 cup)

26 calories	0% of calories from fat
16% of calories from carbohydrate	0 grams of fat
84% of calories from protein	0 grams of fiber

This is an approximate analysis and is based upon a *defatted* chicken stock (see step 4).

Crab and Potato Chowder
SERVES 6

1 tablespoon butter or margarine	1 teaspoon salt
2 leeks, well washed and finely chopped	½ teaspoon dried thyme
2 cups dry vermouth	*1 can (12 or 13 ounces) evaporated skimmed milk
1 cup water	**1 cup skim milk
1½ pounds red potatoes, scrubbed, skin on, cut into bite-sized pieces	1 pound crabmeat
	2–3 tablespoons chopped parsley

1 Melt butter over medium high heat in 3-quart saucepan. Add leeks, turn heat to low, cover, and allow to cook slowly for 3 to 4 minutes or until softened.

2 Add vermouth, water, potatoes, salt, and thyme. Bring to a boil. Turn heat to low, cover, and cook until potatoes are fork tender, about 20 minutes.

3 Add milk and crabmeat. Heat through but do not boil. Sprinkle with chopped parsley and serve.

*If you are lactose intolerant, treat the evaporated skimmed milk with lactase enzyme drops, using two times your usual amount or eliminate the evaporated skimmed milk and use all lactose-reduced milk.
**Use lactose-reduced milk if you are lactose intolerant.

Nutritional information per serving

310 calories
59% of calories from carbohydrate
29% of calories from protein

12% of calories from fat
4 grams of fat
4 grams of fiber

Winter Vegetable Soup
SERVES 4

3 cups defatted chicken stock,
   preferably homemade (see
   page 280)
2 medium carrots, coarsely chopped
2 small parsnips, coarsely chopped
1 medium onion, coarsely chopped
½ pound celery root, coarsely
   chopped

*¼ teaspoon freshly ground nutmeg
½ teaspoon salt (omit if you are
   using canned broth)
1 teaspoon sugar
2 tablespoons chopped fresh dill

1   In 3-quart saucepan, bring stock to boil over medium high heat.
2   Add vegetables, reduce heat to medium low, cover, and simmer for
30 minutes.
3   Remove soup to food processor or blender and puree until smooth.
(Do in batches if necessary.)
4   Return to pan. Add spices, heat through, and serve.

Note: This is a thick soup. Add an additional cup of stock if you would
prefer a thinner soup. For an interesting variation, add 1 cup of cooked
brown rice or barley after pureeing.

Nutritional information per serving

76 calories
71% of calories from carbohydrate
26% of calories from protein

3% of calories from fat
less than 1 gram of fat
3 grams of fiber

Salmon Mousse
SERVES 4

15½-ounce can salmon, reserve
   liquid
1 envelope unflavored gelatin
**1 cup plain nonfat yogurt

1 small onion, quartered
1 stalk celery, cut in 3 pieces
1 tablespoon lemon juice
1 tablespoon fresh parsley, minced

*Nutmeg is a Flag Food for some people.
**Yogurt is usually well tolerated by lactose-intolerant individuals. If you are unable to
tolerate yogurt, take 1 lactase enzyme tablet with the mousse.

1   Drain salmon liquid into cup measure. Add enough cold water to equal ⅔ cup.

2   Pour liquid into small saucepan. Sprinkle gelatin on liquid and let it soften for 5 minutes. Heat liquid until gelatin melts.

3   Remove skin from salmon and crush bones. (The bones are included because they are so soft and are an excellent source of calcium.) In blender, puree salmon, yogurt, onion, and celery.

4   In medium bowl, stir together salmon puree, gelatin mixture, lemon juice, and parsley until thoroughly mixed.

5   Place bowl in refrigerator until mousse is partially set.

6   Coat 4-cup mold with nonstick vegetable oil spray. Pour partially gelled mousse into mold. Chill until firm, about 3 hours.

7   Unmold the mousse by inverting onto a platter lined with lettuce leaves. Serve with crackers or cocktail bread.

Nutritional information per serving

200 calories	31% of calories from fat
14% of calories from carbohydrate	7 grams of fat
55% of calories from protein	1 gram of fiber

Tomato Basil Soup
SERVES 4

This soup is best made at the height of tomato and basil season. It freezes well, so can be eaten all winter long when you want the feel of summer.

2½ cups chicken stock, preferably homemade (see page 280)	1 cup fresh basil leaves, cleaned
1 medium yellow onion, chopped	2 teaspoons honey
2 pounds ripe tomatoes (about 4 medium), peeled and quartered	1 bay leaf
	¼ teaspoon salt, or to taste (omit if you are using canned broth)

1   Bring ½ cup of stock to a boil in a 2-quart nonaluminum saucepan. Add onion and cook over medium heat until soft. If extra liquid is necessary, use a small amount of water.

2   Add tomatoes, basil, honey, and bay leaf. Reduce heat to low, cover, and cook for about 10 minutes, stirring occasionally.

3   Puree mixture in blender or food processor. Press through strainer to remove seeds. Return to saucepan.

4   Add remaining 2 cups of stock and salt if desired. Excellent hot or cold!

Nutritional information per serving

99 calories
69% of calories from carbohydrate
26% of calories from protein

5% of calories from fat
less than 1 gram of fat
5 grams of fiber

Turkey Meatball Soup
SERVES 6 TO 8

This soup is very low in sodium if you use homemade chicken stock. You may want to add a teaspoon of salt to the recipe in step 3. Do not add salt if you are using canned chicken broth.

¾ pound ground turkey
1 tablespoon soy sauce, preferably reduced sodium
1 tablespoon dry sherry
1 tablespoon cornstarch
2 tablespoons finely chopped cilantro
2 tablespoons coarsely chopped water chestnuts (about 6)
¼ cup whole wheat bread crumbs

5 cups defatted chicken stock (see page 280)
3 cups water
1½ cups cooked brown rice
¼ cup sliced water chestnuts (about 12)
3 cups coarsely chopped romaine lettuce or other green
1 tablespoon sesame oil

1   Mix turkey, soy sauce, sherry, cornstarch, cilantro, chopped water chestnuts, and bread crumbs together. Shape into about 20 meatballs.

2   Bring broth and water to boil in large pot. Add meatballs, turn heat to medium, and cook for 5 minutes covered.

3   Add rice, sliced water chestnuts, romaine, and oil. Turn heat down to low. Cover and cook another 10 minutes. Serve hot.

Nutritional information per serving

212 calories
37% of calories from carbohydrate
40% of calories from protein

23% of calories from fat
5 grams of fat
2 grams of fiber

36 *Entrees:*

Fish and Seafood

Baked Tomato-Orange Flounder
Fettucini with Clam Sauce
Flounder in a Flash
Mediterranean Monk Fish
Poached Flounder in Creamy Sauce
Scallops in a Veggie Nest
Snappy Seafood Salad
Sweet and Sour Shrimp
Teriyaki Salmon Kabobs
Tuna Patties

Baked Tomato-Orange Flounder
SERVES 4

Substitute any lean fish of your choice for the flounder. This is a very simple dish, equally suitable for your family or for company.

1 pound flounder filets

SAUCE

¼ cup white wine
1 medium onion, chopped
1 cup canned crushed tomatoes
*¼ cup frozen unsweetened orange
   juice concentrate

3 tablespoons frozen unsweetened
   apple juice concentrate
⅓ cup water
½ teaspoon thyme
slices of orange

*Orange juice may be irritating to the esophagus. Replace with extra apple juice.

1   Preheat oven to 350°.

2   Coat shallow baking pan with nonstick vegetable oil spray. Lay fish filets in pan forming single layer.

3   Pour wine into small saucepan and bring to a boil. Add onion and sauté until transparent.

4   Add tomatoes and simmer 5 minutes.

5   Add orange and apple juice concentrates, water, and thyme and simmer 5 minutes.

6   Pour sauce over fish filets in baking dish and bake for 25 to 30 minutes. Remove to serving platter and garnish with fresh orange slices.

Nutritional information per serving

205 calories
78% of calories from carbohydrate
46% of calories from protein

7% of calories from fat
2 grams of fat
2 grams of fiber

Fettuccini with Clam Sauce
SERVES 4

3 dozen littleneck clams
1 yellow bell pepper, cut in thin strips
3 large shallots, minced
1 leek, white part only, chopped

½ cup white wine or dry vermouth
*½ cup skim milk
1 teaspoon thyme
2 tablespoons minced parsley
12 ounces fettuccini, uncooked

1   Scrub the clams well, discarding any that are open.

2   Combine pepper, shallots, leek, and wine in large heavy skillet with lid. Cover and cook over medium low heat until very tender, about 25 minutes.

3   Transfer mixture to processor or blender. Puree until very smooth (add more wine if necessary). Return the puree to skillet.

4   Stir milk into puree. Boil gently, stirring frequently, about 10 minutes. Add clams and herbs, cover, and let simmer for 5 to 7 minutes. Discard unopened clams.

5   Cook fettuccini in large pot of rapidly boiling water until just tender but still firm to bite. Drain well. Add small amount of sauce to pasta and toss to coat the fettuccini.

6   Divide pasta among 4 plates and top with the remaining sauce.

*If you are lactose intolerant, use lactose-reduced milk.

Nutritional information per serving

462 calories

67% of calories from carbohydrate

27% of calories from protein

6% of calories from fat

3 grams of fat

2 grams of fiber

Flounder in a Flash
SERVES 4

1 large onion, sliced thinly

1 pound flounder filets

SAUCE

*¼ cup plain nonfat or low-fat yogurt

1 tablespoon lemon juice

1 tablespoon Dijon-style mustard

1 tablespoon prepared horseradish

1 Coat broiler pan with nonstick vegetable oil spray. Spread sliced onions over bottom of pan. Place fish filets on top of onions in single layer.

2 Mix together sauce ingredients in small bowl. Spread sauce over fish filets.

3 Broil fish for 5 to 10 minutes (depending on thickness). Serve.

Nutritional information per serving

130 calories

16% of calories from carbohydrate

74% of calories from protein

10% of calories from fat

1 gram of fat

1 gram of fiber

Mediterranean Monk Fish
SERVES 4

2 teaspoons olive oil

1½ pounds monk fish

2 teaspoons dried basil

1 tablespoon capers, drained

about 20 black olives, chopped

2 tomatoes, sliced

1 Preheat oven to 350°.

2 Cut square of aluminum foil large enough to hold the monk fish. Brush oil over the foil.

*Most lactose-intolerant individuals can tolerate yogurt without any problem. If you do not, then take 1 lactase enzyme tablet with this meal.

3   Place fish in center of foil. Rub basil into fish. Top with capers, olives, and tomatoes. Form a seal with the aluminum foil.

4   Bake fish for about 20 to 25 minutes or until it just flakes. Serve.

Nutritional information per serving

265 calories

5% of calories from carbohydrate

61% of calories from protein

34% of calories from fat

10 grams of fat

1 gram of fiber

Poached Flounder in Creamy Sauce
SERVES 4

This is an incredibly easy recipe and yet rich in flavor.

1 pound flounder filet

1 cup dry vermouth

*1½ cups evaporated skimmed milk

¾ teaspoon allspice

1   Place flounder and vermouth in large skillet. Cover and simmer until flounder is cooked, about 8 to 10 minutes.

2   Remove flounder from pan to serving plate and cover to keep warm.

3   Boil cooking liquid until reduced to about ¼ cup. Add evaporated milk and allspice and cook until thickened, stirring continuously.

4   Pour sauce over flounder and serve.

Nutritional information per serving

180 calories

26% of calories from carbohydrate

67% of calories from protein

7% of calories from fat

1 gram of fat

0 grams of fiber

Scallops in a Veggie Nest
SERVES 4

This is a lovely dish to look at and it also tastes great. There is a lot of work involved in slicing the vegetables, so you may want to use this as a company meal.

---

*If you are lactose intolerant, make the evaporated skimmed milk into lactose-free milk by using lactase enzyme drops. Use double the usual amount for 1½ cups of milk and do twenty-four hours in advance. Regular low-lactose milk will not work well in this recipe because it is too thin, but if you do try it, use only ¾ cup.

2 medium carrots, cut into
matchstick-size julienne strips
2 medium red peppers, cut into
matchstick-size julienne strips
1 medium zucchini, skin on, cut into
matchstick-size julienne strips
1 cup dry white wine or dry
vermouth
4 tablespoons lemon juice
3 green onions, white part only,
chopped

¼ cup chopped fresh basil (if
unavailable, use 3½ tablespoons
of chopped fresh parsley and
½ tablespoon of dried basil)
2 tablespoons chopped fresh dill
2 tablespoons dry sherry
2 teaspoons cornstarch
1 pound bay scallops

1 Prepare vegetables and set aside.

2 Bring wine and lemon juice to a boil in a medium-sized saucepan. Add onions and basil and allow to simmer uncovered at medium heat for about 5 minutes to reduce by half.

3 Meanwhile, steam carrots, peppers, and zucchini about 1½ minutes. Turn heat off, toss with dill, and cover to keep warm.

4 Combine sherry and cornstarch. Add to reduced sauce, stirring. Heat to boiling, add scallops, and cook for 3 to 4 minutes until done, stirring occasionally.

5 Arrange vegetables in a nest on each plate and mound scallops in the middle. Pour a little sauce over each serving. Serve hot.

Nutritional information per serving

166 calories
30% of calories from carbohydrate
60% of calories from protein

10% of calories from fat
2 grams of fat
2 grams of fiber

Snappy Seafood Salad
SERVES 6

DRESSING

*½ cup plain nonfat yogurt
½ cup low-fat mayonnaise
1 tablespoon lemon juice

2 teaspoons Dijon-style mustard
2 tablespoons prepared horseradish

*Yogurt is usually well tolerated by lactose intolerant individuals. If you are unable to tolerate yogurt, take 1 lactase enzyme tablet with this meal or replace the yogurt with low-fat mayonnaise. (This will make the salad higher in fat.)

SALAD

1 pound imitation crabmeat or other seafood

½ pound green beans, blanched, cut in 1-inch pieces

2 medium carrots, grated

1 medium onion, chopped

1   In a small bowl combine all dressing ingredients.

2   In a medium bowl, mix together all prepared salad ingredients. Pour the dressing over them and toss.

3   Serve on pita bread or a bed of lettuce.

Variation: Add cooked, cooled pasta to seafood and vegetables and toss with dressing for a main dish pasta salad.

Nutritional information per serving

263 calories

36% of calories from carbohydrate

31% of calories from protein

33% of calories from fat

10 grams of fat

2 grams of fiber

Sweet and Sour Shrimp
SERVES 4

Other types of fish or seafood can be used as substitutes in this recipe. Be prepared—you'll never have leftovers of this tasty dish! Garlic is a great addition to this dish, if you can tolerate it. Add 1 or 2 cloves of finely chopped garlic to the sauce.

SAUCE

¼ cup lemon juice

¼ cup soy sauce (preferably reduced sodium)

¼ cup tomato paste

2 tablespoons honey

6 tablespoons water

MAIN DISH

1 cup white wine

1½ pounds fresh shrimp, shelled and cleaned

2 medium green peppers, cut in 1-inch squares

¾ pound mushrooms, sliced

8-ounce can sliced water chestnuts, drained

1   In a medium bowl, whisk together sauce ingredients until thoroughly mixed. Set aside.

2   Pour wine into large skillet. Bring to a simmer; poach shrimp for about 3 minutes. Remove shrimp from skillet with slotted spoon and place in bowl with sauce.

3   Simmer green peppers and mushrooms in remaining wine until tender. Pour off any wine left in skillet.

4   Add sauce, shrimp, and water chestnuts to skillet and cook over medium heat for several minutes until heated through.

5   Serve over rice or noodles.

Nutritional information per serving

233 calories
44% of calories from carbohydrate
49% of calories from protein

7% of calories from fat
2 grams of fat
2 grams of fiber

Teriyaki Salmon Kabobs
SERVES 6

The directions in this recipe are for a broiler, but it would work equally well on a barbecue grill.

MARINADE

2 tablespoons soy sauce, preferably
  reduced sodium
2 tablespoons dry sherry

3 tablespoons unsweetened
  pineapple juice

KABOB

3 pounds fresh salmon steak, 1-inch
  thick
3 small zucchini, cut crosswise into
  8 pieces each

12 cherry tomatoes, whole
12 mushrooms, whole

1   Combine marinade ingredients in small bowl.

2   Remove fish skin and bones. Cut into 1-inch cubes (about 48 pieces). Place in plastic bag with marinade mixture, close bag, and marinate in refrigerator for 1 to 2 hours.

3   While fish is marinating, steam zucchini until crisp but tender.

4   Coat broiler pan with nonstick vegetable oil spray. Alternately thread fish and vegetables onto 12 skewers using 4 pieces of fish, 2 pieces of zucchini, 1 tomato, and 1 mushroom for each kabob. Lay kabobs on broiler pan.

5   Broil about 3 inches from heat, 3 to 5 minutes per side. Be careful not to overcook fish because it will dry out and fall off skewers.

6   Serve on bed of cooked grain, such as rice or barley.

Nutritional information per serving

240 calories
12% of calories from carbohydrate
55% of calories from protein

33% of calories from fat
9 grams of fat
2 grams of fiber

Tuna Patties
SERVES 3

1 medium zucchini, grated and
   patted dry with paper towel
6½-ounce can waterpacked tuna,
   well drained
3 slices whole wheat bread, made
   into bread crumbs in blender

1 egg or 2 egg whites
1 teaspoon lemon juice
¼ teaspoon cumin
1 tablespoon olive oil

1   Mix zucchini, tuna, and bread crumbs together in medium bowl.

2   Add egg, lemon juice, and cumin. Stir until well mixed.

3   Shape into 3 patties.

4   Heat oil in medium skillet. Cook patties in skillet over medium heat until browned on both sides, about 8 minutes total time.

5   Serve on whole grain roll with lettuce and tomato.

Nutritional information per serving

215 calories
24% of calories from carbohydrate
43% of calories from protein

33% of calories from fat
8 grams of fat
4 grams of fiber

37

Entrees:
Meat

Beef Kabobs
Beef Stew with Cranberries
Marinated and Grilled Flank Steak
Stir-Fry Orange Beef
Veal with Sun-Dried Tomatoes
Very Veggie Meatloaf

Beef Kabobs
SERVES 4

⅔ cup dry red wine
2 teaspoons sugar
4 teaspoons olive or canola oil
4 teaspoons lemon juice
1 teaspoon basil
1 teaspoon thyme

1 pound lean round steak, cut into 24 cubes
2 green or red peppers, cut into 24 squares
1 medium onion, cut into 24 pieces

1 Combine wine, sugar, oil, lemon juice, basil, and thyme in small bowl. Add beef cubes and marinate in refrigerator for several hours or overnight.

2 Remove beef from marinade, reserving marinade.

3 Preheat broiler or grill.

4 Alternately thread meat, peppers, and onions onto 8 skewers, using 3 pieces of each per skewer.

5 Grill or broil about 3 to 4 inches from heat source, basting frequently with reserved marinade. Cook for about 10 minutes or to desired doneness. Serve 2 kabobs per person on a bed of brown rice.

Nutritional information per serving

245 calories	38% calories from fat
14% calories from carbohydrate	10 grams of fat
48% calories from protein	1 gram of fiber

Beef Stew with Cranberries
SERVES 6

While this is an unlikely combination, it works well and is a very interesting beef stew. It's wonderful on a cold January day!

2 pounds lean stew meat, trimmed of all visible fat and cut into 1-inch cubes	2 tablespoons red wine vinegar
	1 tablespoon tomato paste
	½ teaspoon salt, if desired
1½–2 cups burgundy wine	2 tablespoons whole wheat flour
2–3 small cinnamon sticks	1 tablespoon honey
½ teaspoon lightly crushed coriander seeds	1 cup fresh cranberries, washed and finely chopped (most easily done in a food processor or blender)
1 large onion, sliced	

1　Marinate beef in mixture of 1½ cups wine, cinnamon sticks, and coriander all day or overnight. Drain beef, reserving marinade and spices. Add enough extra wine to reserved marinade to total 2 cups.

2　Set heavy 6-quart pot over medium heat. Add meat in batches and cook over medium heat until brown. It is not necessary to add oil. Transfer to plate as each batch is browned.

3　Return meat to pan. Add onion, vinegar, tomato paste, salt, and re-served marinade.

4　Bring to a boil, cover, reduce heat, and simmer slowly for about 1½ hours.

5　Remove ½ cup of sauce and stir into flour until smooth. Return flour mixture to pot. Add honey and cranberries to beef mixture.

6　Increase heat to medium and cook uncovered for 15 additional minutes, stirring frequently.

7　Serve over noodles or rice. (This stew is especially good if refrigerated and reheated the following day. It gives the flavors a chance to blend.)

Nutritional information per serving

292 calories	25% of calories from fat
20% of calories from carbohydrate	8 grams of fat
55% of calories from protein	2 grams of fiber

Marinated and Grilled Flank Steak
SERVES 4

1 pound flank steak, trimmed of all fat

MARINADE

1 can beer (12 ounces)
2 tablespoons Worcestershire sauce
1 tablespoon brown sugar
¼ cup chopped parsley
½ teaspoon dried tarragon

½ teaspoon dried thyme
2 bay leaves
2 green onions, white and green parts, chopped
2 tablespoons red wine vinegar

1 Mix marinade ingredients together and pour over flank steak. Marinate overnight in large sealable plastic bag in refrigerator.

2 Remove steak from marinade. Preheat broiler or grill. Place steak in broiler pan and broil 6 minutes on each side. (Or grill the steak.)

3 Meanwhile, bring marinade to a boil, turn heat to low, and allow to simmer while steak cooks.

4 Carve meat across the grain in paper-thin slices. Spoon some of the sauce over it and pass the remaining sauce separately.

Nutritional information per serving

183 calories
12% of calories from carbohydrate
61% of calories from protein

27% of calories from fat
5 grams of fat
less than 1 gram of fiber

Stir-Fry Orange Beef
SERVES 4

The entire cooking process for this stir-fry takes under 5 minutes. If your vegetables are all set to go, it's a quick delicious meal.

1 pound flank steak, trimmed of fat
*⅔ cup orange juice concentrate
1 tablespoon lime juice
**2 tablespoons mirin
2 tablespoons reduced-sodium soy sauce
½ tablespoon minced fresh ginger

¼ cup dry vermouth
2 teaspoons cornstarch
½ pound carrots, sliced
½ pound snow peas, strings removed
8 ounce can sliced water chestnuts, drained
3 green onions, chopped

*Orange juice can be irritating to the esophagus. It really is essential to this recipe, so there is no replacement.

**Mirin is a sweet rice wine available in Asian markets. It will keep in your refrigerator indefinitely, so buy a bottle to have on hand.

1   Slice flank steak across the grain into thin strips. (It is easier to do this if you put the flank steak in the freezer for a little while before slicing.) Place into large sealable plastic bag.

2   Mix together juices, mirin, soy sauce, ginger, and vermouth. Pour over beef, and marinate overnight.

3   Drain meat, reserving marinade. Whisk cornstarch into marinade.

4   Heat wok or large nonstick skillet over high heat. Add beef and cook for 1 to 1½ minutes to desired doneness. Remove to platter.

5   Add carrots and cook for about 30 seconds, stirring constantly. Add snow peas and water chestnuts, and cook for an additional 15 to 30 seconds.

6   Return beef to pan and add marinade-cornstarch mixture. Bring to a boil and cook for about 1 minute or until sauce is desired thickness. Add green onions, remove from heat, and serve over rice or another grain of your choice.

Nutritional information per serving

312 calories	18% of calories from fat
40% of calories from carbohydrate	6 grams of fat
42% of calories from protein	6 grams of fiber

Veal with Sun-Dried Tomatoes
SERVES 4

½ cup sun-dried tomatoes	⅓ cup chopped shallots
1 tablespoon olive oil	1 teaspoon lemon juice
4 veal scallopini (1 pound total weight)	2 teaspoons fresh parsley, chopped
	2 teaspoons fresh basil, chopped
½ cup dry white wine or vermouth	(½ teaspoon dried)
½ cup sliced mushrooms	salt to taste

1   Soak sun-dried tomatoes in hot water for at least 10 minutes. Drain and slice into strips.

2   Heat oil in large skillet and quickly sauté the veal, about 1 minute on each side. Remove and drain on paper towels.

3   Add wine, mushrooms, tomatoes, and shallots to the skillet. Sauté until vegetables are tender. Sprinkle lemon juice, parsley, and basil over softened vegetables and stir.

4   Add veal to the sauce to reheat. Season with salt if desired.

Nutritional information per serving

260 calories
12% of calories from carbohydrate
41% of calories from protein

47% of calories from fat
13 grams of fat
2 grams of fiber

Very Veggie Meatloaf
SERVES 6

This is a tasty meatloaf as heavy on the vegetables as on the meat. It is good either plain with a marinara sauce (see page 356) or as a sandwich filler.

½ pound potato, peeled and shredded
½ pound onion (1 medium),
   shredded
¼ pound carrot (1 large), shredded
¼ cup chopped parsley
2 tablespoons white wine
Worcestershire sauce

¼ cup bread crumbs, preferably
   whole wheat
1 egg white
1 tablespoon Dijon-style mustard
½ teaspoon dried oregano
½ teaspoon dried basil
1 pound lean ground beef

1 Preheat oven to 350°
2 In large bowl, mix together all ingredients.
3 Press mixture into loaf pan. Bake for 1 hour.

Nutritional information per serving

240 calories
29% of calories from carbohydrate
31% of calories from protein

40% of calories from fat
11 grams of fat
2 grams of fiber

38 *Entrees:*
Meatless

Eggless Salad
Spinach Rice Casserole
Stuffed Bell Peppers
Tofu Stroganoff

Eggless Salad
SERVES 4

This is very similar to egg salad, but it is lower in fat and is cholesterol-free. Although this recipe appears to be high in fat, it is much lower than a mayonnaise-based egg salad.

SALAD

⅔ pound firm tofu, cut in ½-inch cubes
½ large green pepper, diced
1 large stalk celery, diced

1 large carrot, grated
½ medium red onion, diced
*¼ cup sunflower seeds, toasted

DRESSING

⅓ pound firm tofu
2 tablespoons prepared mustard

soy sauce to taste

1 Prepare all salad ingredients as described.
2 Blend together dressing ingredients in blender or food processor.
3 Stir salad and dressing together gently until well mixed.

*Seeds can be gas-producing. You may be able to tolerate this small amount, but if not you may omit them. This will decrease the fat content as well.

4 Serve eggless salad on bread or bed of greens. It is especially good served on whole wheat pita bread and topped with alfalfa sprouts.

Nutritional information per serving

240 calories

16% of calories from carbohydrate

32% of calories from protein

52% of calories from fat

15 grams of fat

1 gram of fiber

Spinach Rice Casserole
SERVES 4

Leftovers of this main dish casserole are good cold for lunch.

1 egg (or 2 egg whites)

*2 cups 1% low-fat cottage cheese

3 cups cooked brown rice

4 cups fresh spinach, torn, uncooked, well drained

2 cups mushrooms, quartered

1 medium onion chopped

1 teaspoon marjoram

**2 tablespoons grated Romano cheese

1 Preheat oven to 375°.

2 Beat egg and cottage cheese together.

3 Stir in rice, spinach, mushrooms, onion, and marjoram until well blended.

4 Pour mixture into 9 × 13-inch baking dish that has been coated with nonstick vegetable oil spray. Sprinkle with grated cheese.

5 Bake for 30 minutes.

Nutritional information per serving

320 calories

60% of calories from carbohydrate

29% of calories from protein

11% of calories from fat

4 grams of fat

8 grams of fiber

*If you have a lactose intolerance, look for low-lactose cottage cheese or take 2 lactase enzyme tablets with this meal.

**This small amount of Romano cheese should be well tolerated in all but the most severely lactose-intolerant individuals. The cheese can be left off for those individuals.

Stuffed Bell Peppers
SERVES 4

4 large bell peppers
*½ cup dry bulgur wheat
3 tablespoons chopped onion
1 tablespoon vegetable oil,
  preferably olive or canola
½ pound tofu, cut into small cubes
1½ cups tomato puree
2 tablespoons green pepper, finely
  chopped

2 tablespoons celery, finely chopped
1 tablespoon brown sugar
1 tablespoon oregano
¼ teaspoon allspice
¼ teaspoon cloves (optional)
1 cup *cooked* brown rice
1 tablespoon grated carrots

1 Preheat oven to 350°.

2 Wash and core peppers. Steam for 20 minutes.

3 Soak bulgur in ⅓ cup warm water. Set aside.

4 In large skillet, sauté onion in oil until softened.

5 Add tofu. Stir until evenly browned.

6 Add 1 cup of tomato puree, diced green pepper, celery, brown sugar, herbs, and spices. Heat mixture until bubbly. Reduce heat to a simmer and cook for about 15 minutes.

7 Add rice and bulgur. Stir.

8 Fill each pepper with stuffing.

9 Place in casserole and top with the reserved ½ cup tomato puree. Pour about ¼ inch water in bottom of pan.

10 Bake for 30 minutes. Remove from oven and sprinkle grated carrots on top of stuffed peppers.

Nutritional information per serving

297 calories
66% of calories from carbohydrate
13% of calories from protein

21% of calories from fat
7 grams of fat
4 grams of fiber

*Bulgur wheat is available in health food or bulk food stores.

Tofu Stroganoff
SERVES 4

Try this delicious lower fat version of a classic main dish!

MARINADE

1 pound firm tofu
¼ cup soy sauce, preferably low
  sodium

*½ teaspoon garlic powder
*⅓ teaspoon black pepper
⅓ teaspoon cumin

MAIN DISH

1 tablespoon cornstarch
**1 cup plain nonfat yogurt
1 teaspoon olive oil
1 medium onion, minced
½ pound mushrooms, sliced

½ teaspoon basil
*dash nutmeg
4 cups uncooked flat noodles
¼ cup white wine

1   At least 3 hours prior to meal, begin marinating tofu; it can be marinated overnight. Cut tofu into ½-inch cubes and place in small deep bowl. Add soy sauce, spices, and enough water to cover. Mix well and put into refrigerator until ready to prepare main dish.

2   Begin heating water to cook noodles in large pot. Drain tofu of marinade. Whisk cornstarch into yogurt.

3   Heat oil in large nonstick frying pan. Cook onion in oil for 2 to 3 minutes, add tofu and mushrooms, and cook 2 to 3 minutes more. Add basil and nutmeg. Reduce heat, cover, and cook about 10 minutes. Begin cooking noodles.

4   When mushrooms are tender, add wine and yogurt-cornstarch mixture. Heat through over low heat. When noodles are done, drain in colander.

5   Serve stroganoff over noodles.

Nutritional information per serving

550 calories
52% of calories from carbohydrate
25% of calories from protein

23% of calories from fat
14 grams of fat
4 grams of fiber

---

*Garlic powder, black pepper, and nutmeg are gastric irritants. You may omit them if you are unable to tolerate them.

**Yogurt is usually well tolerated by lactose-intolerant individuals. If you are unable to tolerate yogurt, take 1 lactase enzyme tablet with this meal.

39

Entrees:
Poultry

Chicken and Herbs Baked in Foil

Chicken Breasts in Creamy Mustard Sauce

Chicken Fajitas

Chicken-Vegetable Stir-Fry

Chicken with Mushrooms and Sun-Dried Tomatoes

Creole Topped Potato

Fruited Chicken Salad

Ground Turkey in Zucchini Shells

Lemonade Chicken

Marinated and Grilled Chicken Breast

Oriental Barbecued Chicken

Chicken and Herbs Baked in Foil
SERVES 4

4 chicken breast halves, boned and
   skinned
1 teaspoon olive oil
¼ cup chopped fresh dill

*¼ cup chopped fresh mint
4 scallions, diced
1 lemon, thinly sliced

1   Preheat oven to 350°.
2   Brush each chicken breast with ¼ teaspoon of olive oil. Place each breast on a large piece of aluminum foil.

*Mint commonly causes gastric distress and heartburn. If you are unable to tolerate mint, replace it with fresh coriander (also called cilantro or Chinese parsley).

3　Mix together dill, mint, and scallions. Divide mixture and spread equally over chicken breasts.

4　Top each breast with 2 to 3 lemon slices. Fold foil over, making a tight seal.

5　Bake for 30 minutes. Remove from foil and serve.

Nutritional information per serving

230 calories	23% of calories from fat
7% of calories from carbohydrate	6 grams of fat
70% of calories from protein	less than 1 gram of fiber

Chicken Breasts in Creamy Mustard Sauce
SERVES 4

4 chicken breast halves, each about 6 ounces, skinned, boned, trimmed
3 tablespoons flour, preferably whole wheat
½ teaspoon dried marjoram
½ teaspoon dried thyme
*½ teaspoon fresh ground black pepper

1 teaspoon butter or margarine
½ cup dry vermouth or white wine
1 cup defatted chicken stock, preferably homemade (see page 280)
2 tablespoons Dijon-style mustard
**¼ cup evaporated skimmed milk
Fresh thyme sprigs

1　Pound chicken breasts between sheets of waxed paper to the thickness of ¼ inch.

2　Combine flour, herbs, and spices. Transfer 1 tablespoon of mixture to small bowl and reserve. Rub remainder into chicken.

3　Coat skillet with nonstick vegetable oil spray. Add butter and melt. Add chicken and cook until brown, about 2 minutes per side. Transfer to plate.

4　Add vermouth to skillet and boil until reduced to a glaze, scraping up any browned bits, about 1 minute. Mix in stock and mustard and boil for 2 to 3 minutes.

5　Mix evaporated skimmed milk into reserved flour. Whisk in ¼ cup of the hot stock/mustard mixture and return to pan. Simmer until thickened and smooth, stirring constantly for about 3 minutes.

*Black pepper is a gastric irritant. If you are unable to tolerate it, replace the black pepper with ½ teaspoon of chervil.

**A lactose-intolerant individual should be able to tolerate the small amount of lactose in one serving. However, if you are severely lactose-intolerant, either treat the evaporated skimmed milk with lactase enzyme drops (use two times your usual amount) or take 1 lactase enzyme tablet with this meal.

6   Return chicken to skillet and cook at medium low heat until opaque, about 1 minute per side.

7   Serve chicken with extra sauce on the side. Garnish with fresh thyme sprigs.

Nutritional information per serving

290 calories	21% of calories from fat
11% of calories from carbohydrate	7 grams of fat
68% of calories from protein	0 grams of fiber

Chicken Fajitas
SERVES 4

2 whole chicken breasts, boned and skinned
*1 cup tomato juice
2 tablespoons lime juice
1 tablespoon reduced-sodium soy sauce
2 tomatoes, coarsely chopped
4 scallions, coarsely chopped
1 bunch cilantro, chopped
1 red or green bell pepper, coarsely chopped
8 flour tortillas
1 cup mock sour cream (see page 357)

1   Cut the chicken across the grain into thin strips. It is easier to do this if the chicken is slightly frozen. Place the chicken in a nonaluminum bowl.

2   Pour tomato juice, lime juice, and soy sauce over chicken strips and allow to marinate several hours or overnight. (If you can tolerate it, 2 cloves of finely chopped garlic is a great addition to the marinade.)

3   Meanwhile, prepare tomatoes, scallions, cilantro, and pepper. Arrange on serving platter and refrigerate.

4   Preheat broiler. Drain marinade from chicken. Place marinade in small, nonaluminum saucepan, bring to a boil, and allow to simmer while chicken is cooking.

5   Broil chicken strips in a single layer, 4 inches from heat source, for about 3 to 5 minutes or until done. Turn for the last minute of cooking.

6   Seal tortillas in aluminum foil and place in bottom of oven to heat while you broil the chicken (or place in 350° oven for 5 to 10 minutes).

7   To serve, place chicken strips, vegetables, and marinade sauce (if desired) in center of tortilla. Top with mock sour cream. Roll or fold tortilla and eat as a sandwich.

*Tomato juice can be irritating to the esophagus. It can be replaced with chicken stock.

Nutritional information per serving

450 calories	17% of calories from fat
39% of calories from carbohydrate	9 grams of fat
44% of calories from protein	2 grams of fiber

Chicken-Vegetable Stir-Fry
SERVES 4

½ cup defatted chicken stock or broth (see page 280)

1 whole chicken breast (10 to 12 ounces), boned, skinned, and cut into bite-sized pieces

MARINADE

¼ cup dry white wine
¼ cup reduced-sodium soy sauce
8 ounce can of sliced or chunk pineapple (undrained) in its own juice, pureed

*2 garlic cloves, finely minced
1 teaspoon fresh ginger, finely minced

VEGETABLES

**1 bunch broccoli, stalks peeled and sliced on diagonal; florets cut into bite-size pieces
¼ pound snow peas, strings removed
2 red peppers, cut into julienne strips
1 yellow pepper, cut into julienne strips

2 teaspoons cornstarch
½ teaspoon vegetable oil, preferably canola or olive oil
½ pound whole wheat pasta twists

1 Heat chicken stock to boiling in small skillet. Add chicken pieces and poach until done, about 4 to 5 minutes.
2 Combine marinade ingredients. Add chicken and cooking broth and marinate overnight in refrigerator.
3 Heat 2 to 3 quarts of water for pasta.
4 Prepare vegetables.
5 Remove chicken from marinade, reserving marinade.
6 Remove ½ cup of marinade and mix with cornstarch. Set aside.
7 Put oil into wok or large skillet and spread it with a paper towel. Heat wok.

*Garlic is gas-producing. If you are unable to tolerate the garlic, it may be omitted.
**Broccoli is gas-producing. Substitute ½ pound of green beans if you are unable to tolerate the broccoli.

8   Put pasta into boiling water. Cook until done (about 7 minutes), stirring as necessary, while you stir-fry the vegetables.

9   Add broccoli to wok and stir-fry for about 2 minutes. Add snow peas and stir-fry for about 1 minute. Add pepper and stir-fry for about 30 seconds. Add chicken for another 30 seconds. If additional liquid is necessary, add a small amount of reserved marinade.

10   Remove vegetable-chicken mixture to large bowl or platter. Add the reserved marinade to wok and bring to a boil. Add the cornstarch-marinade mixture and stir until it reaches the desired thickness.

11   Return the chicken-vegetable mixture to the wok and heat through.

12   Meanwhile, drain the pasta.

13   Serve chicken-vegetable mixture over pasta.

Nutritional information per serving

423 calories	11% of calories from fat
52% of calories from carbohydrate	5 grams of fat
37% of calories from protein	8 grams of fiber

Chicken with Mushrooms and Sun-Dried Tomatoes
SERVES 4

This is a wonderful company meal, yet so simple you'll want to prepare it for your family.

1 cup chicken stock, preferably homemade (see page 280)
½ cup dry sherry
2 whole chicken breasts, skinned, boned, and split
¾ pound mushrooms, sliced
⅓ cup finely chopped onion
⅓ cup chopped parsley

2 ounces sun-dried tomatoes (12 to 15), soaked in 2 cups of boiling water for 5 minutes, drained and chopped. Reserve ½ cup of soaking liquid.
½ teaspoon dried basil
2 teaspoons Dijon-style mustard
Fresh basil sprigs

1   Bring ½ cup of chicken stock and sherry to a boil in large skillet. Add chicken and cook for about 15 seconds on each side. Add mushrooms, onion, and parsley, turn heat to low, cover, and simmer for about 5 minutes or until chicken is cooked through. Remove chicken to platter.

2   Add remaining ½ cup of chicken stock, tomatoes, ½ cup of reserved tomato liquid, basil, and mustard. Bring to a boil and cook for 5 to 8 minutes or until liquid is almost completely reduced.

3 Spread mushroom-tomato mixture over a serving platter and place chicken on top. Garnish with fresh basil sprigs.

Nutritional information per serving

275 calories
18% of calories from carbohydrate
65% of calories from protein

17% of calories from fat
5 grams of fat
4 grams of fiber

Creole Topped Potato
SERVES 4

This is a wonderful main dish potato.

4 medium-sized baking potatoes,
  well scrubbed and dried
2 teaspoons vegetable oil, preferably
  olive or canola oil
¼ cup chopped onion
½ cup chopped green pepper

½ pound ground turkey
⅛ teaspoon dried basil
1 tablespoon white wine or dry
  vermouth
½ cup tomato puree
*4 ounces grated cheddar cheese

1 Preheat oven to 375°.

2 Pierce potatoes with fork tines. Wrap in foil and bake 1 hour.

3 While potatoes are baking, heat oil in large pot. Add onion and green pepper and cook until tender, about 10 minutes, stirring often. If additional liquid is necessary, use wine or vermouth.

4 Add ground turkey and cook until no longer pink.

5 Add basil, wine, and tomato puree. Bring to boil, lower heat, and simmer covered for 30 minutes.

6 Remove potatoes from oven, unwrap, and slice lengthwise. Top each potato half with about ¼ cup of creole mixture and ½ ounce of cheese. Serve.

Nutritional information per serving

453 calories
49% of calories from carbohydrate
24% of calories from protein

27% of calories from fat
14 grams of fat
5 grams of fiber

*You may tolerate a small amount of cheese if you are lactose-intolerant, but if not, the cheese may be omitted, or you may take 1 lactase enzyme tablet.

Fruited Chicken Salad
SERVES 4

The Grape Nuts in this recipe provide an interesting and low-fat alternative to nuts.

2 cups cooked chicken, cubed
2 medium oranges, each section cut
   into 3 or 4 pieces
½ cup diced celery
*½ cup plain nonfat yogurt

½ cup low-fat mayonnaise
1 tablespoon honey
1 tablespoon Dijon-style mustard
½ cup Grape Nuts cereal
Salad greens

1   Stir together chicken, oranges, and celery in medium-size bowl.

2   In small bowl, mix together yogurt, mayonnaise, honey, and mustard until well blended.

3   Pour yogurt dressing over chicken salad and toss until well mixed.

4   Just before serving, stir in Grape Nuts.

5   Serve on a bed of greens. Especially tasty served on a bed of fresh spinach leaves.

Nutritional information per serving

305 calories
37% of calories from carbohydrate
32% of calories from protein

31% of calories from fat
11 grams of fat
2 grams of fiber

Ground Turkey in Zucchini Shells
SERVES 4

4 medium zucchini
½ pound ground turkey
1 medium onion, chopped
½ cup bread crumbs (preferably
   whole wheat)

1 egg or 2 egg whites
½ teaspoon thyme
**¼ cup grated Romano cheese

---

*Most lactose-intolerant individuals can tolerate yogurt without any problem. If you do not, you may take 1 lactase enzyme tablet with this meal or use all low-fat mayonnaise. The use of low-fat mayonnaise will increase the fat content of this recipe.

**This small amount of cheese should be tolerated by all but the most severely lactose-intolerant individual. If you are unable to tolerate the cheese, take 1 lactase enzyme tablet with this meal.

1 Preheat oven to 350°.

2 Boil whole zucchini until just tender, about 8 minutes.

3 While zucchini are boiling, cook ground turkey and onion in skillet. To prevent sticking, put turkey in cold skillet and begin cooking over low heat. After turkey is cooked, remove from heat and drain off liquid.

4 Cut cooked zucchini in half lengthwise. Scoop out pulp and mash it with a fork. Reserve zucchini shells.

5 Stir mashed zucchini pulp, bread crumbs, egg, and thyme into turkey mixture. Mix well.

6 Spoon mixture evenly into zucchini shells. Sprinkle with grated cheese.

7 Place shells in baking dish and bake in 350° oven for 25 to 30 minutes.

Nutritional information per serving

235 calories	26% of calories from fat
33% of calories from carbohydrate	7 grams of fat
41% of calories from protein	3 grams of fiber

Lemonade Chicken
SERVES 4

3 pounds chicken pieces, skinned	¼ cup reduced-sodium soy sauce
*¾ cup (6 ounces) lemonade concentrate, defrosted	¼ teaspoon ground ginger

1 Skin chicken and place in glass ovenproof pan.

2 Mix lemonade, soy sauce, and ginger together. Pour over chicken. Marinate all day or overnight. Remove chicken from marinade.

3 Preheat broiler. Broil about 5 inches from heat source, about 15 minutes per side. Baste chicken often (about 10 times total while cooking). Serve.

*Nutritional information per serving***

340 calories	37% of calories from fat
14% of calories from carbohydrate	14 grams of fat
49% of calories from protein	0 grams of fiber

*Lemonade can be irritating to the esophagus.

**The nutrient analysis was done using chicken thighs and legs. The calorie and fat content would be lowered by using white meat (i.e., breast meat).

Marinated and Grilled Chicken Breast
SERVES 4

You'll find this to be a little different from the typical grilled chicken. It's a quick summer meal that can be prepared outside on the grill, but works just as well under your broiler.

2 whole chicken breasts, boned,
    skinned, and split

MARINADE

4 tablespoons reduced-sodium soy
    sauce
2 tablespoons brown sugar

4 tablespoons dry vermouth
2 tablespoons white wine
Worcestershire sauce

BASTING SAUCE

½ cup apricot preserves
¼ cup white vinegar

1 tablespoon white wine
Worcestershire sauce

1   Mix marinade ingredients together in glass bowl or large sealable plastic bag. Add chicken breasts and marinate overnight.

2   In small saucepan, bring basting sauce ingredients to a boil. Turn heat to low and simmer uncovered, stirring occasionally, for 3 minutes.

3   Preheat broiler or grill. Coat broiler pan with nonstick vegetable oil spray. Remove chicken from marinade and discard marinade.

4   Broil or grill 4 inches from heat, basting at least 3 times on each side. Cook for about 5 to 6 minutes per side or until cooked through. Serve immediately.

Nutritional information per serving

336 calories
39% of calories from carbohydrate
49% of calories from protein

12% of calories from fat
5 grams of fat
0 grams of fiber

Oriental Barbecued Chicken
SERVES 4

This is excellent hot, but even better cold for picnics.

3 pounds chicken pieces with skin
    and fat removed

MARINADE

*2 garlic cloves, peeled and finely
  chopped
½ inch slice ginger, peeled and
  minced
3 scallions, white and green parts,
  chopped

2 tablespoons hoisin sauce
2 tablespoons catsup
2 tablespoons reduced-sodium
  soy sauce
3 tablespoons rice wine vinegar

1   Place chicken in 11 × 8-inch glass baking pan. Mix all ingredients for marinade together and pour over chicken. Cover with aluminum foil. Marinate overnight in refrigerator. Turn chicken over once.

2   Preheat oven to 450°. Bake covered for 20 minutes, basting as necessary. Turn oven down to 350°, turn chicken, baste well. Cook another 20 minutes, basting as necessary.

Nutritional information per serving**

256 calories
9% of calories from carbohydrate
55% of calories from protein

36% of calories from fat
10 grams of fat
0 grams of fiber

*Garlic is gas-producing. Omit the garlic if you are unable to tolerate it.
**To decrease the fat content further, use only chicken breasts. This recipe was analyzed using breasts, thighs, and legs. The dark meat of poultry is higher in fat than white meat.

40

Side Dishes:
Grains and Starches

Barley Delight

Beautiful Bow Tie Pasta

Cinnamon Rice

Cold Barley Salad

Cold Bulgur Wheat Salad

Italian-style Couscous

Kasha and Corn

Rice Salad

Wheat Berry Salad

Whole Grain Pasta Salad

Barley Delight
SERVES 4

3 cups water	**½ cup plain nonfat yogurt
1 cup barley	¼ teaspoon nutmeg
*½ cup raisins	***¼ cup sesame seeds, toasted

1   Bring 3 cups water and 1 cup barley to a boil. Reduce heat to a simmer, cover, and cook for 35 to 40 minutes or until water is absorbed.

*Raisins are gas-producing. You could replace the raisins with dried currants or another dried fruit of your choice. If you are unable to tolerate nutmeg, it can be replaced with cinnamon.

**Yogurt is usually well tolerated by lactose-intolerant individuals. Take 1 lactase enzyme tablet with this meal if you are unable to tolerate yogurt.

***Seeds are gas-producing. Omit the seeds if you are unable to tolerate them, although they may be well tolerated in this small amount.

2   Stir in raisins, yogurt, and nutmeg. Mix well.
3   Sprinkle with sesame seeds just before serving.

Nutritional information per serving

296 calories
76% of calories from carbohydrate
10% of calories from protein

14% of calories from fat
5 grams of fat
3 grams of fiber

Beautiful Bow Tie Pasta
SERVES 6

16 ounces bow tie pasta, cooked al
  dente
2 tablespoons olive oil
*½ cup wine vinegar
½ cup crumbled feta cheese (about 4
  ounces)
1 cup snow peas, cleaned and cut in
  half lengthwise, blanched for 1
  minute
1 large sweet red pepper, julienned,
  blanched for 1 minute

1 large yellow pepper, julienned,
  blanched for 1 minute
1 carrot cut into coins, blanched for
  2 minutes
½ large purple onion, cut into rings,
  blanched for 2 minutes
1 large red tomato, diced
¼ cup finely chopped parsley
¼ cup coarsely chopped fresh basil
**fresh black pepper

1   Cook pasta al dente, drain, and run under cold water.
2   In small bowl combine the oil, vinegar, and feta cheese and whisk
briskly.
3   Combine pasta, vegetables, herbs, and dressing in large bowl and
toss gently until all are combined. Top with freshly grated black pepper.

Nutritional information per serving

400 calories
64% of calories from carbohydrate
14% of calories from protein

22% of calories from fat
10 grams of fat
4 grams of fiber

*Many people with a lactose intolerance are able to tolerate small amounts of cheese. If
you are unable to tolerate the feta cheese, take 1 lactase enzyme tablet with this meal or omit
the cheese and use 4 tablespoons of olive oil.
**Omit the black pepper if you find it to be a gastric irritant. (Most people will need to
omit it.)

Cinnamon Rice
SERVES 6

This is a very simple yet interesting variation on rice. Try to use brown rice as it is significantly higher in fiber.

2 cups raw brown rice	2 cinnamon sticks
6 cups water	1 tablespoon lemon juice

1 Mix all ingredients together in 3-quart saucepan and bring to a boil.
2 Reduce heat to low, cover, and cook until all the liquid is absorbed, about 45 minutes.

Nutritional information per serving

232 calories	5% of calories from fat
87% of calories from carbohydrate	1 gram of fat
8% of calories from protein	6 grams of fiber

Cold Barley Salad
SERVES 6

1 cup raw barley	1½ tablespoons olive oil
1½ cups chicken stock, preferably homemade (see page 280)	3 stalks celery, diced
	3 small carrots, sliced thinly
1½ cups water	*1 medium red onion, diced
3 tablespoons balsamic vinegar	

1 Cook barley in broth and water until barley is tender and liquid is absorbed.
2 Stir vinegar and olive oil into hot barley. Chill until serving time.
3 Stir celery, carrot, and onion into cooled barley and serve.

Nutritional information per serving

182 calories	20% of calories from fat
70% of calories from carbohydrate	4 grams of fat
10% of calories from protein	3 grams of fiber

---

*If you are unable to tolerate raw onion, omit it. Try scallions if you tolerate them better.

Cold Bulgur Wheat Salad
SERVES 4

2 cups water, boiling
*1 cup bulgur wheat, dry
1 cucumber, peeled and diced
1 tomato, diced
6 scallions, chopped

1 cup fresh parsley, chopped
4 tablespoons lemon juice
1 tablespoon soy sauce
1 tablespoon olive oil

1 Pour boiling water over bulgur. Soak for 1 hour. Drain off any excess water.

2 Stir remaining ingredients into bulgur and chill until serving.

Nutritional information per serving

216 calories
74% of calories from carbohydrate
10% of calories from protein

16% of calories from fat
4 grams of fat
3 grams of fiber

Italian-Style Couscous
SERVES 4

1 cup sliced mushrooms
½ cup dry white wine or dry
    vermouth
1 teaspoon dried basil

½ cup water
1 tomato, peeled and chopped
**1 cup whole wheat couscous, dry

1 Marinate mushrooms in wine for 30 minutes.

2 Add basil and cook mushrooms in marinade until tender.

3 Add water and tomato and bring to boil. Remove from heat, stir in couscous, cover, and let stand for 5 minutes. Serve.

Nutritional information per serving

168 calories
86% of calories from carbohydrate
10% of calories from protein

4% of calories from fat
less than 1 gram of fat
2 grams of fiber

*Bulgur wheat is a cracked wheat that has been steamed, dried, and cracked into small pieces. It is available in health food stores, bulk food stores, and specialty food stores.

**Couscous is available in health food or bulk food stores. Look for whole wheat couscous, which is higher in fiber. Couscous is finely cracked wheat that has been steamed and dried. Its quick cooking time (5 minutes) makes it a great alternative to rice and other grains.

Kasha and Corn
SERVES 4

1 cup kasha (buckwheat)
1 medium onion, chopped
1 tablespoon olive oil
2 cups chicken stock, preferably
   homemade (see page 280)

*1 cup corn, whole kernel
¼ cup fresh parsley, chopped

1   Sauté kasha and onion in oil until onion is translucent.

2   Add stock and bring to a boil. Cover and simmer until kasha is tender, about 15 minutes.

3   Stir in corn and parsley, heat through, and serve.

Nutritional information per serving

183 calories
60% of calories from carbohydrate
15% of calories from protein

25% of calories from fat
5 grams of fat
4 grams of fiber

Rice Salad
SERVES 4

Although this salad may appear to be high in fat, it contains much less oil than you typically find in a salad. The usual proportion of oil to vinegar in a dressing is 3 parts oil to 1 part vinegar.

SALAD

3 cups cooked brown rice, cooled
1 cup cooked wild rice, cooled
1 large green pepper, sliced

2 medium carrots, scraped and sliced
   on diagonal
¼ cup parsley, chopped

DRESSING

5 tablespoons red wine vinegar
3 tablespoons olive oil
2 teaspoons Dijon-style mustard

¼ teaspoon dried tarragon
pinch of basil
pinch of thyme

1   Combine salad ingredients in large serving bowl.

2   Whisk ingredients for dressing together. Pour over salad. Refrigerate several hours before serving.

*Corn can be gas-producing. If you are unable to tolerate corn, replace it with green peas.

Nutritional information per serving

302 calories
60% of calories from carbohydrate
7% of calories from protein

33% of calories from fat
11 grams of fat
8 grams of fiber

Wheat Berry Salad
SERVES 4

1½ cups water
*½ cup hard wheat berries (often called winter wheat)
1 cinnamon stick
1 celery stalk, diced
1 medium apple, cored and coarsely chopped, skin on

**¼ cup raisins
½ teaspoon vanilla
½ teaspoon ground coriander
***¼ cup plain low-fat or nonfat yogurt

1 Bring water to a boil. Add wheat berries and cinnamon stick and return to boil. Reduce heat to simmer, cover, and cook about 2 hours or until berries are tender. Drain if necessary and cool.

2 Add celery, apple, raisins, spices, and yogurt. Stir to combine. Refrigerate until ready to serve. Leave cinnamon stick in salad until ready to serve, but remove before serving.

Nutritional information per serving

195 calories
86% of calories from carbohydrate
10% of calories from protein

4% of calories from fat
1 gram of fat
7 grams of fiber

---

*Wheat berries can be found in health food and bulk food stores. They are delicious and worth the effort to find them and to cook them. Cook extra and freeze them for future use.

**Raisins are gas-producing. Omit them if you are unable to tolerate them.

***Lactose-intolerant individuals can usually tolerate yogurt. This is a very small amount per portion and should not cause any problems. If you would prefer, you may use low-fat mayonnaise.

Whole Grain Pasta Salad
SERVES 6

*1 cup broccoli florets
¾ cup carrots, sliced into coins
1 small zucchini, unpeeled, cut into
  1-inch chunks
½ cup mushrooms, halved

1¼ cups cherry tomatoes, halved
1¼ cups whole wheat pasta,
  preferably corkscrew, cooked al
  dente (about 3 cups cooked)

DRESSING

**½ cup plain low-fat yogurt
¼ cup red wine vinegar
***2 tablespoons grated Parmesan
  cheese

1 tablespoon low-fat mayonnaise
1 tablespoon parsley

1 Place broccoli and carrots in a vegetable steamer and steam for 5 minutes. Add zucchini and steam for 3 more minutes.

2 Combine steamed vegetables, mushrooms, tomatoes, and pasta in large bowl.

3 In container of blender or food processor, combine the dressing ingredients. Cover and process at low speed until smooth.

4 Add dressing to pasta and toss gently to coat. Chill at least 1 hour before serving.

Nutritional information per serving

150 calories
70% of calories from carbohydrate
17% of calories from protein

13% of calories from fat
2 grams of fat
4 grams of fiber

*If you are unable to tolerate broccoli, replace it with green beans or another vegetable that you can tolerate.

**Yogurt is usually well tolerated, even if you are lactose-intolerant. If you do not tolerate yogurt, take 1 lactase enzyme tablet with this salad or replace the yogurt with the same amount of low-fat mayonnaise. Remember that the salad will be higher in fat with low-fat mayonnaise.

***This small amount of Parmesan cheese should be tolerated except in the case of a severe lactose intolerance. You may omit the cheese if desired.

41

Side Dishes:

Salads and Vegetables

Apple Salad

Applejack Acorn Squash

Asparagus Salad

Boiled Potatoes with Apples

Broiled Tomato Halves

Carrot Salad

Cucumber-Radish Salad

Dilly Carrots

Eggplant in Rich Tomato Sauce

Green Beans Italian Style

Green Salad

Grilled Zucchini

Lemony Potatoes

Potato Salad

Snow Pea Salad

Spinach Salad

Steamed Broccoli with Orange Sauce

Sweet Potato Casserole

Vegetable Kabob

Veggie Stir-Fry

Apple Salad
SERVES 4

4 celery stalks, diced
8 ounce can of sliced water
  chestnuts, drained
4 tart apples, sliced (either red or
  green are attractive)
2 tablespoons low-fat mayonnaise

*6–8 tablespoons plain nonfat or
  low-fat yogurt
1 teaspoon lemon juice
½ teaspoon ground cinnamon
¼ teaspoon ground ginger

1   Place celery, water chestnuts, and apples in medium-sized serving bowl.
2   In small bowl, mix together mayonnaise, yogurt, lemon juice, and spices. Pour over the apple mixture.
3   Chill and serve.

Nutritional information per serving

132 calories
78% of calories from carbohydrate
6% of calories from protein

16% of calories from fat
3 grams of fat
4 grams of fiber

Applejack Acorn Squash
SERVES 4

2 medium acorn squash
¼ cup applejack, apple brandy, or
  another apple-flavored liqueur

2 tablespoons brown sugar
2 teaspoons butter or margarine

1   Preheat oven to 350°.
2   Cut squash in half and remove seeds. Place on baking sheet.
3   Mix applejack and brown sugar together. Spoon into center of each squash half, dividing the mixture evenly.
4   Put ½ teaspoon of butter in center of each squash.
5   Bake for 1 hour or until soft, basting occasionally.

Nutritional information per serving

157 calories
84% of calories from carbohydrate
5% of calories from protein

11% of calories from fat
2 grams of fat
4 grams of fiber

*Yogurt is usually well tolerated by lactose-intolerant individuals. If you would prefer not to use the yogurt, you may replace with additional low-fat mayonnaise, but this will be higher in fat.

Asparagus Salad
SERVES 4

Although the percentage of fat in this salad appears high, the grams of fat are actually low because the total calories are so low.

1 pound asparagus, washed
1½ tablespoons white rice vinegar
1½ tablespoons dry vermouth

2 teaspoons sesame oil
¼ teaspoon salt, if desired
2 teaspoons white rice vinegar

1 Cut each asparagus spear in 3 to 4 pieces each. Cut on the diagonal, rolling the spear halfway around after each cut.

2 Heat vinegar (1½ tablespoons) and vermouth in medium skillet. Bring to a bare simmer. Add asparagus and sauté for about 2 to 3 minutes. Remove from heat.

3 Place asparagus into serving bowl. Add oil, salt, and additional vinegar. Toss and chill.

Nutritional information per serving

49 calories
38% of calories from carbohydrate
21% of calories from protein

41% of calories from fat
3 grams of fat
1 gram of fiber

Boiled Potatoes with Apples
SERVES 4

2 large baking potatoes, sliced
     ½ inch thick
1 medium onion, diced
1 cup water

½ teaspoon salt
2 tart apples, chopped (do not peel)
1 teaspoon cider vinegar

1 In medium saucepan simmer potatoes and onion in salted water for 10 minutes.

2 Add apples and cook for an additional 10 minutes.

3 Drain any remaining water and gently stir in vinegar. Serve.

Nutritional information per serving

160 calories
91% of calories from carbohydrate
7% of calories from protein

2% of calories from fat
less than 1 gram of fat
5 grams of fiber

Broiled Tomato Halves
SERVES 4

2 large tomatoes
4 tablespoons whole wheat bread
  crumbs

1 teaspoon oregano
2 teaspoons balsamic vinegar

1 Preheat broiler.

2 Cut tomatoes in half.

3 Mix together bread crumbs, oregano, and vinegar. Divide evenly and spread over tomato halves.

4 Broil 4 inches from heat source for about 5 minutes or until top is browned.

Nutritional information per serving

38 calories
75% of calories from carbohydrate
14% of calories from protein

11% of calories from fat
less than 1 gram of fat
1 gram of fiber

Carrot Salad
SERVES 4

1 pound carrots, peeled and sliced on
  diagonal
½ cup chopped parsley
3 tablespoons raspberry vinegar
4 teaspoons olive oil

2 teaspoons Dijon-style mustard
1 teaspoon sugar
¼ teaspoon ground cinnamon
lettuce

1 Steam carrots until crisp-tender, about 5 to 7 minutes.

2 Toss carrots and parsley together in medium-sized serving bowl.

3 Whisk together remaining ingredients in small bowl. Pour over carrots and parsley.

4 Refrigerate for several hours before serving. Serve on a bed of curly lettuce.

Nutritional information per serving

97 calories
53% of calories from carbohydrate
6% of calories from protein

41% of calories from fat
5 grams of fat
4 grams of fiber

Cucumber-Radish Salad
SERVES 4

1 cucumber, peeled and deseeded
½ pound radishes
½ cup cilantro, chopped

4 tablespoons white rice vinegar
2 tablespoons mirin
½ tablespoon sesame seed oil

1   Slice cucumbers and radishes paper thin. Mix with chopped cilantro in a serving bowl.

2   Mix remaining ingredients together and pour over vegetables. Chill 1 to 2 hours in refrigerator before serving.

Nutritional information per serving

42 calories
56% of calories from carbohydrate
7% of calories from protein

37% of calories from fat
2 grams of fat
3 grams of fiber

Dilly Carrots
SERVES 4

6 medium carrots, scraped and sliced
½ cup grapefruit juice

¼ teaspoon dried dill

1   Steam carrots until almost tender, about 5 to 7 minutes.

2   Heat grapefruit juice to boiling in small skillet. Add carrots and cook at medium high heat until the juice is nearly evaporated, about 2 to 3 minutes.

3   Add dill, stir, and serve hot.

Nutritional information per serving

60 calories
88% of calories from carbohydrate
8% of calories from protein

4% of calories from fat
less than 1 gram of fat
4 grams of fiber

Eggplant in Rich Tomato Sauce
SERVES 4

If you hate to open a can of tomato paste when only 1 or 2 tablespoons are called for in a recipe, here's the solution: the remainder can be frozen in tablespoon portions in small plastic bags.

1 teaspoon olive oil
1 medium onion, chopped
1 medium eggplant, peeled and cut
  into 2 × ½ × ½-inch strips
1 medium green pepper, coarsely diced

2 tablespoons soy sauce
2 tablespoons tomato paste
1 tablespoon lemon juice
¾ cup water

1   Heat oil in saucepan and cook onion for 1 to 2 minutes over medium heat.

2   Add eggplant and green pepper and cook, stirring frequently, until eggplant is almost tender, about 10 minutes. Add water as necessary to prevent sticking.

3   Add remaining ingredients and stir until well mixed. Cover and cook until flavors are well blended and eggplant is soft, about 5 minutes. Serve.

Nutritional information per serving

58 calories
65% of calories from carbohydrate
14% of calories from protein

21% of calories from fat
2 grams of fat
3 grams of fiber

Green Beans Italian Style
SERVES 4

2 cups green beans, cut in 1-inch
  pieces
½ cup onion, chopped
1 cup chopped tomato

1 teaspoon oregano
½ cup chicken stock, preferably
  homemade (see page 280)

Put all ingredients in saucepan. Cook over medium heat until green beans are tender, about 10 minutes. Serve.

Nutritional information per serving

40 calories
70% of calories from carbohydrate
21% of calories from protein

9% of calories from fat
less than 1 gram of fat
2 grams of fiber

Green Salad
SERVES 4

You'll find this to be a very interesting and delicious salad. It is time-consuming but worth the effort!

4 small heads of Belgian endive, washed and torn into bite-sized pieces
1 cup sorrel, washed and stems removed, torn into bite-sized pieces
½ cup chopped fennel
10–12 basil leaves, chopped
1 tablespoon finely chopped lemon peel

4 teaspoons lemon juice
4 teaspoons sparkling water or club soda
4 teaspoons white vinegar
4 teaspoons olive oil
¾ cup fresh or unsweetened frozen, thawed, and well-drained blueberries

1　Mix endive, sorrel, fennel, basil, and lemon peel together in large salad bowl.

2　In medium bowl, whisk together lemon juice, water, vinegar, and oil. Add ½ cup of blueberries and mash with a spoon. Strain and discard pieces of blueberry.

3　Pour dressing over salad and garnish with remaining blueberries.

Nutritional information per serving

65 calories
33% of calories from carbohydrate
6% of calories from protein

61% of calories from fat
5 grams of fat
2 grams of fiber

Grilled Zucchini
SERVES 4

2 whole zucchini
2 teaspoons olive oil
1½ teaspoons oregano

½ teaspoon salt (if desired)
*¼ teaspoon black pepper

1　Cut zucchini into quarters lengthwise. You will have 8 long pieces of zucchini.

2　Mix together oil, oregano, salt, and pepper. Brush each zucchini section lightly.

*Black pepper is a gastric irritant. Omit the pepper if you find it to be irritating, and use dried basil instead.

3   Place on heated grill, pulp side down, and grill for 5 to 8 minutes or until soft but not mushy. Serve immediately.

Nutritional information per serving

36 calories	54% of calories from fat
33% of calories from carbohydrate	2.4 grams of fat
13% of calories from protein	2 grams of fiber

Lemony Potatoes
SERVES 4

12 small new potatoes, cleaned and unpeeled	*1 teaspoon grated lemon peel
	1 tablespoon chopped fresh parsley
½ cup defatted chicken stock, preferably homemade (see page 280)	*¼ cup lemon juice
	1 teaspoon cornstarch

1   Boil potatoes until tender.

2   In small saucepan, heat stock, lemon peel, and parsley.

3   Mix lemon juice with cornstarch until thoroughly blended. Add this to broth, stirring constantly over low heat until slightly thickened.

4   Place potatoes in serving dish and pour lemon sauce over top. Toss lightly to coat all potatoes.

Nutritional information per serving

125 calories	1% of calories from fat
90% of calories from carbohydrate	less than 1 gram of fat
9% of calories from protein	2 grams of fiber

Potato Salad
SERVES 4

1½ pounds small red-skinned potatoes	2 teaspoons low-fat mayonnaise
**½ cup 1% low-fat cottage cheese	1½ teaspoons Dijon-style mustard
***¼ cup plain nonfat or low-fat yogurt	¼ cup chopped onion
	¼ cup chopped fresh parsley
½ teaspoon dried dill	2 tablespoons minced green pepper (optional)

*Lemon may be irritating to the esophagus.

**If you are lactose-intolerant, purchase low-lactose cottage cheese or take 1 lactase enzyme tablet with this meal.

***Yogurt is usually well tolerated by lactose-intolerant individuals. If you cannot tolerate yogurt, replace with an additional ¼ cup of low-fat mayonnaise. This will increase the recipe's fat content.

1 Steam unpeeled potatoes until fork tender. Do not overcook.

2 While potatoes are steaming, place the cottage cheese, yogurt, dill, mayonnaise, and mustard in the blender and blend until smooth.

3 Drain potatoes when cooked. Cut them into bite-sized pieces, taking care not to tear the skins.

4 Combine potatoes, onion, parsley, and green pepper in bowl. Pour dressing over top and toss lightly.

Nutritional information per serving

190 calories
78% of calories from carbohydrate
16% of calories from protein

6% of calories from fat
1 gram of fat
2 grams of fiber

Snow Pea Salad
SERVES 4

SALAD

½ pound snow peas, washed and
   strings removed
*½ pound (about 20) young corn
   spears, sliced on diagonal

¼ cup finely chopped fresh
   coriander (cilantro)
¼ cup finely chopped fresh parsley

DRESSING

1 teaspoon brown sugar
¼ cup rice wine vinegar

1 teaspoon soy sauce
1 tablespoon sesame oil

1 Mix peas, corn, coriander, and parsley together in medium-sized serving bowl.

2 Mix dressing ingredients together in small bowl. Pour over vegetables.

3 Refrigerate for at least 1 hour before serving.

Nutritional information per serving

109 calories
58% of calories from carbohydrate
11% of calories from protein

31% of calories from fat
4 grams of fat
4 grams of fiber

*Available in Asian food stores or the specialty food section of your grocery store. They are more digestible and cause less gas and discomfort than regular corn.

Spinach Salad
SERVES 4

Although this salad appears to be high in fat, it is actually much lower than a typical salad as the amount of oil is less than usual. The salad will be lower in fat if you omit the walnuts.

8 cups fresh spinach leaves, washed and torn
*1 grapefruit, sectioned, membranes removed
**¼ cup walnuts, chopped

1 tablespoon olive oil
1 tablespoon wine vinegar or balsamic vinegar
1 tablespoon lemon juice
1½ teaspoons honey

1   Place spinach in salad bowl. Arrange grapefruits and walnuts on the spinach.

2   In small bowl, whisk together oil, vinegar, lemon juice, and honey.

3   Pour dressing over salad. Toss and serve.

Nutritional information per serving

130 calories
35% of calories from carbohydrate
13% of calories from protein

52% of calories from fat
8 grams of fat
4 grams of fiber

Steamed Broccoli with Orange Sauce
SERVES 4

***1 pound broccoli, stalks peeled and sliced on diagonal, florets cut into bite-sized pieces
****½ cup orange juice
¼ cup dry white wine

½ medium onion, chopped
¼ teaspoon thyme
1 teaspoon cornstarch
1 teaspoon cold water

1   Steam broccoli until tender.

2   While broccoli is cooking, place orange juice, wine, onion, and thyme in saucepan and simmer until onion is translucent.

*Grapefruit may be irritating to the esophagus.
**Nuts are often gas-producing. You may be able to tolerate this small amount, but the recipe will work equally well without the nuts.
***Broccoli can be gas-producing. You may substitute any other vegetable that you find easier to tolerate, such as green beans or carrots.
****Orange juice may be irritating to the esophagus.

3   Mix cornstarch with cold water. Add cornstarch mixture to orange juice mixture. Cook until thickened, stirring constantly.

4   Place cooked broccoli spears in serving dish. Pour orange sauce over broccoli and serve.

Nutritional information per serving

50 calories	6% of calories from fat
70% of calories from carbohydrate	less than 1 gram of fat
24% of calories from protein	4 grams of fiber

Sweet Potato Casserole
SERVES 4

2 cups cooked, mashed sweet potatoes	2 tablespoons brown sugar
1 cup crushed pineapple, drained	*¼ teaspoon ground cloves

1   Preheat oven to 400°.
2   Stir together all ingredients.
3   Coat baking dish with nonstick vegetable oil spray and add sweet potato mixture.
4   Bake for 25 minutes and serve.

Nutritional information per serving

235 calories	2% of calories from fat
93% of calories from carbohydrate	less than 1 gram of fat
5% of calories from protein	3 grams of fiber

Vegetable Kabob
SERVES 5

KABOBS

20 cherry tomatoes	2 large green peppers, cut in 20
20 whole mushrooms	square pieces

*Cloves can be replaced with allspice.

SAUCE

*¼ cup plain nonfat yogurt	1 teaspoon lemon juice
**2 teaspoons tahini	¼ teaspoon coriander

1 Arrange vegetables on skewer in the following order: tomato, mushroom, pepper, tomato, mushroom, pepper. Repeat to total 10 skewers.

2 Coat broiler pan with nonstick vegetable oil spray. Lay kabobs on pan.

3 Broil kabobs about 3 minutes per side.

4 While vegetables are broiling, mix sauce ingredients together, stirring until smooth.

5 Serve kabobs and sauce separately, allowing each person to drizzle sauce over vegetables as desired.

Nutritional information per serving (2 kabobs and 1 tablespoon sauce)

52 calories	24% of calories from fat
55% of calories from carbohydrate	2 grams of fat
21% of calories from protein	3 grams of fiber

Veggie Stir-Fry
SERVES 4

1 tablespoon olive oil	1½ cups mushrooms, sliced
1 medium onion, thinly sliced	½ teaspoon basil
1 medium red potato, unpeeled, cut in half lengthwise, then thinly sliced crosswise	4 cups spinach leaves, washed and well drained
	soy sauce to taste

1 Heat oil in work or large skillet. Cook onion and potato over medium high heat, stirring frequently. Add water to wok as needed to prevent sticking.

2 When potatoes are partially cooked, add mushrooms and basil. Continue stirring as vegetables cook.

---

*Yogurt is usually well tolerated by lactose-intolerant individuals. If you are unable to tolerate yogurt, you could take 1 lactase enzyme tablet with the kabobs, or use a sauce of tahini, lemon juice, and coriander.

**Tahini is a sesame seed paste available in specialty food stores, Middle Eastern markets, and health food stores.

3   When potatoes and mushrooms are almost cooked, add spinach and soy sauce. Cook until spinach is done and remove from heat. Serve.

Nutritional information per serving

115 calories	30% of calories from fat
60% of calories from carbohydrate	4 grams of fat
10% of calories from protein	4 grams of fiber

Banana Bran Bread

Blueberry Orange Bread

Easy Corn Bread

Oat Biscuits

Oatmeal Raisin Muffins

Pumpkin Muffins

Banana Bran Bread

YIELD: 16 SLICES

½ cup unprocessed wheat bran
*½ cup buttermilk
2 tablespoons softened margarine
½ cup sugar
1 whole egg
2 egg whites
2 medium ripe bananas, mashed

1½ teaspoons vanilla
½ cup unbleached white flour
½ cup whole wheat flour
1 tablespoon baking powder
½ teaspoon baking soda
½ teaspoon salt
½ teaspoon ginger

1 Preheat oven to 350°.

2 Prepare loaf pan by lightly greasing with margarine or coating with nonstick vegetable oil spray.

3 In small bowl, soak bran in buttermilk for 15 minutes.

4 In medium bowl, cream the margarine, sugar, and eggs. Add mashed banana, vanilla, and bran mixture and mix well.

5 In large bowl, sift together dry ingredients and spices. Add wet ingredients to dry ingredients and mix until combined. Do not overmix.

6 Pour into a 9 × 5 × 3-inch loaf pan and bake for 50 minutes.

*Buttermilk is usually well tolerated by lactose-intolerant individuals because it is cultured. The total amount of buttermilk is also very small in this recipe.

Nutritional information per serving (1 slice)

92 calories

71% of calories from carbohydrate

10% of calories from protein

19% of calories from fat

2 grams of fat

2 grams of fiber

Blueberry Orange Bread

YIELD: 16 SLICES

If you are using frozen blueberries, it is important to drain them well. Start draining them several hours before you plan to make the bread.

2 tablespoons butter or margarine

¼ cup boiling water

½ cup orange juice

1 tablespoon finely chopped orange rind

1 egg

1 cup sugar

1 cup unbleached white flour

1 cup whole wheat flour

1 teaspoon baking powder

¼ teaspoon baking soda

½ teaspoon salt

1 cup fresh or thawed, well-drained, frozen blueberries

1   Preheat oven to 325°.

2   Melt butter in boiling water in small bowl. Add juice and rind.

3   In large bowl, beat egg with sugar until light and fluffy.

4   Sift flour, baking soda, baking powder, and salt together into small bowl.

5   Add dry ingredients alternately with orange liquid to the egg and sugar mixture. Mix blueberries in gently.

6   Bake in 9 × 5 × 3-inch loaf pan that has been coated with non-stick vegetable oil spray.

7   Bake for 1 hour and 10 minutes. Turn out onto rack to cool. Slice when completely cool.

Nutritional information per serving (1 slice)

133 calories

79% of calories from carbohydrate

7% of calories from protein

14% of calories from fat

2 grams of fat

2 grams of fiber

Easy Corn Bread
YIELD: 9 PIECES

1 cup yellow cornmeal
1 cup whole wheat flour
¼ cup granulated sugar
1 tablespoon baking powder

½ teaspoon salt
2 egg whites
3 tablespoons vegetable oil
*1 cup skim milk

1 Preheat oven to 400°.

2 Coat a 9-inch-square, 2½-inch-deep baking pan with nonstick vegetable oil spray.

3 In medium bowl, stir together the cornmeal, flour, sugar, baking powder and salt until well mixed.

4 In small bowl, beat together egg whites and oil until blended. Stir in the milk. Very gently, stir the egg-milk mixture into the dry ingredients until well blended but not overmixed. Spoon batter into prepared pan, smoothing and spreading the top out toward the edges.

5 Bake for 18 to 20 minutes, or until the bread is tinged with brown and is springy on top. Cut into pieces and serve while warm.

Nutritional information per serving (1 piece)

168 calories
62% of calories from carbohydrate
11% of calories from protein

27% of calories from fat
5 grams of fat
2 grams of fiber

Oat Biscuits
YIELD: 1 DOZEN

This is significantly lower in fat than a typical biscuit.

1 cup unbleached white flour
3 tablespoons sugar
1 tablespoon baking powder
½ teaspoon salt

¼ cup rolled oats
⅓ cup oat bran
2 tablespoons margarine
*¾ cup skim milk

1 Preheat oven to 425°.

2 Coat a 9-inch-round baking pan with nonstick vegetable oil spray.

3 Sift flour, sugar, baking powder, and salt into a medium bowl. Add oats and oat bran. Cut in the margarine with two butter knives and blend until mixture is crumbly.

*Use lactose-reduced milk if you are lactose-intolerant.

4 Make a well in the center of the flour mixture. Pour in the skim milk. Stir quickly, but gently, just until dough comes together. The dough should be moist but pliable.

5 Turn out the dough onto a lightly floured sheet of waxed paper. Fold the waxed paper over the dough and gently pat to a thickness of about ¾ inch.

6 Cut biscuits, using a floured 2-inch-round biscuit cutter or glass. Place on prepared pan.

7 Bake for 15 minutes or until golden brown. Serve immediately.

Nutritional information per serving (1 biscuit)

83 calories	23% of calories from fat
66% of calories from carbohydrate	2 grams of fat
11% of calories from protein	1 gram of fiber

Oatmeal Raisin Muffins
YIELD: 1 DOZEN

1 cup rolled oats	1¼ teaspoon baking powder
*¾ cup buttermilk	½ teaspoon baking soda
2 tablespoons softened margarine	½ teaspoon salt
2 egg whites	½ teaspoon cinnamon
⅓ cup brown sugar	**⅛ teaspoon ground nutmeg
⅓ cup orange juice concentrate	***1 cup seedless raisins
1 cup whole wheat flour	

1 Preheat oven to 400°.

2 Prepare muffin tins with paper liners or coat with nonstick vegetable oil spray.

3 In medium bowl, soak rolled oats in buttermilk for 15 minutes.

4 In medium bowl, cream margarine, egg whites, brown sugar, and orange juice concentrate. When thoroughly mixed, add to oat mixture.

5 In large bowl, mix dry ingredients and spices.

6 Add wet ingredients and raisins to dry ingredients, mixing only enough to thoroughly combine. Do not overmix.

7 Bake for 15 to 20 minutes.

*Buttermilk is usually well tolerated by lactose-intolerant individuals because it is cultured. If you are unable to tolerate buttermilk, you can treat it with lactase enzyme drops twenty-four hours before making this recipe.

**Omit the nutmeg if you are unable to tolerate it.

***Raisins can be gas-producing. If you prefer to omit the raisins, increase the brown sugar to ½ cup.

Nutritional information per serving (1 muffin)

155 calories	15% of calories from fat
75% of calories from carbohydrate	3 grams of fat
10% of calories from protein	3 grams of fiber

Pumpkin Muffins
YIELD: 1 DOZEN

2 tablespoons margarine	1 cup unbleached white flour
½ cup brown sugar	2 teaspoons baking powder
1 egg	½ teaspoon baking soda
1 egg white	1 teaspoon cinnamon
*1 cup buttermilk	¼ teaspoon ground ginger
½ cup canned pumpkin	**¼ teaspoon ground nutmeg
1 cup whole wheat flour	**¼ teaspoon ground cloves

1   Preheat oven to 400°.

2   Prepare muffin tins with paper liners or coat with nonstick vegetable oil spray.

3   In medium bowl, cream margarine, brown sugar, egg, and egg white. Add buttermilk and pumpkin and mix well.

4   In large bowl, combine dry ingredients and spices. Mix well to ensure adequate distribution of the leavening agents and spices.

5   Add wet ingredients to dry ingredients. Mix until combined, but do not overmix.

6   Fill muffin tins three-quarters full and bake for about 25 minutes.

Nutritional information per serving (1 muffin)

144 calories	17% of calories from fat
72% of calories from carbohydrate	3 grams of fat
11% of calories from protein	2 grams of fiber

*Buttermilk is usually well tolerated by lactose-intolerant individuals because it is cultured. If you are unable to tolerate buttermilk, you can treat it with lactase enzyme drops twenty-four hours before making these muffins.
**These spices can be eliminated from recipe if they are irritating for you.

43 *Breakfast Dishes*

Berry Banana Smoothie
Brown Rice Cereal
Buttermilk Wheat Pancakes
Frosted Melon Cooler
Fruit Cup
Granola
Hot Buckwheat Cereal
Lemon Pancakes
Orangy French Toast
Strawberry Pancakes
Tomato, Mushroom, and Basil Omelet

Berry Banana Smoothie
SERVES 1

*½ cup plain nonfat yogurt
**½ cup skim milk
1 small ripe banana, cut in chunks
⅓ cup strawberries, cut in half
   (blueberries or raspberries would
   also work well)

1 teaspoon maple syrup
3 ice cubes

Combine all ingredients in blender and process until smooth and thick.
Serve.

*Yogurt is usually well tolerated by lactose-intolerant individuals. If you cannot tolerate yogurt, take 1 lactase enzyme tablet with this drink.
**Use low-lactose milk if you are lactose-intolerant.

Nutritional information per serving

245 calories	4% of calories from fat
77% of calories from carbohydrate	1 gram of fat
19% of calories from protein	4 grams of fiber

Brown Rice Cereal
SERVES 4

This is a great way to use up leftover rice, especially on a cold winter morning.

4 cups cooked brown rice	2 peaches, sliced, or 1 cup canned
2 tablespoons maple syrup	peaches in their own juice
*1 cup skim milk	

1   Combine all ingredients in medium saucepan.

2   Bring to a boil, turn heat to medium, and cook to desired thickness, about 8 minutes. Serve warm.

Nutritional information per serving

302 calories	4% of calories from fat
86% of calories from carbohydrate	1 gram of fat
10% of calories from protein	7 grams of fiber

Buttermilk Wheat Pancakes
SERVES 4

⅔ cup unbleached white flour	½ teaspoon salt
1⅓ cups whole wheat flour	**2 cups buttermilk (or a little more,
1 teaspoon baking powder	if needed)
½ teaspoon baking soda	4 teaspoons vegetable oil

1   Stir dry ingredients together in a medium bowl until thoroughly mixed.

2   Beat the buttermilk and oil together until blended. Gently stir buttermilk mixture into dry ingredients until thoroughly blended but not overmixed. If the batter seems too thick, thin it with a bit more buttermilk until a pourable but still fairly thick consistency is achieved.

*Use low-lactose milk if you are lactose-intolerant.

**Buttermilk is usually well tolerated by lactose-intolerant individuals because it is cultured. If you are unable to tolerate buttermilk you can treat it with lactase enzyme drops twenty-four hours before making these pancakes.

3 Lightly oil and preheat a griddle. Pour batter onto hot griddle and cook until bubbles form on the top surface and the bottoms are browned (about 60 to 70 seconds). Turn over with a spatula and cook about 1½ more minutes or until cooked through and nicely browned. Serve warm with maple syrup or fruit.

Nutritional information per serving

300 calories	19% of calories from fat
66% of calories from carbohydrate	6 grams of fat
15% of calories from protein	6 grams of fiber

Frosted Melon Cooler
SERVES 1

1 cup cantaloupe, fresh or frozen (thawed)	¼ cup apple juice concentrate
1 cup ice	¼ cup water

Combine all ingredients in blender and whip until frothy. Serve.

Nutritional information per serving

168 calories	4% of calories from fat
92% of calories from carbohydrate	less than 1 gram of fat
4% of calories from protein	2 grams of fiber

Fruit Cup
SERVES 6

1 medium apple, cored and diced (peeled if desired)	½ cup blueberries, fresh or frozen
1 medium pear or peach, cored, pitted, and diced	¼ cup frozen lemonade concentrate (any other juice concentrate would also be acceptable)
1 banana, peeled and sliced	***¾ cup plain low-fat or nonfat yogurt
*10 ounce can of mandarin oranges, drained	
**½ cup seedless grapes (halved if desired)	

*Oranges may be irritating to the esophagus; omit if you are unable to tolerate them.

**Grapes are a gas-producing fruit. You may want to substitute 1/2 cup of melon for the grapes.

***Yogurt is often well tolerated by lactose-intolerant individuals. If you are unable to tolerate yogurt, take 1 lactase enzyme tablet with this salad.

1   Prepare fruits and place in a large bowl. (The fiber content will be higher if the skins are left on the fruit.)

2   Mix lemonade concentrate with yogurt. Pour over fruit and toss lightly.

Nutritional information per serving

110 calories

87% of calories from carbohydrate

7% of calories from protein

6% of calories from fat

1 gram of fat

3 grams of fiber

Granola

YIELD: 5 CUPS

Granola is traditionally high in fat because it usually has more oil or margarine than this recipe, as well as nuts and coconut.

2 tablespoons margarine

2 tablespoons water

¼ cup honey

1 teaspoon cinnamon

3 cups rolled oats

1 cup Grape Nuts

*½ cup raisins

1   Preheat oven to 350°. While oven is preheating, melt margarine in 9 × 13-inch baking pan. Remove from oven.

2   Stir water, honey, and cinnamon into margarine until well blended.

3   Stir oats and Grape Nuts into margarine mixture until grains are well coated.

4   Bake for 15 minutes until oats are lightly browned. Stir twice during baking time to prevent uneven browning.

5   Remove from oven and stir in raisins. Cool. Serve with nonfat or lactose-reduced milk or with fruit juice.

Nutritional information per serving (½ cup)

202 calories

73% of calories from carbohydrate

10% of calories from protein

17% of calories from fat

4 grams of fat

3 grams of fiber

*Raisins are gas-producing. If you are unable to tolerate raisins, use chopped dried apples or apricots instead.

Hot Buckwheat Cereal
SERVES 2

This is a wonderful, hearty breakfast for those mornings when you need a lot of energy. It's great before a day of skiing.

5 cups water	1½ teaspoons minced orange peel
1 cup whole buckwheat (kasha)	1½ teaspoons ground cinnamon
2 apples, unpeeled, diced	

1 Bring water to boil in 3-quart saucepan. Add buckwheat, stirring, and return to boil. Reduce heat to medium and cook uncovered for about 8 minutes, stirring occasionally.

2 Stir in diced apples, orange peel, and cinnamon. Continue to cook about 3 to 5 more minutes or until most of the liquid has evaporated.

3 Serve topped with skimmed milk or low-lactose skimmed milk. (If you would prefer not to use any milk at all, only cook the buckwheat an additional 2 to 3 minutes after adding the apples. It will then be a thinner consistency.)

Nutritional information per serving

260 calories	6% of calories from fat
85% of calories from carbohydrate	2 grams of fat
9% of calories from protein	8 grams of fiber

Lemon Pancakes
YIELD: 18 PANCAKES

PANCAKES

1 cup unbleached white flour	2 egg yolks
1 cup whole wheat flour	*2½ cups skim milk
2½ tablespoons sugar	2 tablespoons melted margarine
1½ tablespoons baking powder	grated rind of 1 lemon
½ teaspoon salt	2 egg whites, stiffly beaten
¼ cup unprocessed wheat bran	

1 In large bowl, sift flour, sugar, baking powder, and salt. Add bran and mix.

*If you are lactose-intolerant, use lactose-reduced milk.

2   In medium bowl, beat egg yolks until creamy and stir in milk, margarine, and lemon rind.

3   Stir egg yolk mixture into flour mixture using as few strokes as possible.

4   Fold in egg whites thoroughly.

5   Drop batter onto hot griddle coated with nonstick vegetable oil spray. Bake until bubbly on surface. Turn and brown on the other side.

6   Serve with lemon-honey topping.

LEMON-HONEY TOPPING*
YIELD: 2 CUPS

1 tablespoon cornstarch	1 cup honey
¾ cup water	**dash nutmeg
¼ cup lemon juice	

1   Whisk cornstarch into water and lemon juice.

2   Heat until thickened, stirring constantly.

3   Add honey and nutmeg. Stir.

4   Serve hot over pancakes.

Nutritional information per serving (3 pancakes, 3 tablespoons topping)

376 calories	15% of calories from fat
74% of calories from carbohydrate	6 grams of fat
11% of calories from protein	4 grams of fiber

Orangy French Toast***
SERVES 6

TOPPING

1 cup mandarin oranges in light syrup	¾ cup maple syrup

FRENCH TOAST BATTER

2 whole eggs	½ teaspoon vanilla
2 egg whites	1 tablespoon Grand Marnier
2 cups orange juice	1 pound loaf of day-old French
****1½ cups skim milk	bread cut into 1½-inch diagonal
¼ cup sugar	slices

*This topping should not be used by individuals with esophageal irritation.
**Nutmeg can be replaced with cinnamon.
***Individuals with esophageal irritation should not make this recipe.
****If you are lactose-intolerant, use lactose-reduced milk.

1   Place topping ingredients in saucepan and let simmer over low heat.

2   Separate eggs and beat whites (4) until thick but not stiff.

3   Whisk egg yolks, juice, milk, sugar, vanilla, and Grand Marnier together. Fold in the thickened whites.

4   Cut bread. Add bread to the egg mixture and let soak for 10 minutes on each side.

5   Coat medium skillet with nonstick vegetable oil spray. Heat over medium heat. Add bread slices to skillet and cook on each side until golden brown.

6   Serve topped with orange syrup.

Nutritional information per serving

478 calories
80% of calories from carbohydrate
11% of calories from protein

9% of calories from fat
5 grams of fat
2 grams of fiber

Strawberry Pancakes
SERVES 4

1 egg or 2 egg whites
*1¼ cups buttermilk
1 tablespoon melted butter or
   margarine
¾ cup whole wheat flour, sifted
½ cup unbleached white flour, sifted
¼ cup unprocessed wheat bran

1 teaspoon sugar
2 teaspoons baking powder
½ teaspoon baking soda
½ teaspoon salt
1 cup sliced strawberries, frozen or
   fresh

1   In large bowl, beat egg with electric mixer at high speed.

2   Add buttermilk and margarine or butter and beat for 1 minute.

3   Add remaining ingredients except berries and mix by hand, until just blended.

4   Add berries and mix.

5   Cook on hot griddle using ¼ cup batter for each pancake. You may have to coat griddle with nonstick vegetable oil spray.

6   Top pancakes with your favorite syrup, honeyed yogurt, or cottage cheese.

---

*Buttermilk is usually well tolerated by lactose-intolerant individuals because it is cultured. If you cannot tolerate buttermilk, or if you are severely lactose-intolerant then add lactase enzyme drops to the milk twenty-four hours before making this recipe.

Nutritional information per serving (3 pancakes)

235 calories	21% of calories from fat
65% of calories from carbohydrate	5 grams of fat
14% of calories from protein	2 grams of fiber

Tomato, Mushroom, and Basil Omelet
SERVES 2

2 teaspoons olive oil	2 egg yolks
½ medium onion, chopped	4 egg whites
½ cup chopped fresh mushrooms	1 tablespoon seltzer water
1 small tomato, diced	fresh chopped parsley
1½ tablespoon chopped fresh basil or ½ teaspoon dried	

1   Coat a nonstick skillet with a nonstick vegetable oil spray. Add the olive oil and heat. Sauté the onion until soft. Add the mushrooms, tomato, and basil and cook another 1 to 2 minutes. Remove from the heat.

2   Beat the egg yolks and egg whites with seltzer water.

3   Coat another nonstick skillet with nonstick vegetable oil spray and heat. Add eggs. Cook, stirring a few times and swirling the pan so that it is evenly coated with eggs, until the eggs are almost completely cooked.

4   Top the egg with the vegetable mixture. Tilt the pan to a 45-degree angle from the burner and using a fork push one edge of the omelet so that it rolls over the filling and into an oval shape. Continue cooking over low heat for about 1 minute. Tilt the pan so that the omelet rolls onto a serving plate.

5   Serve immediately, garnished with chopped parsley.

Nutritional information per serving

165 calories	56% of calories from fat
18% of calories from carbohydrate	10 grams of fat
26% of calories from protein	2 grams of fiber

44 *Desserts*

Apple Cake
SERVES 8 TO 9

1 tablespoon softened margarine	¾ cup whole wheat flour
¾ cup brown sugar	1½ teaspoon baking powder
*¼ cup skim milk	¼ teaspoon baking soda
1 egg	1½ teaspoon cinnamon
1 cup unsweetened applesauce	1 medium apple, peeled, cored, and
¼ cup unprocessed wheat bran	chopped
¾ cup unbleached white flour	¼ cup confectioners' sugar

1   Preheat oven to 350°.

2   Coat 8 × 8-inch baking pan with nonstick vegetable oil spray.

*Use low-lactose milk if you are lactose-intolerant.

3 In small bowl, cream together margarine and brown sugar. Add milk, egg, and applesauce. Mix well.

4 In large bowl, combine dry ingredients and cinnamon and mix well to ensure even distribution of the leavening agents.

5 Add wet ingredients to dry ingredients. Mix. Add apple and mix just until distributed.

6 Pour batter into pan and bake for 50 minutes or until firm.

7 Sift confectioners' sugar over top after cake is completely cooled.

Nutritional information per serving

200 calories	10% of calories from fat
83% of calories from carbohydrate	2 grams of fat
7% of calories from protein	3 grams of fiber

Apricot Apples
SERVES 6

6 medium Granny Smith apples, washed, peeled, and cored	¾ cup apricot jam
	3 tablespoons apricot brandy
1 cup firmly packed light brown sugar	*¼ cup slivered almonds

1 Preheat oven to 375°.

2 Place apples in 9 × 13-inch glass baking dish.

3 In small bowl, combine sugar and jam.

4 Place 1 to 2 tablespoons of sugar mixture in the center of each apple, filling halfway (you will have some left over).

5 Add ½ inch of water to baking dish.

6 Bake apples 20 minutes, basting with cooking liquid occasionally.

7 Add brandy to the remaining sugar mixture. Brush apples with sugar and brandy mixture.

8 Continue baking the apples about 20 minutes more or until soft.

9 Top apples with almonds and bake for 2 more minutes or until almonds are toasted.

10 Transfer apples to plates. Pour cooking liquid into small heavy saucepan and boil to thicken, if necessary. Pour sauce over apples. Serve warm or at room temperature.

*Nuts are often gas-producing. You may be able to tolerate this small amount as a garnish however.

Nutritional information per serving

350 calories
92% of calories from carbohydrate
1% of calories from protein

7% of calories from fat
3 grams of fat
3 grams of fiber

Banana Dream Pie
YIELD: ONE 8-INCH PIE (SERVES 8)

CRUST

1½ cups graham cracker crumbs
½ cup All Bran cereal
½ cup orange juice

1 tablespoon melted margarine or
  butter

FILLING

*1 cup skim milk
1 envelope unflavored gelatin
**¾ cup part-skim ricotta cheese

2 teaspoons vanilla
3 medium-sized *ripe* bananas
¼ cup sugar

GARNISH

2 kiwi fruit, peeled and sliced

8–10 fresh strawberries, sliced

1　Blend crust ingredients. Press crust over bottom and sides of 8-inch pie pan. Bake in 350° oven for 10 minutes. Cool.

2　Place ½ cup cold skim milk in small saucepan. Sprinkle gelatin on top. Let soak for 5 minutes. Heat and stir until gelatin dissolves.

3　In food processor or blender, combine gelatin/milk mixture with remaining ½ cup milk and other filling ingredients. Blend until smooth and creamy.

4　Pour into crust and chill for 1 hour. Remove and garnish with sliced kiwi and strawberries. *Note:* The top of the banana cream will discolor slightly from exposure to the air so the pie will have a better appearance if the garnish covers the entire top. Other garnish alternatives are fresh raspberries or low-fat yogurt.

5　Return to refrigerator to set for another 3 hours.

*Use lactose-reduced milk if you are lactose-intolerant.
**If you are mildly lactose-intolerant, you should tolerate the amount of ricotta cheese in one serving. However, if you are severely lactose-intolerant, take 1 lactase enzyme tablet with this pie.

Nutritional information per serving

226 calories
69% of calories from carbohydrate
12% of calories from protein

19% of calories from fat
5 grams of fat
4 grams of fiber

Banana-Rhubarb Compote
SERVES 4

2 cups frozen rhubarb
*⅓ cup orange juice
⅓ cup honey

2 medium-sized bananas, sliced
**½ cup vanilla low-fat yogurt
***4 teaspoons minced walnuts

1   In medium saucepan combine rhubarb, orange juice, and honey. Cover and cook for 10 minutes.
2   Add sliced bananas, cover, and heat until bananas are warmed and softened.
3   Serve in individual dessert dishes with 2 tablespoons of vanilla yogurt on top, sprinkled with 1 teaspoon of finely chopped walnuts.

Nutritional information per serving

320 calories
90% of calories from carbohydrate
4% of calories from protein

6% of calories from fat
2 grams of fat
4 grams of fiber

Blueberry-Apple Crumble
SERVES 6

FILLING

2 tablespoons granulated sugar
1 tablespoon whole wheat flour
¼ teaspoon ground cinnamon
2 cups fresh or frozen blueberries
  (thaw before using)

1 large tart apple, skin on, finely
  chopped

---

*The small amount of orange juice shouldn't present a problem for individuals with esophogeal irritation.
**Yogurt is usually well tolerated by lactose-intolerant individuals. If you cannot tolerate yogurt or prefer not to use it, sprinkle a small amount of confectioners' sugar on top as a garnish.
***Most people find nuts to be gas-producing. You may be able to tolerate a small amount as a garnish. If not, omit them.

TOPPING

⅓ cup whole wheat flour
⅔ cup rolled oats
½ cup packed brown sugar

1½ tablespoons vegetable oil
1–2 tablespoons water or apple juice
   (if necessary)

1 Preheat oven to 375°

2 To prepare the filling, stir together the granulated sugar, flour, and cinnamon in a 1½-quart baking dish. Stir in the blueberries and chopped apple until they are coated with the flour-sugar mixture. Set aside.

3 To prepare the topping, stir together the flour, oats, and brown sugar in a small bowl until well mixed. Stir in the oil until thoroughly incorporated. Mixture should clump together slightly so use the additional water or juice as necessary. Sprinkle the topping over the blueberry mixture.

4 Bake the crumble, uncovered, for 25 to 30 minutes or until bubbly at the edges and cooked through. Serve warm or at room temperature.

Nutritional information per serving

217 calories
78% of calories from carbohydrate
5% of calories from protein

17% of calories from fat
4 grams of fat
4 grams of fiber

Carrot Brownies
YIELD: 24 SQUARES

1 cup brown sugar
2 tablespoons margarine
1 egg
2 egg whites
1 teaspoon vanilla
*½ cup orange juice
1½ cups unbleached white flour

½ cup rolled oats
½ teaspoon baking powder
½ teaspoon baking soda
2 cups finely grated carrots
1 cup confectioners' sugar
**skim milk

1 Preheat oven to 350°.

2 Coat a 9 × 13-inch baking pan with nonstick vegetable oil spray.

3 Mix sugar and margarine together in large bowl.

4 Add eggs, vanilla, and orange juice; beat.

*The small amount of orange juice shouldn't present a problem for individuals with esophageal irritation.
**Use low-lactose milk if you are lactose-intolerant, although you will use such a small amount that it should not have any effect.

5   Stir in dry ingredients and mix well. Stir in carrots.

6   Spread mixture into baking pan. Bake 30 to 35 minutes or until firm when pressed.

7   Place confectioners' sugar in small bowl and add just enough skim milk to thicken. Drizzle over brownies while still warm.

Nutritional information per serving (1 square)

106 calories

82% of calories from carbohydrate

7% of calories from protein

11% of calories from fat

1 gram of fat

1 gram of fiber

Chocolate Angel Cake
SERVES 10

1 cup sifted flour

1 cup sugar

¼ cup cocoa, unsweetened

½ teaspoon salt

1½ cups egg whites (approximately 6 medium)

1 teaspoon cream of tartar

1 teaspoon vanilla confectioners' sugar

1   Preheat oven to 325°.

2   Sift flour, sugar, cocoa, and salt *ten* times into a medium bowl. This step is essential to the success of the recipe.

3   With electric mixer, beat egg whites until frothy, add cream of tartar, and beat again by hand.

4   Fold in dry ingredients, and add vanilla.

5   Turn into an ungreased 10 × 4-inch tube pan.

6   Bake for about 1 hour and 15 minutes or until cake springs back when lightly touched. Invert pan for about 1 hour. Remove from pan and cook on rack.

7   If desired, sift confectioners' sugar over top before serving.

Nutritional information per serving

130 calories

86% of calories from carbohydrate

11% of calories from protein

3% of calories from fat

less than 1 gram of fat

less than 1 gram of fiber

Oatmeal Drop Cookies
YIELD: 3 DOZEN

1 cup unbleached white flour
½ cup sugar
½ teaspoon baking powder
¼ teaspoon baking soda
½ teaspoon salt
½ teaspoon cinnamon
1 cup oats, regular or quick cooking

½ cup oat bran
*½ cup raisins
¼ cup vegetable oil
1 whole egg
2 egg whites
**⅓ cup skim milk
***¼ cup chopped walnuts

1 Preheat oven to 400°.

2 Sift flour, sugar, baking powder, baking soda, salt, and cinnamon together. Add oats and oat bran. Mix. Add raisins and mix.

3 In small bowl, beat oil, eggs, and milk until blended. Add wet ingredients to dry ingredients and mix until thoroughly blended.

4 Add walnuts and stir.

5 Drop by heaping teaspoonful onto ungreased baking sheet about 1½ inches apart.

6 Bake 10 to 12 minutes.

Nutritional information per serving (2 cookies)

129 calories
57% of calories from carbohydrate
10% of calories from protein

33% of calories from fat
5 grams of fat
2 grams of fiber

Patriotic Pizzazz****
SERVES 4

This is a very elegant dessert, suitable for company.

1 pint strawberries
¼ cup confectioners' sugar
2 cups lemonade

2½ cups blueberries
*****¼ cup vanilla low-fat yogurt
fresh mint

*Raisins can be gas-producing. You may want to substitute diced, peeled apples. Dice apples in ¼-inch cubes and reduce the milk to ¼ cup.

**Use low-lactose milk if you are lactose-intolerant.

***Nuts can be gas-producing. They may be tolerated in these small amounts, but can be omitted if desired.

****Individuals with esophageal irritation should not make this recipe.

*****Yogurt is usually well tolerated by lactose-intolerant individuals. If you are unable to tolerate yogurt, take 1 lactase enzyme tablet with this dessert.

1   Wash and hull strawberries, drain thoroughly, and cut into small pieces.

2   Put strawberries and sugar in a food processor or blender and puree until smooth.

3   Add enough lemonade to the strawberry puree to make 2 cups of liquid. Pour liquid into a plastic freezer container, cover, and put in the freezer. When the mixture begins to freeze around the sides of the container, after about 20 minutes, remove from the freezer and scrape the frozen bits into the center of the container to break up ice crystals. Return to freezer and freeze until firm but not solid, about 45 minutes.

4   While strawberry ice is setting, wash blueberries, drain thoroughly, place in food processor or blender, and puree. Strain and discard any seeds or skins.

TO ASSEMBLE DESSERT:

1   Pour about ⅓ of blueberry puree onto each of 4 chilled dessert plates, forming an even pool.

2   Place yogurt into a pastry bag with a round tip.

3   Pipe about a tablespoon dollop of yogurt in the center of the puree. Draw a toothpick through the yogurt at regular intervals, alternating from the edge of the puree to the center and then from the center of the dish to the edge, creating a web design.

4   Place 3 small scoops of the strawberry ice on the outside of the puree. Garnish with a fresh sprig of mint placed in the center of each scoop of ice.

5   Repeat to make 4 servings. Serve immediately.

Nutritional information per serving

167 calories
88% of calories from carbohydrate
8% of calories from protein

4% of calories from fat
less than 1 gram of fat
4 grams of fiber

Peanut Butter Bars
YIELD: 12 BARS, 2¼ × 2½ INCHES EACH

½ cup peanut butter
½ cup honey
2 tablespoons water
1 egg yolk
2 egg whites

½ cup dry rolled oats
½ cup Grape Nuts cereal (not flakes)
1 teaspoon cinnamon
2 teaspoons baking powder
¼ teaspoon baking soda

½ teaspoon vanilla extract · · · · · · · · · · *½ cup seedless raisins
½ cup unbleached white flour

1 Preheat oven to 350°.
2 Coat 8 × 8-inch baking pan with nonstick vegetable oil spray.
3 In medium-sized bowl, beat peanut butter, honey, water, egg yolk, egg whites, and vanilla until smooth.
4 In large bowl, combine flour, oats, Grape Nuts, cinnamon, baking powder, and baking soda.
5 Add wet ingredients to dry ingredients and beat until combined.
6 Add raisins and stir to combine. Pour into baking pan and bake for about 20 minutes or until set.

Nutritional information per serving (1 bar)

182 calories
59% of calories from carbohydrate
12% of calories from protein

29% of calories from fat
6 grams of fat
2 grams of fiber

Refrigerator Chip Cookies
YIELD: 3 DOZEN

Although these cookies are not low in calories, they have less than half the fat of a typical cookie and more fiber.

2 eggs
1 cup brown sugar, firmly packed
3 tablespoons vegetable oil
½ teaspoon vanilla
¾ cup unbleached white flour

1 cup whole wheat flour
¾ teaspoon baking powder
¼ cup mini chocolate chip morsels, semisweet

1 Beat eggs. Add brown sugar, oil, and vanilla. Beat.
2 Sift flour and baking powder into large bowl.
3 Add wet ingredients to dry and mix well (texture will be crumbly). Add chips and mix.
4 Shape with hands into a 2-inch-round roll. Wrap in waxed paper and refrigerate until firm.
5 Preheat oven to 375°.

*Raisins may be omitted if you find them to be gas-producing.

6   Remove roll from refrigerator when firm and slice thin, into approximately 36 slices.

7   Bake on ungreased cookie sheet for 5 to 8 minutes or until golden brown.

Nutritional information per serving (2 cookies)

128 calories

67% of calories from carbohydrate

7% of calories from protein

26% of calories from fat

4 grams of fat

1 gram of fiber

45 *Miscellaneous*

Basic Vinaigrette Dressing
Cooked Salad Dressing
Marinara Sauce
Mock Sour Cream

Basic Vinaigrette Dressing
YIELD: 1 CUP

This very basic, easy-to-prepare dressing is something you will always want to keep on hand. When refrigerated, it will stay good indefinitely and tastes much better than bottled salad dressings. Use this on your tossed salads, grain-based salads, and for basting or marinating your meats or poultry. The typical proportion of oil to vinegar in a salad dressing is 3 parts oil to 1 part vinegar. In order to keep the fat content lower, this proportion has been altered. If you have difficulty getting accustomed to more vinegar and less oil, start with a 1 to 1 ratio and make the change gradually. Use any type of oil or vinegar to change the flavor of this recipe, but always use the best quality!

10 tablespoons balsamic vinegar
6 tablespoons extra virgin olive oil
4 teaspoons Dijon-style mustard
½ teaspoon dried tarragon

pinch of basil
pinch of thyme
*1 garlic clove, whole

Whisk ingredients together and store in covered jar in refrigerator. Garlic should be left whole to flavor the dressing. Remove the garlic before serving.

*Garlic can be gas-producing. If you are unable to tolerate it, the dressing is good even without the garlic.

Nutritional information per serving (2 tablespoons)

92 calories
6% of calories from carbohydrate
0% of calories from protein

94% of calories from fat
10 grams of fat
0 grams of fiber

Cooked Salad Dressing

YIELD: 1¼ CUPS

1 tablespoon cornstarch
1 teaspoon sugar
*1 small garlic clove, finely chopped

1 cup cold water
¼ cup catsup
3 tablespoons red wine vinegar

1   Combine cornstarch, sugar, garlic, and water in small saucepan and blend until cornstarch dissolves. Add catsup and vinegar.

2   Stir over medium heat at a slow boil until thickened. If you are not using garlic, add your herb(s) at this point and cook another minute. Remove from heat, place in small bowl, and refrigerate.

Nutritional information per serving (2 tablespoons)

10 calories
100% of calories from carbohydrate
0% of calories from protein

0% of calories from fat
0 grams of fat
0 grams of fiber

Marinara Sauce**

YIELD: 3½ CUPS STRAINED, 4 CUPS UNSTRAINED

1 tablespoon olive oil
¼ cup chopped onion
¼ cup chopped celery
*1 garlic clove, finely minced
3 cups whole canned tomatoes

6 ounces tomato paste
4 ounces water
2 tablespoon fresh parsley
1 tablespoon dried basil
1 tablespoon sugar

1   Heat oil in large saucepan. Sauté onion, celery, and garlic until softened.

2   Place remaining ingredients in food processor or blender and puree until smooth.

3   Add tomato ingredients to saucepan, cover, and simmer over very low heat for 45 minutes to 1 hour.

*Garlic can be gas-producing. If you are unable to tolerate the garlic, replace it with 1 teaspoon of one or more dried herbs of your choice, such as basil, dill, oregano, or tarragon.

**Individuals with esophageal irritation should not make this recipe.

4 Serve the sauce as it is or, if you prefer, strain it to remove the seeds.

Note: If you have fresh basil on hand, omit the dried basil and add 3 basil leaves just before you cover to simmer.

Nutritional information per serving (½ cup)

58 calories
59% of calories from carbohydrate
12% of calories from protein

29% of calories from fat
2 grams of fat
1 gram of fiber

Mock Sour Cream
YIELD: ABOUT 1¼ CUPS

*1 cup 1% low-fat cottage cheese
*2 tablespoons skim milk

1 tablespoon lemon juice

1 Combine all ingredients in blender. With blender on high speed, blend the mixture until smooth, about 2 minutes.
2 Chill in refrigerator for several hours before serving.

Nutritional information per serving (2 tablespoons)

18 calories
20% of calories from carbohydrate
67% of calories from protein

13% of calories from fat
less than 1 gram of fat
0 gram of fiber

Note: The same amount of regular sour cream has 62 calories and 6 grams of fat (87% of the calories are from fat).

*Use lactose-reduced products if you are lactose intolerant.

Appendix I

Clear-Liquid Diet

Modified from the Thomas Jefferson University Nutritional Manual

General Description	Food Allowed	Indications
Includes foods that are	Clear broth	*Typically ordered as initial diet in feeding progression for patients*
• liquid at body temperature	Clear fruit ades without fruit pulp	
• very low in fiber	Clear fruit juice (e.g., apple, cranberry, grape, and citrus juices) without fruit pulp	• who have undergone surgery
• lactose free		• who have undergone certain diagnostic procedures
• virtually fat-free	Clear, noncarbonated soft drinks (e.g., Kool-Aid or Gatorade)	
Typically provides approximately		• who have been without oral or enteral nutritional intake for extended period
• 2000 ml fluid	Coffee (regular or decaffeinated)	
• 400–600 calories		• who have been experiencing nausea, vomiting, or diarrhea
• 5–7 grams low-quality protein	Gelatin	
	Ice popsicle	*May be ordered*
• <1 gram dietary fiber	Ice tea	• to minimize pancreatic exocrine secretion or biliary contraction for
• <1 gram fat per day	Lemon juice	
	Salt	
	Soda	

General Description	Food Allowed	Indications
	Sugar	patients with certain gastrointestinal (GI) disorders (e.g., acute diverticulitis or acute cholecystitis)
	Sugar substitute	
	Tea (regular, decaffeinated, or herbal)	
	Ice water	• for bowel preparation before certain medical or surgical procedures

Appendix II

Low-Residue Diet

The low-residue diet is a useful adjunct in the treatment of diarrheas and gastrointestinal inflammation of varied origin such as Crohn's disease and ulcerative colitis.

A low-residue diet is one which will leave minimal residue in the colon after digestion and absorption have taken place. A low residue diet is useful in any condition where the presence of bulky stool in the large intestine would strain the bowel. Low- or non-residue diets tend to help the diseased colon by easing obstruction, distention, edema, inflammation of the bowel wall.

Lean red meat, chicken, fish, eggs, rice, gelatin, strained fruit juices, sugar, and other refined carbohydrates leave minimal residues. Milk, whether boiled or raw, produces a residue of medium bulk, whereas cottage cheese does not. Fruits and vegetable, rich fatty foods, potatoes, soft-boiled eggs, butter, lard, Swiss cheese, and lactose produce large residues.

Indigestible carbohydrates and proteins as found in fruits and vegetables (especially when raw), uncooked cereals, bran, skins, seeds, nuts, and fried foods are omitted, as are strong spices and condiments, relishes, and onions.

Recipe Index

Index